AF545010

Hemodiafiltration

....

Contributions to Nephrology

Vol. 158

Series Editor

Claudio Ronco, Vicenza

Hemodiafiltration

Volume Editors

Claudio Ronco, *Vicenza*
Bernard Canaud, *Montpellier*
Pedro Aljama, *Cordoba*

42 figures, 5 in color, and 11 tables, 2007

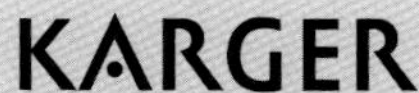

Basel · Freiburg · Paris · London · New York ·
Bangalore · Bangkok · Singapore · Tokyo · Sydney

Contributions to Nephrology
(Founded 1975 by Geoffrey M. Berlyne)

Claudio Ronco
Department of Nephrology
St. Bortolo Hospital
I-36100 Vicenza (Italy)

Bernard Canaud
Department of Nephrology
Dialysis and Intensive Care
University Hospital Lapeyronie
F-34295 Montpellier (France)

Pedro Aljama
Department of Nephrology
University Hospital Reina Sofía
E-14004 Cordoba (Spain)

Library of Congress Cataloging-in-Publication Data

Hemodiafiltration / volume editors, Claudio Ronco, Bernard Canaud, Pedro Aljama.
p. ; cm. – (Contributions to nephrology, ISSN 0302-5144 ; v. 158)
Includes bibliographical references and indexes.
ISBN 978-3-8055-8288-9 (hard cover : alk. paper)
1. Blood–Filtration. 2. Hemodialysis. I. Ronco, C. (Claudio), 1951– II. Canaud, Bernard. III. Aljama, Pedro. IV. Series.
[DNLM: 1. Hemodiafiltration–methods. W1 CO778UN v.158 2007 / WJ 378 H4883 2007]
RC901.7.H47H43 2007
617.4'61059–dc22

2007024039

Bibliographic Indices. This publication is listed in bibliographic services, including Current Contents® and Index Medicus.

Disclaimer. The statements, options and data contained in this publication are solely those of the individual authors and contributors and not of the publisher and the editor(s). The appearance of advertisements in the book is not a warranty, endorsement, or approval of the products or services advertised or of their effectiveness, quality or safety. The publisher and the editor(s) disclaim responsibility for any injury to persons or property resulting from any ideas, methods, instructions or products referred to in the content or advertisements.

Drug Dosage. The authors and the publisher have exerted every effort to ensure that drug selection and dosage set forth in this text are in accord with current recommendations and practice at the time of publication. However, in view of ongoing research, changes in government regulations, and the constant flow of information relating to drug therapy and drug reactions, the reader is urged to check the package insert for each drug for any change in indications and dosage and for added warnings and precautions. This is particularly important when the recommended agent is a new and/or infrequently employed drug.

www.karger.com
Printed in Switzerland on acid-free and non-aging paper (ISO 9706) by Reinhardt Druck, Basel
ISSN 0302–5144
ISBN 978–3–8055–8288–9

Contents

Membranes and Hardware for Hemodiafiltration

Technical Aspects and Fluids in Hemodiafiltration

Hemodiafiltration Techniques

Clinical Aspects of Hemodiafiltration

Preface

Exactly 40 years after the first contribution of Lee W. Henderson on the potential use of convection as a blood-cleansing modality and exactly 30 years after H. Leber published his first paper on a new dialysis modality called 'hemodiafiltration', this book is a tribute to the genius and creativity in the field of artificial organs. But the book is not just a homage to the brilliant idea or to the important investigators, it is a real updated review of the evolution, the advances and the recent results achieved by hemodiafiltration in the clinical arena as renal replacement modality. For this reason, this comprehensive review, made possible by a series of outstanding scientists and physicians, represents today an important source of information and a valuable tool for implementing hemodiafiltration in the daily practice. For a long time, results were limited, and evidence was scanty and insufficient to expand the application of hemodiafiltration; recently however, large studies and important clinical investigations have produced enough evidence for a clinical application of hemodiafiltration on a broader scale and even on a routine basis in some centers.

The present book is a collection of papers that include historical notes and a journey through the evolution of different forms of hemodiafiltration, made possible by technological developments in the field of membranes, machines and fluids.

The subsequent group of papers describe the theoretical rationale for hemodiafiltration with a detailed analysis of the involved mass separation processes and the hydraulic properties of the dialyzers. In this section, fluid mechanics and crossfiltration in hollow-fiber hemodialyzers are described in detail.

A special section has been devoted to the description of different hemodiafiltration techniques; in each chapter, a specific technique is analyzed, and the particular transport mechanism and related technology are reported.

Finally, the clinical effects of hemodiafiltration are described in a series of chapters that conclude the book.

At the end of this important enterprise, we are proud of our effort to unify the knowledge about hemodiafiltration. The book includes different technologies and therefore offers the readers a complete overview of the technical and clinical possibilities provided by the technique in its widest concept. It is not a case that the three editors come from three different European countries where hemodiafiltration has found large application and interesting clinical results. Joining our efforts has been mutually rewarding, but also a precise warranty that a multinational view has been conveyed in the main message of the book.

We are indebted to Karger for the prompt and efficient publication of the book that allows physicians and investigators to have a comprehensive overview of hemodiafiltration from its molecular basis to the most practical application. Thus, we hope that this book will represent an important aid for beginners and for experts, for scientists and for physicians, for students and for senior faculty members, creating the bridges that today's translational research is intended to build.

Claudio Ronco
Bernard Canaud
Pedro Aljama

Ronco C, Canaud B, Aljama P (eds): Hemodiafiltration.
Contrib Nephrol. Basel, Karger, 2007, vol 158, pp 1–8

The Birth of Hemodiafiltration

L.W. Henderson

Sorbent Therapeutics Inc., Vernon Hills, Ill., USA

It should be duly noted that there have been several relevant writings on the origin of the filtration technologies to treat end-stage renal disease (ESRD) [1–7]. In this chapter, I will provide a brief précis of this work on the early history of the use of convection, rather than diffusion, to cleanse uremic blood. I will then focus on the 'birth' of 'hemodiafitration' as a clinical tool for the treatment of ESRD.

Preconception: Précis of Earlier Work

Lysaght [4] notes that ultrafiltration of whole blood for analytical purposes dates to 1928 with the work of Brull [8]. However, the first application of ultrafiltration for the purpose of removing uremic toxins may be ascribed to Malinow and Korzon [9] who, in 1947, described the use of an 0.8-m^2 cellophane ultrafilter in uremic dogs that was intended to 'duplicate glomerular function' and prolong their life. The blood flow of 100 ml/min and pressure of 500 mm Hg yielded only 15–20 ml/min of ultrafiltrate, which was duly replaced with intermittent intravenous injections of Krebs-Ringer solution. Approximately 7 liters of fluid was exchanged over an 8-hour time period, and blood urea nitrogen fell from 175 to 75 mg/dl. The report in 1944 of the rotating-drum diffusion-based dialyzer by Kolff et al. [10] eclipsed these early findings with convective transport. Others, such as Alwall [11] in Sweden, conducted ultrafiltration with a stationary drum hemodialysis device. The aim of these studies, however, was to remove excess body water and was not aimed at the removal of uremic toxins. As such, no replacement fluid was used, and the potential for convective blood cleansing was therefore sharply limited. In the mid-1940s, Kolff and Alwall opened the era of hemodialysis treatment for acute renal failure. The era of hemodialysis for ESRD was introduced by Quinton, Dillard and Scribner with their introduction of the arteriovenous shunt in 1960 [12]. This era persists today.

Gestation: Examination of More Recent Work

The next deliberate use of ultrafiltration to mimic glomerular blood cleansing in patients with ESRD was reported by myself, Bluemle and colleagues in 1967 [13]. My interest in convective transport came from work with the peritoneal membrane. Here, ultrafiltration with hypertonic glucose solutions clearly resulted in the transport of urea and other small-molecular-weight plasma water constituents into the peritoneal cavity [14]. I was not at this time aware of the prior work by Malinow and Kurzon [9]. I was sharing the laboratory of my mentor and colleague, Lewis W. Bluemle Jr., at the University of Pennsylvania. Bluemle held a contract with a division of the National Institutes of Health, the National Institute of Arthritis and Metabolic Diseases (NIAMD), to explore novel membranes for hemodialysis [5]. At that time, Alan Michaels, the President of the then recently founded Amicon Corporation, came to Philadelphia to discuss with Bluemle and myself a new series of membranes that his new corporation was able to produce. The result was a 10-year collaboration involving funding from the NIAMD and joint research between the University of Pennsylvania laboratories (Henderson and colleagues), Amicon (notably Cheryl Ford and Michael Lysaght) and the Massachusetts Institute of Technology (Clark Colton).

Noteworthy parallel investigative activities using convective transport came from Dorson and Markovitz [15], who reported an in vitro pulsatile ultrafiltration system in 1968, and of course the elegant clinical studies of Edward Quellhorst in 1972 [16] using the Hospal AN69 membrane.

Birth: Nomenclature, Membranes and Equipment

The first name applied to the convective technology aimed at cleansing uremic blood was 'diafiltration' in 1967. The name appeared to acknowledge the potential roles of both diffusion (dialysis) and convection (filtration). However, 6 years later (1973), Ben Burton of the NIAMD suggested that 'hemofiltration' was a more apt designation, as solute kinetic studies had shown little in the way of diffusive transport with this technique. The name stuck. The work reported from the University of Pennsylvania was all conducted in the predilution mode, because bench studies with postdilution were interpreted to be less flexible in application, owing to the limitations imposed by high filtration fractions and the lower efficiency of removal of toxic solutes loosely bound to protein [17]. It should be noted with appropriate respect that W. Leber, working in Giessen, Germany, was the first investigator to deliberately couple diffusion and convection in what is now termed 'hemodiafiltration', which technique he presented in an unpublished report at a conference in Gstaad, Switzerland, in 1977. His subsequent untimely death in a traffic accident sadly ended his contributions to the convective technologies.

Membranes

Unlike the existing Cuprophan® cellulosic membranes of the day that dominated the field of dialysis, the membranes from Amicon were made from precipitated polyelectrolyte. These membranes were neutral in charge and could be cast in a wide range of hydraulic permeabilities. Unlike the homogeneous structure of Cuprophan, the Amicon membranes were asymmetrical, with a thin 1- to 2-μm skin supported by a thick spongy stroma. The stroma was exceedingly open and offered no real resistance to fluid flow. This structure may be found in the polysulfone membranes in common use today. By traditional standards of dialysis, the Amicon membrane was too thick (200 μm) and presented a significant barrier to diffusion [18]. However, the skin was thin and sufficiently porous to permit inulin (5,200 Da, the traditional index solute for measuring glomerular filtration rate) to pass through unrestrained with the ultrafiltered plasma, similar to the glomerular basement membrane (i.e. a sieving coefficient = 1.0). It was, however, far more permeable to water than was the Cuprophan membrane. Of note was the commercial presence of the dialysis membrane from Rhone Poulenc (Hospal), which was synthetic in origin (polyacrylonitrile) and quite comparable in hydraulic permeability to the Amicon polyelectrolyte membrane [18]. It was tighter in pore structure, sieving inulin at 0.7 rather than unity. The ready availability of this membrane in Europe boosted the investigative efforts of Quellhorst and others in exploring convective transport. Interestingly, it carried a net negative surface charge, causing the solute clearance profile to differ from that of the neutral membrane from Amicon [19].

Equipment

The very high water permeability of these polyelectrolyte membranes (200–300 ml/min depending on the transmembrane pressure) made it necessary to design and build fluid-cycling equipment of exceptional precision. Figure 1 shows the original paired pump principle employed in the early animal work and clinical trials. Reciprocating pistons, driven by a common shaft and cam, presumably rendered the ultrafiltrate into the same volume of diluting fluid. This volumetric approach, however, had problems with degassing the ultrafiltrate,

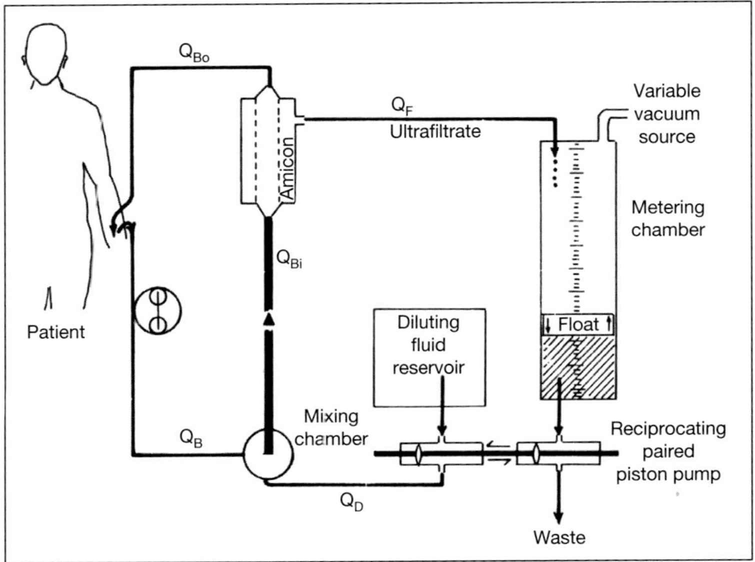

Fig. 1. Diagram of the paired-pump volumetrically based system employed for the first patient trials. Errors incurred by differential pressures in the pumping chambers resulted in degassing errors that subsequently led to abandoning this method for a gravimetrically based system. Q_B = Blood flow rate; i = inlet; o = outlet; Q_D = dialysate flow rate; Q_F = ultrafiltration flow rate.

causing unacceptable fluid balance errors. Subsequently, gravimetrically based machines proved to be more accurate and are now widely available.

Postpartum: Clinical Research and Adjunctive Technologies

Clinical Research in Europe and the USA

The difference between the regulatory climates of Europe and the USA was a significant factor affecting the development of hemodiafiltration. In the USA in the late 1960s and, more particularly, in the early 1970s, the need for independent review of experimental procedures involving patients was recognized, and Institutional Review Boards were put in place. Even prior to this recognition, there was a strong concern held by those of us investigating the new convective cleansing modality for uremic blood. We feared that some critical, but as yet unknown, plasma substance of medium molecular weight, that could be vital to the life and/or well-being of the study subject, would be swept into the drain with the effluent ultrafiltrate. Therefore, when moving from animal work to the first human study subject, the ultrafiltration technique was not fully applied. Rather, a 'creeping substitution' protocol was instituted, in which an initial combined therapy with a small hemofilter and a standard Travenol twin-coil dialyzer was applied for 30 min of the 4-hour hemodialysis. Following a week free of adverse events, the application of the parallel ultrafiltration was increased in duration to 60 min, and then to 90 min, etc. As no adverse events were encountered, we eventually applied a full-scale hemofilter once per week in the thrice weekly treatment schedule, but watched for clinical signs of vital solute deficiency in whichever way it might manifest itself. This caution, encouraged by the regulatory climate in the USA, led us to focus on the details of the experimental technique, resulting in the development of the fundamental mathematical relationships for hemodiafiltration [20, 21] and the relatively slow, deliberate movement to large clinical trials.

Europe, on the other hand, was not constrained by these formal requirements. There was a lively discussion at a 1977 meeting in Europe where a number of investigators interested in the convective technologies participated. The subject under discussion was the reprocessing of spent dialysate. Upon my return to the USA, I began a series of experiments with uremic sheep. The following year, I duly reported my results with the REDY cartridge [22], only to find that a European investigator was reporting his initial clinical experience with this technique. These patients subsequently displayed crippling osteopathy which was felt to be due to the high aluminum concentration in the reprocessed dialysate. This observation was critical to the formulation change of the cartridge and to the benefit of all subsequent users. Furthermore, it was this freedom of investigators and expectation of patient study in Europe that permitted Quellhorst to move directly into the clinical application of hemodiafiltration with the Hospal AN69 polyacrylonitrile membrane, reporting brilliant results in his series of 100 study subjects and their clinical response over a 10-year time frame [23].

In short, the regulatory climate at the time led to our investigative interest in transport kinetics while Europe was applying the technique clinically.

Adjunctive Technologies

The birth of hemodiafiltration spawned several useful technologies that are worthy of comment. The continuous therapies used to treat acute renal failure were the result of work by Silverstein et al. [24] and particularly by Kramer et al. [25]. Online production of sterile pyrogen-free electrolyte solution was made possible by the availability of the Amicon membrane technology. The lack of necessity for heat sterilization reduced the cost of using the prepackaged replacement solution required for the filtration-based technologies [26]. It even provided the potential for using sterile pyrogen-free dialysate in routine hemodialysis for those who wished to do so. Precise fluid-monitoring machines

Table 1. Prevalence of hemodiafiltration use by country in DOPPS II and DOPPS III: percent of patients receiving hemodiafiltration in the initial prevalent cross-section

Country	DOPPS II		DOPPS III	
	n	%	n	%
Australia/New Zealand	513	6.6	421	4.8
Belgium	538	5.6	482	13.1
Canada	601	0.2	523	0.0
France	528	12.9	486	17.1
Germany	571	10.0	558	5.9
Italy	576	19.1	500	16.0
Japan	1,805	0.0	1,826	4.7
Spain	613	2.8	504	6.0
Sweden	547	13.2	542	20.1
UK	565	5.0	263	8.7
USA	2,260	0.5	1,652	0.1

Hemodiafiltration is defined as patients receiving ≥5 liters of replacement fluid during dialysis [28].

began to be used as a requirement for performing hemofiltration. They are now generally available for hemodialysis as well as for the convective technologies. Apart from the two original membranes (from Amicon and from Rhone Poulenc) mentioned above, there are now many high-hydraulic-permeability membranes composed of either cellulosic or synthetic materials for use in hemodiafiltration or other high-flux applications.

Infancy

It is noteworthy that, while we are still in the era of maintenance hemodialysis, there are reports of the increasing use of convective technologies. Europe leads the world in this regard (table 1) [Port F., DOPPS studies I and II, pers. commun.] and, as reported by Canaud et al. [27], high-volume convective therapy is associated with a marked (36%) reduction in mortality compared with conventional hemodialysis. The USA, with its regulatory restrictions and fiscal constraints on provision of care, now trails badly. Use of high-flux membranes in which passive (internal) hemodiafiltration occurs is widespread, even in the USA; however, as noted in the National Institutes of Health study of dialysis dose and membrane flux (HEMO-I), this degree of convective transport fails to confer the benefit of improved survival [28]. Treatment time as a prescription variable is now under experimental examination (National Institutes of Health: Frequent Hemodialysis Network Trials, 2007; HEMO-II). Longer weekly treatment duration and greater frequency of application offer the broader solute clearance profile achieved with hemodiafiltration. I am advised that high-volume hemodiafiltration (>20 l/treatment), coupled with increased frequency and/or duration of treatment (e.g. overnight), will be needed to match the divine prototype in terms of longevity and quality of life [Hova J.A., pers. commun.].

References

1 Henderson LW: Present status of hemofiltration; in Chang TMS (ed): Artificial Kidney, Artificial Liver and Artificial Cells. New York, Plenum Publishers, 1978, pp 39–46.
2 Henderson LW: Historical overview and principles of hemodiafiltration. Dial Transplant 1980;9:220–221.
3 Henderson LW: The beginning of hemofiltration; in Schaefer K, Koch K, Quellhorst E, von Herrath D (eds): Hemofiltration. Contrib Nephrol. Basel, Karger, 1982, pp 1–19.
4 Lysaght M: The history of hemofiltration; in Henderson LW, Quellhorst EA, Baldamus CA, Lysaght MJ (eds): Hemofiltration. Berlin, Springer, 1986, pp. 1–13.
5 Bluemle LW Jr: Early days of hemofiltration. ASAIO Trans 1987;33:54–56.
6 Cameron S: History of the Treatment of Renal Failure by Dialysis. Oxford, Oxford University Press, 2002, pp 239–244.
7 Henderson LW: The beginning of clinical hemofiltration: a personal account. ASAIO J 2003;49:513–517.
8 Brull L: Réalisation de l'ultrafiltration in vivo. Biol C R 1928;99:105–107.
9 Malinow MR, Korzon W: An experimental method for obtaining an ultrafiltrate of the blood. J Lab Clin Med 1947;32:461–471.
10 Kolff WJ, Berk HTHJ, Ter Welle M, van der Leg JW, van Dijk EC, van Noordwijk J: The artificial kidney: a dialyser with great area. Acta Med Scand 1944;117:121–134.
11 Alwall N: Apparatus for dialysis of the blood in vivo. Acta Med Scand 1947;128:317–325.
12 Quinton WE, Dillard DH, Scribner BH: Cannulation of blood vessels for prolonged hemodialysis. Trans Am Soc Artif Intern Organs 1960;6:104–111.
13 Henderson LW, Besarab A, Michaels A, Bluemle LW Jr: Blood purification by ultrafiltration and fluid replacement (diafiltration). Trans Am Soc Artif Intern Organs 1967;13:216–226.
14 Henderson LW: Peritoneal ultrafiltration dialysis: enhanced urea transfer using hypertonic peritoneal dialysis fluid. J Clin Invest 1966;45:950–955.
15 Dorson W, Markovitz M: A pulsating ultrafiltration artificial kidney. Chem Eng Prog Symp Ser 1968;64:85–89.
16 Quellhorst E, Fernandez E, Scheler F: Treatment of uremia using an ultrafiltration-filtration system. Proc Eur Dial Transplant Assoc 1972;9:584–587.
17 Henderson LW: Pre- vs post-dilution hemofiltration. Conference on nondialytic management of uremia. Clin Nephrol 1979;11:120–124.
18 Colton CK, Lysaght MJ: Membranes for hemodialysis; in Jacobs C, Kjellstrand CM, Koch KM, Winchester JF (eds): Replacement of Renal Function by Dialysis. New York, Kluwer Academic Publishers, 1966, pp 103–113.
19 Leypoldt JK, Frigon RP, Henderson LW: Macromolecular charge effects hemofilter solute sieving. Trans Am Soc Artif Intern Organs 1986;32:384–387.
20 Colton CK, Henderson LW, Ford CA, Lysaght MJ: Kinetics of hemodiafiltration. I. In vitro transport characteristics of a hollow-fiber blood ultrafilter. J Lab Clin Med 1975;85:355–371.

21 Henderson LW, Colton CK, Ford C: Kinetics of hemodiafiltration. II. Clinical characteristics of a new blood cleansing modality. J Lab Clin Med 1975;85:372–391.
22 Henderson LW, Parker HR, Schroeder JP, Frigon R, Sanfelippo ML: Continuous low flow hemofiltration with sorbent regeneration of ultrafiltrate. Trans Am Soc Artif Intern Organs 1978;24:178–184.
23 Quellhorst E: Long term follow up in chronic hemofiltration. Int J Artif Organs 1983;6:115–120.
24 Silverstein ME, Ford CA, Lysaght MJ, Henderson LW: Treatment of severe fluid overload by ultrafiltration. N Engl J Med 1974;291:747–751.
25 Kramer P, Wigger W, Rieger J, Mathaei D, Scheler F: Arteriovenous hemofiltration: a new and simple method for the treatment of overhydrated patients resistant to diuretics. Klin Wochenschr 1977;55:1121.
26 Henderson LW, Beans E: Successful production of sterile pyrogen-free electrolyte solution by ultrafiltration. Kidney Int 1978;14:522–525.
27 Canaud B, Bragg-Gresham JL, Marshall MR, Desmueles S, Gillespie BW, Depner T, Klassen P, Port F: Mortality risk for patients receiving hemodiafiltration versus hemodialysis: European results from the DOPPS. Kidney Int 2006;69:2087–2093.
28 Eknoyen G, Beck GJ, Cheung AK, Daugirdas JT, Greene T, Kusek JW, Allon M, Bailey J, Delmez JA, Depner TA, Dwyer JT, Levey AS, Levin NW, Milford E, Ornt DB, Rocco MV, Schulman G, Schwab ST, Teehan BP, Toto R: Effect of dialysis dose and membrane flux in maintenance hemodialysis. N Engl J Med 2002;347:2010–2019.

Lee W. Henderson, MD, FACP
480 Clapboard Hill Road
Guilford, CT 06437 (USA)
Tel. +1 203 458 2847, E-Mail hndrsnlee@aol.com

Ronco C, Canaud B, Aljama P (eds): Hemodiafiltration.
Contrib Nephrol. Basel, Karger, 2007, vol 158, pp 9–19

Evolution of Hemodiafiltration

Claudio Ronco

Department of Nephrology, St. Bortolo Hospital, Vicenza, Italy

Abstract

The evolution of hemodiafiltration (HDF) has become possible by the advances in the construction of dialysis membranes. The availability of a high-flux membrane, partially hydrophilic with high sieving coefficients and a reduced wall thickness has made it possible to conveniently combine diffusion and convection for blood purification. The second important step has been the development of accurate ultrafiltration control systems. Machines capable of managing large amounts of fluid turnover allowed safe and effective HDF. Some new dialysis machines are specifically designed to perform HDF with adequate embedded software. The third step regards the production of large amounts of ultrapure dialysate and replacement fluid. For years replacement fluid was produced in bags, while recently, online production has enabled high volume exchanges in HDF. All these advances, together with the creativity of several groups, have spurred new interest in HDF and have led to the development of various HDF techniques, which are successfully applied to uremic patients with important clinical benefits.

In 1967, Henderson et al. [1] published the rationale for a new blood-cleansing modality based on ultrafiltration and fluid replacement: they defined the new method 'diafiltration'. Years later, thanks to the contribution of Clark Colton and other collaborators, the same senior author published a systematic characterization of the new blood purification modality [2]. The new term 'hemodiafiltration' (HDF) was however used for the first time by Leber et al. [3] in Germany. The combination of diffusion and convection to achieve an efficient and adequate blood purification was proposed as a new method full of potential for blood purification [4]. From that moment, a series of developments took place until the modern days. These developments represent the evolution of HDF from its original conception to the most updated and recent modalities of its application.

As in its original description, HDF is an extracorporeal renal replacement technique utilizing a highly permeable membrane, in which diffusion and convection are conveniently combined to enhance solute removal in a wide spectrum of molecular weights. Ultrafiltration exceeds the desired fluid loss in the patient, and therefore replacement fluid must be administered to achieve the target fluid balance. Different modalities of HDF are applied in clinical practice today; however, the common denominator of such a therapy is the combination of diffusion and convection to achieve solute and volume control.

Evolution of Hemodiafiltration Technology

Dialysis in its beginning was mostly a diffusive process. The possibility of using convection in extracorporeal therapies was substantially limited by the low hydraulic permeability of cellulosic membranes. In fact, Cuprophan®, like all cellulosic membranes, was considerably hydrophilic with a wall thickness in the range of 10–20 μm and therefore good for diffusion, but its porosity was insufficient to provide high water fluxes and elevated sieving coefficients.

On the other hand, original synthetic fibers had an internal skin layer surrounded by a microporous structure with a total thickness of 75–100 μm. The polymer was hydrophobic, and its hydraulic permeability and sieving capacity were high and thus adequate for convection, but the efficiency in diffusion was poor due to the marked thickness. Thus high-flux membranes were only used for hemofiltration with consequent limitations in terms of small-solute clearance. A further and decisive evolution in the field of membranes has been represented by the new generation of synthetic polymers with a combined hydrophilic-hydrophobic structure and a reduced wall thickness. Such membranes are constituted of polyethersulfone, polyamide, polymethylmethacrylate, polyacrylonitrile and other polymers mixed in various proportions with hydrophilic compounds such as polyvinylpyrrolidone. Thus, only after the advent of these membranes could the use of therapies such as HDF be adequately developed with an optimization of the combination of diffusion and convection [5].

The first convective therapy made commercially available was performed with a closed dialysate delivery system called Rhodial 75. This system was instrumental in supporting the theory of middle molecules [6, 7]. The system had to rely on a closed tank of dialysate to overcome the excessive ultrafiltration provided by the flat polyacrylonitrile RP6 dialyzer. Subsequently, the technology for controlling ultrafiltration was developed in conjunction with the evolution of hemofiltration and the expanded production of high-flux dialyzers [8]. The real advance was obtained when ultrafiltration control systems were routinely applied to standard dialysis machines. In those years, closed and open (single-pass) volumetric systems were developed together with other approaches such as gravimetric or fluximetric ultrafiltration control mechanisms. The main difference between two widely used approaches was that in one case the system was acting as flow equalizer and a separate pump was providing net ultrafiltration; in the other case, the system was a differential flow-measuring device and the difference between the outlet and inlet flow was governing transmembrane pressure in the filter. Once the problem of ultrafiltration control had been solved, it became evident that a balancing system for fluid replacement was needed to perform a safe and accurate HDF. Thus, machines started to be equipped with specific balancing systems to manage up to 9 liters of fluid reinfusion and up to 15 liters of ultrafiltration per session. Different companies implemented various strategies to solve the technicality of HDF, and the treatment became widely available even to those centers where partial access to technology had previously limited the implementation of HDF. A further step in development was then made when online filtration of fresh dialysis fluid through a redundant filtration cascade made large quantities of ultrapure fluid available, ready to be reinfused in the patient during HDF.

Until few years ago, HDF was performed using replacement fluids in bags. Originally fluids contained acetate or lactate while only recently could a bicarbonate-based solution be utilized. A significant advance in the field of HDF was made when biofiltration (a soft form of HDF) was launched on the market. The system provided circuits, lines and a 3-liter bag in a single package making HDF a ready-to-use treatment. Subsequently, as the confidence of the operators became greater, larger surface area dialyzers and larger amounts of fluid were made available in the package leading to a standardization around 9 liters of reinfusion. A further advance was made when acetate was completely eliminated from the solution as in the case of acetate-free biofiltration. Further modifications were suggested in the replacement fluid composition and even a complete regeneration of the endogenous ultrafiltrate by sorbents was proposed and clinically utilized in a 2-chamber HDF technique called paired filtration dialysis/HDF with endogenous reinfusion (HFR).

The advances made in the field of membranes, machines and solutions was paralleled by a significant improvement of the dedicated software so that HDF became an easy procedure, automatically managed by the machine and easily controlled by nurses through a friendly user interface [7–13]. The typical and most recent example for this is the modern Fresenius 5008 machine which has a built-in design specifically oriented towards HDF and online HDF [14].

Evolution of Hemodiafiltration Techniques

As previously stated, HDF is a combination of hemodialysis and hemofiltration. The combination of convection with a high-flux thin membrane allows

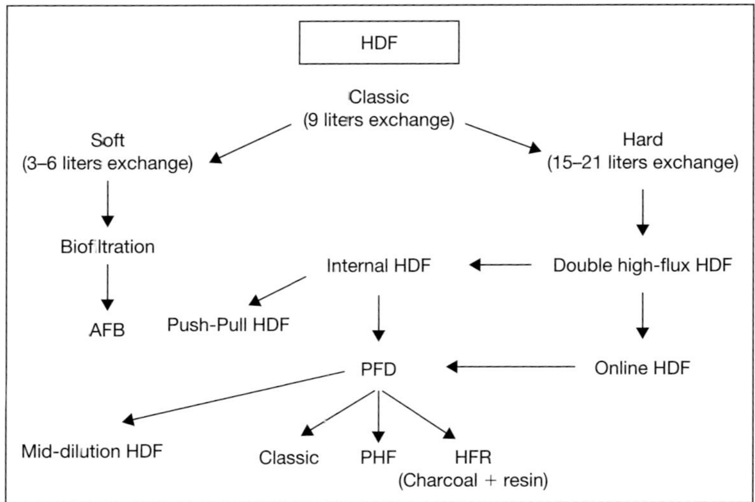

Fig. 1. HDF evolution tree: the evolution of HDF from the original technique to the different modifications. AFB = Acetate-free biofiltration; PFD = paired filtration dialysis; PHF = paired HDF.

for the simultaneous removal of small and large solutes. The relative contribution of convection to the overall solute removal increases progressively with the increasing molecular weight. The above concepts have been implemented in clinical practice leading to different forms of HDF. A flow chart of the HDF evolution into different techniques is reported in figure 1 [8, 9].

The following lines intend to describe a series of techniques utilized over the years to perform HDF; the layout of the relevant circuits is schematically reported in figure 2.

Classic Hemodiafiltration

This technique is based on an average reinfusion rate of 9 l/session typically in postdilution. Fluids are contained in commercial bags. A blood flow higher than 300 ml/min is required to allow the production of sufficient rates of ultrafiltration at acceptable transmembrane pressure regimes. The equipment requires an ultrafiltration control system and a reinfusion pump operated by a

Fig. 2. The different HDF techniques. A = Arterial port; V = venous port; R = replacement fluid; UF = ultrafiltrate; UFC = UF control; Do = dialysate outlet; Di = dialysate inlet; filtr. = filtration; P_1 = pump 1; P_2 = pump 2. ***a*** Classic HDF. ***b*** Soft HDF or biofiltration. ***c*** Hard (high-volume) HDF. ***d*** Online HDF. ***e*** Internal HDF (high-flux dialysis). ***f*** Paired filtration dialysis. ***g*** HDF with HFR. ***h*** Mid-dilution HDF. ***i*** Double high-flux HDF. ***j*** Push-pull HDF.

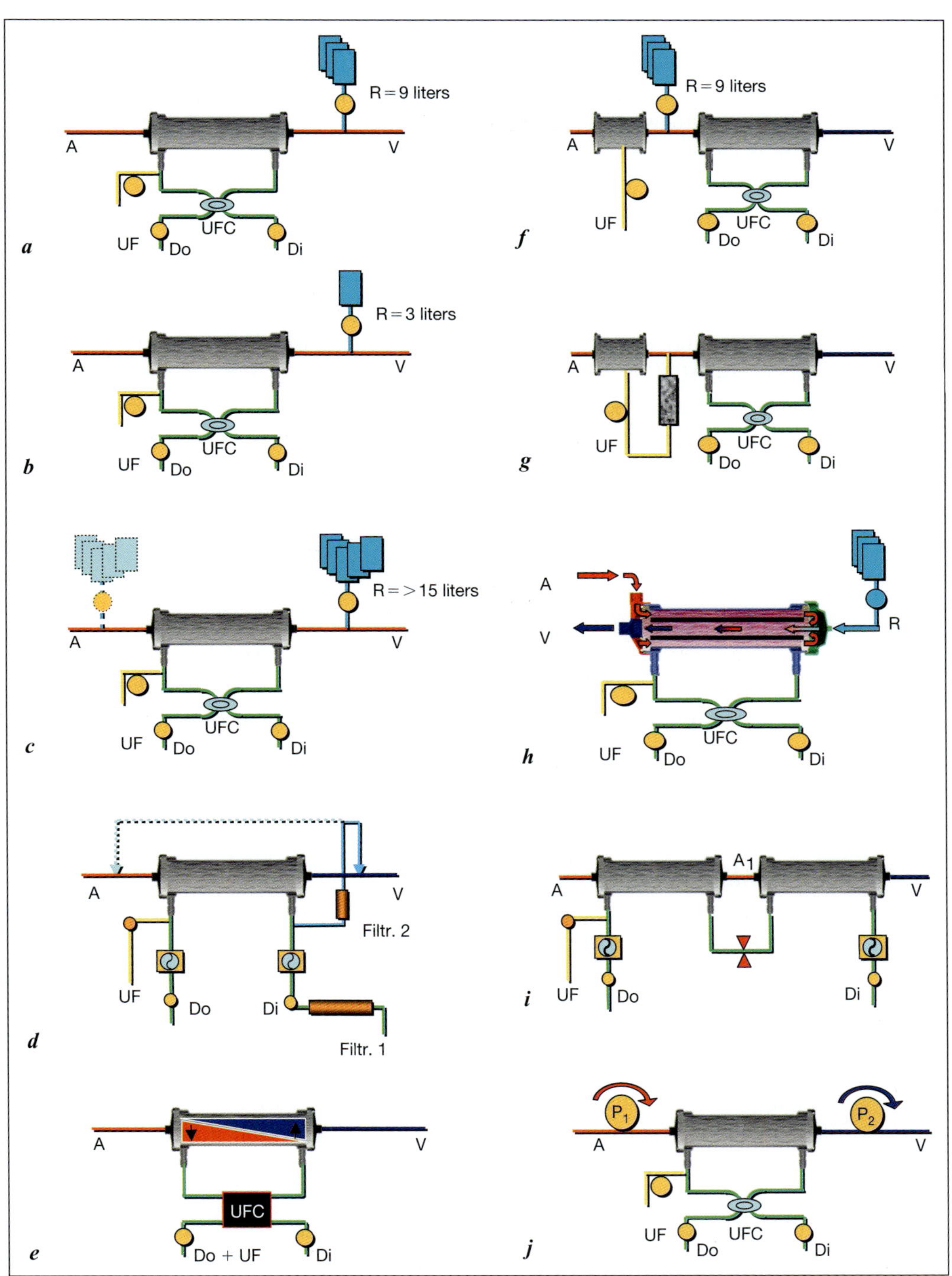
a
R = 9 liters
A
V
UF
Do
UFC
Di
b
R = 3 liters
A
V
UF
Do
UFC
Di
c
R = > 15 liters
A
V
UF
Do
UFC
Di
d
A
V
Filtr. 2
UF
Do
Di
Filtr. 1
e
A
V
UFC
Do + UF
Di
f
R = 9 liters
A
V
UF
UFC
Do
Di
g
A
V
UF
UFC
Do
Di
h
A
V
R
UF
UFC
Do
Di
i
A
A1
V
UF
Do
Di
j
P1
P2
A
V
UF
UFC
Do
Di

scale continuously weighing reinfusion bags. This technique has been used for many years before online modalities were available. In some cases, the amount of reinfusion was as low as 3 l/session (soft HDF) as in the case of biofiltration (a ready-to-use proprietary technique from Hospal, France) or up to 15 l/session as in the case of the so-called hard HDF [8].

Acetate-Free Biofiltration

This is a special form of HDF in which even small traces of acetate were completely eliminated both from dialysate and replacement fluid. The average amount of replacement was normally titrated based on the bicarbonate level of the patient and varied between 6 and 9 l/session [10]. This technique is derived by the soft HDF called biofiltration in which only 3 liters of convection were scheduled. Later, the technique became widely diffused and it became known for the improved hemodynamic tolerance and its effects on treatment efficiency [11]. A special software was implemented to guide the dialysis session making specific profiles of ultrafiltration rate and sodium concentration in the dialysate, not blindly as in the past, but driven by signals coming from the patient and integrated in a biofeedback software technology.

High-Volume Hemodiafiltration

This form of HDF consists in a classic HDF in which however the amount of fluid exchange is 15 l/session or more. Because of the high ultrafiltration rate, high blood flows are required and replacement solution is sometimes infused in predilution mode. This partially decreases the efficiency of the therapy although it allows for an optimal blood flow distribution in the hemodialyzer and a lower protein concentration polarization and the blood membrane interface [12].

Online Hemodiafiltration

The high cost of commercially prepared fluids in bags and the improved technology of dialysate preparation and fluid filtration has allowed it in recent years to develop a novel technique called 'online HDF' [13]. In this technique, a certain amount of freshly prepared ultrapure dialysate is taken from the dialysate inlet line and processed with multiple filtration steps before being used as a replacement fluid. With such a technique, large amounts of inexpensive replacement solution are made available and HDF can be carried out with a very high fluid turnover (up to 30–40 l/session) utilizing pre- and postdilution or even simultaneous pre-/postdilution in different proportions. Specific adjustments had to be made in the past generation of machines, whilst the latter machines are conceived to perform online HDF with adequate embedded software and system controls [14]. The quality of the reinfusion fluid is excellent, and it is guaranteed by the redundancy of the filtration system.

Internal-Filtration Hemodiafiltration

There is a common belief that when a high-flux hemodialyzer is used with a minimal net ultrafiltration, the process is purely diffusive as in the case of low-flux dialyzers. This is an incorrect statement, and the treatment features high amounts of convection although this is masked by the internal kinetics of crossfiltration. As blood moves into the dialyzer, the pressure regime in local regions along the length of the fibers continuously changes. As a consequence, water fluxes in hollow-fiber hemodialyzers are characterized by a postitive transmembrane pressure and direct filtration in the regions near the arterial inlet and a negative transmembrane pressure and reverse filtration (backfiltration) in the region near the venous outlet. In some circumstances this mechanism can be enhanced: by applying a constriction in the middle of the fiber bundle, by operating an obstruction to dialysate flow in the dialysate compartment or by reducing the inner diameter of the fibers, internal filtration can reach values of 40–50 ml/min with a 1.8-m^2 dialyzer operated at zero net filtration [15, 16]. As hydraulic conditions tend to favor an increase in ultrafiltration, the ultrafiltration control system of the machine controls the net fluid balance by modifying the pressures in the system thus increasing the relative amount of backfiltration. Although this in general is defined high-flux dialysis, when specific measures or dialyzer designs are applied to enhance the mechanism of filtration/backfiltration, this form of therapy can be defined as internal HDF [17].

Paired Filtration Dialysis

This technique of HDF has been conceived in Italy for the first time [18]. It is based on two filters placed in series: the first is a hemofilter and removes fluid and solutes by convection; the second is a hemodialyzer in which diffusion is prevalently utilized. Replacement fluid is infused in between the two units. The meaning of this therapy is to minimize the interactions between convection and diffusion, to prevent backfiltration in the hemodialyzer and finally to make ultrafiltrate available for online measurements as a surrogate of plasma water [19]. Recently further evolution of this concept has led to the HFR and paired HDF techniques. HFR is a paired filtration dialysis where the ultrafiltrate produced is purified by adsorption through a resin/charcoal unit and utilized subsequently as a replacement fluid [20]. The paired HDF is another modification of the technique in which the fist unit is used to backfilter some fresh dialysate acting as ultrapure online filtered replacement fluid [21].

Mid-Dilution Hemodiafiltration

This technique is made possible by the use of special filters with two longitudinal compartments in series. Blood flows in the first compartment producing a certain amount of ultrafiltration; at the end of the compartment, instead of having a venous port, there is a chamber designed to receive the replacement fluid infusion. In this chamber, the hemoconcentrated blood – due to the ultrafiltration process – is reconstituted to the original dilution and it is redirected countercurrently in the second blood compartment. Blood then leaves the dialyzer beside the arterial entry. Dialysate in this system flows 50% countercurrently to blood and 50% cocurrently [22].

Double High-Flux Hemodiafiltration

This technique utilizes two high-flux dialyzers in series. Filtration takes place in the proximal unit while backfiltration takes place in the distal unit. High blood flows (>500 ml/min) have been utilized for this technique, and its high efficiency has allowed treatments under 2 h/session [23].

Push-Pull Hemodiafiltration

This technique utilizes the mechanism of filtration and backfiltration alternating the rotation of a prefilter pump (while the postfilter pump is stopped) producing filtration, and the rotation of the postfilter pump (while the prefilter pump is stopped) producing a negative pressure in the blood compartment and thus backfiltration [24]. This technique can also be operated by a similar alternate flow regime in the dialysate compartment instead of the blood compartment.

Evolution of Dialysate Filtration Techniques

The use of high-flux dialyzers with a high surface area and large amounts of crossfiltration requires a careful analysis of the quality of every fluid involved in the process. Thus, water treatment systems, dialysate concentrates and dialysate filtration procedures for online replacement fluid production must be continuously controlled and screened for quality. Online preparation of sterile and pyrogen-free solutions for infusion during HDF is based on the use of water and concentrates that are ultrapure and are mixed and distributed in a well-designed and maintained flow path [25]. Ultrafilters with known retention capacity are placed in strategic positions and dimensioned to remove bacteria and endotoxins, which gives a satisfactory purity assurance level. Microbiological safety of online HDF has been shown in long-term clinical studies, with a notable absence of cytokine-inducing activity and pyrogenic reactions in patients despite the infusion of large volumes of fluid in every session [26, 27].

The combination of biocompatible membranes and ultrapure fluid is beneficial in reducing bioactivation of circulating leukocytes induced by blood-hemodialyzer interaction. The high ultrafiltration rates also result in protein-coating of the membrane, rendering it even more biocompatible.

Arteriovenous Hemodiafiltration and Continuous Venovenous Hemodiafiltration for Acute Cases

HDF was firstly described in acute cases in 1985 [28]. In those times, hemofilters were designed with a single port for ultrafiltrate, and the Vicenza group suggested a modification by adding a second port to the Amicon filters so that dialysate fluid could be circulated countercurrently to blood. This first description was characterized by an arteriovenous circuit with no pumps. At the same time, dialysate was infused and drained from the filter by gravity. Only subsequently pumped circuits started to be used in the acute settings and continuous venovenous hemofiltration/HDF started to appear in the clinical arena. In particular continuous venovenous HDF was made possible by the advent of a machine specific for continuous renal replacement therapy (Prisma) featuring 4 pumps and thus allowing a separate management of dialysate flow and ultrafiltration/reinfusion flow. Today all machines are equipped with circuitry and software that allow a simple and safe management of continuous HDF [29].

Conclusions

The evolution of technology for HDF has made this technique simpler and safer. Furthermore, modifications of the original basic HDF layout have allowed to explore new treatment modalities that however retain the basic principles of combining diffusion and convection. The emerging evidence that these therapies may be superior to classic hemodialysis in terms of morbidity and mortality further encourages the progress of application of HDF and derived techniques. We think that this represents a classic example of translational research where a continuous interaction between bench experiments and clinical testings is paralleled by an intelligent merging of clinical questions and technological responses.

References

1 Henderson LW, Besarab A, Michaels A, Bluemle LW Jr: Blood purification by UF and fluid replacement (diafiltration). Trans Am Soc Artif Intern Organs 1967;17:216–221.

2 Henderson LW, Colton CK, Ford C: Kinetics of HDF. II. Clinical characterization of a new blood cleansing modality. J Lab Clin Med 1975;85:372–375.

3 Leber H, Wizemann V, Goubeaud G, Rawer P, Schutterle G: Hemodiafiltration: a new alternative to hemofiltration and conventional hemodialysis. Artif Organs 1978;2:150–153.

4 Henderson LW: Biophysics of UF and hemofiltration; in Maher JF (ed): Replacement of Renal Function by Dialysis: A Textbook of Dialysis, ed 3. Dordrecht, Kluwer Academic Publishers, 1989, pp 300–326.

5 Hoenich N, Ronco C: Dialyzer evaluation; in Winchester J, Koch K, Jacobs C, Kjiellestrand C (eds): Replacement of Renal Function by Dialysis. Dordrecht, Kluwer Academic Publishers, 1996, pp 256–270.

6 Babb AL, Farrel PC, Uvelli DA, Scribner BH: Hemodialyzer evaluation by examination of solute molecular spectra. Trans Am Soc Artif Intern Organs 1972;18:98–105.

7 Babb AL, Strand MJ, Uvelli DA, et al: Quantitative description of dialysis treatment: a dialysis index. Kidney Int 1975;7(suppl 2):23–28.

8 Ronco C, La Greca G: The role of technology in hemodialysis; in Ronco C, La Greca G (eds): Hemodialysis Technology. Contrib Nephrol. Basel, Karger, 2002, vol 137, pp 1–12.

9 Maduell F: Hemodiafiltration. Hemodial Int 2005;9:47–55.

10 Pacitti A, Casino FG, Pedrini L, Santoro A, Atti M: Prescription and surveillance of the acetate-free biofiltration sessions: the bicarbonate cycle. Int J Artif Organs 1995;18:722–725.

11 Ronco C, Brendolan A, Milan M, Rodighiero MP, Zanella M, La Greca G: Impact of biofeedback-induced cardiovascular stability on hemodialysis tolerance and efficiency. Kidney Int 2000;58: 800–808.

12 Pedrini LA, Cozzi G, Faranna P, Mercieri A, Ruggiero P, Zerbi S, Feliciani A, Riva A: Transmembrane pressure modulation in high-volume mixed hemodiafiltration to optimize efficiency and minimize protein loss. Kidney Int 2006;69:573–579.

13 Canaud B, Levesque R, Krieter D, Desmeules S, Chalabi L, Moragues H, Morena M, Cristol JP: On-line hemodiafiltration as routine treatment of end-stage renal failure: why pre- or mixed dilution mode is necessary in on-line hemodiafiltration today? Blood Purif 2004;22(suppl 2):40–48.

14 Ronco C, Bowry S, Tetta C: Dialysis patients and cardiovascular problems: can technology help solve the complex equation? Blood Purif 2006;24:39–45.

15 Ronco C, Brendolan A, Feriani M, Milan M, Conz P, Lupi A, Berto P, Bettini MC, La Greca G: A new scintigraphic method to characterize ultrafiltration in hollow fiber dialyzers. Kidney Int 1992; 41:1383–1393.

16 Ronco C, Brendolan A, Lupi A, Bettini MC, La Greca G: Enhancement of convective transport by internal filtration in a modified experimental hemodialyzer. Kidney Int 1998;54:979–985.

17 Fiore GB, Guadagni G, Lupi A, Ricci Z, Ronco C: A new semiempirical mathematical model for prediction of internal filtration in hollow fiber hemodialyzers. Blood Purif 2006;24:555–568.

18 Botella J, Ghezzi P, Sanz-Moreno C, Milan M, Conz P, La Greca G, Ronco C: Multicentric study on paired filtration dialysis as a short, highly efficient dialysis technique. Nephrol Dial Transplant 1991;6:715–721.

19 Arrigo G, Tetta C, Santoro A, Ghezzi P, Ronco C, Colasanti G, La Greca G, Zucchelli P, D'Amico G: Continuous urea monitoring in hemodialysis: a model approach to forecast dialytic performance: results of a multicenter study. J Nephrol 2001;14:481–487.

20 Ursino M, Coli L, Magosso E, Capriotti P, Fiorenzi A, Baroni P, Stefoni S: A mathematical model for the prediction of solute kinetics, osmolarity and fluid volume changes during hemodiafiltration with on-line regeneration of ultrafiltrate (HFR). Int J Artif Organs 2006;29:1031–1040.

21 Mandolfo S, Corsi A, Wratten ML, Sereni L, Imbasciati E: Evaluation of hygiene and safety controls for on-line paired hemodiafiltration (PHF). Int J Artif Organs 2006;29:160–165.

22 Santoro A, Conz PA, De Cristofaro V, Acquistapace I, Gaggi R, Ferramosca E, Renaux JL, Rizzioli E, Wratten ML: Mid-dilution: the perfect balance between convection and diffusion; in Ronco C, Brendolan A, Levin NW (eds): Cardiovascular Disorders in Hemodialysis. Contrib Nephrol. Basel, Karger, 2005, vol 149, pp 107–114.

23 Miller JH, von Albertini B, Gardner PW, Shinaberger JH: Technical aspects of high flux hemodiafiltration for adequate short (under 2 hours) treatment. Trans Am Soc Artif Intern Organs 1984; 30:377–380.

24 Miwa M, Shinzato T: Push/pull hemodiafiltration: technical aspects and clinical effectiveness. Artif Organs 1999;23:1123–1126.

25 Ledebo I: On-line preparation of solutions for dialysis: practical aspects versus safety and regulations. J Am Soc Nephrol 2002;13(suppl 1):S78–S83.

26 Canaud B, Bosc JY, Leray-Moragues H, et al: On-line haemodiafiltration: safety and efficacy in long-term clinical practice. Nephrol Dial Transplant 2000;5(suppl 1):S60–S67.

27 Guth HJ, Gruska S, Kraatz G: On-line production of ultrapure substitution fluid reduces TNF-alpha- and IL-6 release in patients on hemodiafiltration therapy. Int J Artif Organs 2003;26:181–187.
28 Ronco C, Bragantini L, Brendolan A, Dell'Aquila R, Fabris A, Chiaramonte S, Feriani M, Laquaniti L, La Greca G: Arteriovenous hemofiltration (AVHDF) combined with continuous arteriovenuous hemofiltration (CAVH). Trans Am Soc Artif Intern Organs 1985;31:349–352.
29 Ronco C, Ricci Z, Bellomo R, Baldwin I, Kellum J: Management of fluid balance in CRRT: a technical approach. Int J Artif Organs 2005;28:765–776.

Claudio Ronco, MD
Department of Nephrology, St. Bortolo Hospital
IT–36100 Vicenza (Italy)
Tel. +39 0444753650, Fax +39 0444753949, E-Mail cronco@goldnet.it

Ronco C, Canaud B, Aljama P (eds): Hemodiafiltration.
Contrib Nephrol. Basel, Karger, 2007, vol 158, pp 20–33

Solute Removal by Hollow-Fiber Dialyzers

William R. Clark[a,b], *Eduardo Rocha*[c], *Claudio Ronco*[d]

[a]Gambro Inc., Lakewood, Colo., and [b]Nephrology Division, Indiana University School of Medicine, Indianapolis, Ind., USA; [c]Nephrology Department, Universidade Federal do Rio de Janeiro, Rio de Janeiro, Brazil; [d]Nephrology Department, St. Bortolo Hospital, Vicenza, Italy

Abstract

Renal replacement therapy performed for end-stage renal disease patients now occurs almost exclusively with hollow-fiber dialyzers. Because renal replacement therapy utilizing such a device requires goals to be set with regard to the rate and extent of solute removal, a thorough understanding of the mechanisms by which solute removal occurs is necessary. This chapter provides an overview of solute removal by hollow-fiber dialyzers. In the first part of the chapter, the major characteristics of hollow-fiber membranes influencing solute removal are discussed. Within this section, the chemical composition and physical characteristics of commonly used dialysis membranes and the features determining their solute permeability properties are reviewed. The remainder of the chapter emphasizes the major determinants of hollow-fiber dialyzer performance.

Renal replacement therapy performed for end-stage renal disease patients now occurs almost exclusively with hollow-fiber dialyzers. Because renal replacement therapy utilizing such a device requires goals to be set with regard to the rate and extent of solute removal, a thorough understanding of the mechanisms by which solute removal occurs is necessary. This chapter provides an overview of solute removal by hollow-fiber dialyzers. In the first part of the chapter, the major characteristics of hollow-fiber membranes influencing solute removal are discussed. Within this section, the chemical composition and physical characteristics of commonly used dialysis membranes and the features determining their solute permeability properties are reviewed. The remainder of the chapter emphasizes the major determinants of hollow-fiber dialyzer performance.

Hollow-Fiber Membranes: Classification by Material

Cellulosic Membranes

The relatively long duration of popularity of cellulosic membranes can be explained largely by their particular suitability for a diffusion-based procedure like hemodialysis (HD) [1]. The underlying hydrogel structure of these membranes and their tensile strength allow the combination of low wall thickness (see below) and high porosity to be attained in the fiber spinning process [2]. These characteristics allow the attainment of high rates of diffusive membrane transport and efficient removal of small, water-soluble uremic solutes, such as urea and creatinine [3, 4]. Another characteristic feature of these membranes is symmetry with respect to composition, implying an essentially uniform resistance to mass transfer over the entire wall thickness.

Synthetic Membranes

Synthetic membranes were developed essentially in response to concerns related to the narrow scope of solute removal and the pronounced complement activation associated with unmodified cellulosic dialyzers. The AN69® membrane, a copolymer of acrylonitrile and an anionic sulfonate group, was first employed in flat sheet form in a closed-loop dialysate system in the early 1970s [5]. Since that time, a number of other synthetic membranes have been developed, including polysulfone [6], polyamide [7], polymethylmethacrylate [8], polyethersulfone [9] and polyarylethersulfone/polyamide [10]. Largely related to the interest in hemofiltration as an end-stage renal disease therapy in the late 1970s and early in the following decade, along with the inability to use low-flux unmodified cellulosic dialyzers for this therapy, these membranes were initially formulated with high water permeability [11]. The large mean pore size and thick wall structure of these membranes allowed the high ultrafiltration rates necessary in hemofiltration to be achieved at relatively low transmembrane pressures. However, with the waning of interest in hemofiltration as a chronic dialysis therapy in the mid-1980s, dialyzers with these highly permeable membranes were used subsequently in the diffusive mode as high-flux dialyzers. This latter mode continues to be the most common application of these membranes, although they are increasingly being employed for chronic hemodiafiltration now [12]. Synthetic membranes have wall thicknesses of at least 20 μm and may be structurally symmetric (e.g. AN69, polymethylmethacrylate) or asymmetric (e.g. polysulfone, polyamide, polyethersulfone, polyamide/polyarylethersulfone). In the latter category, a very thin 'skin' (approx. 1 μm) contacting the blood compartment lumen acts primarily as the membrane's separative element with regard to solute removal.

Properties of Hemodialyzer Membranes Influencing Solute Removal

Membrane Diffusive Permeability

Membrane wall thickness is one important determinant of diffusive transport [13]. The relatively thin-walled structure of cellulosic membranes (usually 6–15 μm) is largely responsible for their particular suitability in the setting of diffusive HD. The other major determinant of dialyzer membrane diffusive transport is porosity, also known as pore density. Based on the cylindrical pore model described above, membrane porosity is directly proportional to both the number of pores and the square of the pore radius (r^2). Therefore, the smaller dependence of membrane porosity on pore size, relative to the case of water permeability, implies a relatively greater importance of pore number in determining diffusive permeability. That the major determinants of flux (r^4) and diffusive permeability (number of pores, r^2 and wall thickness) differ so significantly implies that the two properties can be independent of one another for a particular HD membrane. Such is the case for cellulosic high-efficiency dialyzers, which typically have very high diffusive permeability values for small solutes but low water permeability.

Nondiffusive Membrane Considerations

A membrane represented by the cylindrical pore model described above deviates from an actual membrane used for clinical HD in that the latter actually has a distribution of pore sizes. Ronco et al. [4] have recently discussed the manner in which pore size distribution may differ among HD membranes and the manner in which this distribution influences a membrane's sieving properties (fig. 1). The membrane represented by curve A has a large number of relatively small pores while the membrane represented by curve B has a large number of relatively large pores. Based on the relatively narrow pore size distributions, the solute sieving coefficient versus molecular weight profile for both membranes has the desirable sharp cut-off, similar to that of the native kidney. However, the molecular-weight cut-off for membrane A (approx. 10 kDa) is consistent with a high-efficiency membrane while that of membrane B (approx. 60 kDa) is consistent with a high-flux membrane. In addition, primarily due to the large number of pores, both membranes would be expected to demonstrate favorable diffusive transport properties. On the other hand, membrane C exhibits a pore size distribution that is unfavorable from both a diffusive transport and sieving perspective. The relatively small number of pores accounts for the poor diffusive properties. In addition, the broad distribution of pores explains not only the 'early' drop-off in sieving coefficient at relatively low molecular weight but also the 'tail' effect at high molecular weight. This latter phenomenon is highly undesirable as it may lead to unacceptably high albumin losses

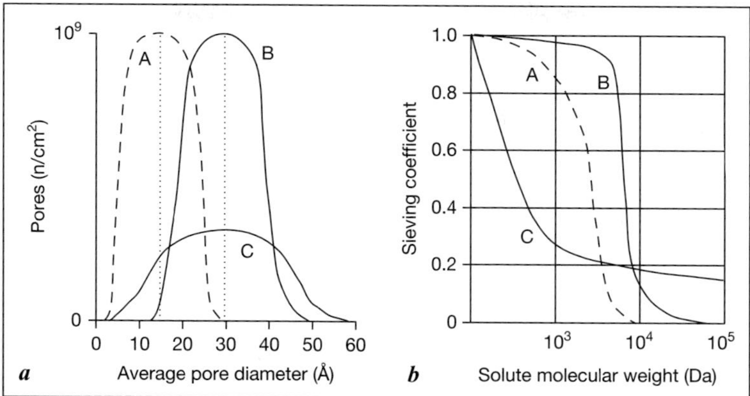

Fig. 1. Pore size distribution and sieving coefficient profiles for three hypothetical membranes A, B and C. ***a*** Relationship between number of pores and pore size. ***b*** Sieving coefficient as a function of solute molecular weight. Reprinted with permission from Ronco et al. [14].

across the membrane. In actual practice, all highly permeable membranes have measurable albumin sieving coefficient values such that the design of this type of membrane involves striking a balance between optimized large-molecular-weight toxin removal and minimal albumin losses.

Another convection-related mechanism by which large uremic toxins can be removed relates to fluid flow within the filter. Under normal operating conditions of high-flux dialysis, the large axial pressure drop that occurs in such highly permeable membranes typically results in pressures in a certain portion of the distal (venous) end of the fiber that are less than the corresponding dialysate compartment pressure. This results in the routine occurrence of backfiltration of dialysate during high-flux HD [15]. Although the combination of significant backfiltration and contaminated dialysate raises concerns related to 'backtransfer', this internal filtration ('Starling's flow') mechanism can significantly augment removal of larger molecules. In fact, under normal operating conditions of high-flux HD, this mechanism is typically the predominant mechanism by which large-solute removal occurs. Attempts at accentuating this internal filtration mechanism, either through a decrease in hollow-fiber inner diameter or manipulations in dialysate compartment pressure, have been described recently [16].

Adsorption (membrane binding) is another mechanism by which hydrophobic compounds like peptides and proteins may be removed during HD. Although adsorption during HD is a relatively poorly understood phenomenon, certain membrane characteristics play an important role. First, adsorption primarily occurs within the pore structure of the membrane rather than at the nominal surface contacting the blood only [17]. Therefore, the open pore structure of high-flux membranes affords more adsorptive potential than do low-flux counterparts. Second, synthetic membranes, many of which are fundamentally hydrophobic, are generally much more adsorptive than hydrophilic cellulosic membranes [18].

Characterization of Dialyzer Performance: The Concept of Solute Clearance

Whole-Blood Clearance

By definition [19], solute clearance (K) is the ratio of mass removal rate (N) to blood solute concentration (C_B):

$$K = N/C_B. \quad (1)$$

For a hemodialyzer, mass removal rate is simply the difference between the rate of solute mass (i.e. product of flow rate and concentration) presented to the dialyzer in the arterial blood line and the rate of solute mass leaving the dialyzer in the venous blood line. This mass balance applied to the dialyzer results in the classical (i.e. arteriovenous) whole-blood dialyzer clearance equation [20]:

$$K_B = [(Q_{Bi} \cdot C_{Bi}) - (Q_{Bo} \cdot C_{Bo})]/C_{Bi} + Q_F \cdot (C_{Bo}/C_{Bi}) \quad (2)$$

In this equation, K_B is whole-blood clearance, Q_B is blood flow rate, C_B is whole-blood solute concentration, and Q_F is net ultrafiltration rate. [The subscripts 'i' and 'o' refer to the inlet (arterial) and outlet (venous) blood lines.]

It is important to note that diffusive, convective and possibly adsorptive solute removals occur simultaneously in HD. For a nonadsorbing solute like urea, diffusion and convection interact in such a manner that total solute removal is significantly less than what is expected if the individual components are simply added together. This phenomenon is explained in the following way. Diffusive removal results in a decrease in solute concentration in the blood compartment along the axial length (i.e. from blood inlet to blood outlet) of the hemodialyzer. As convective solute removal is directly proportional to the blood compartment concentration, convective solute removal decreases as a function of this axial concentration gradient. On the other hand, hemoconcentration resulting from ultrafiltration of plasma water causes a progressive increase in plasma protein concentration and hematocrit (Hct) along the axial length of the dialyzer. This hemoconcentration and resultant hyperviscosity cause an increase in diffusive mass transfer resistance and a decrease in solute transport by this mechanism. The effect of this interaction on overall solute removal has been analyzed rigorously by numerous investigators. The most useful quantification has been developed by Jaffrin [21]:

$$K_T = K_D + Q_F \cdot Tr \quad (3)$$

In this equation, K_T is total solute clearance, K_D is diffusive clearance under conditions of no net ultrafiltration, and the final term is the convective component of clearance. The latter term is a function of the ultrafiltration rate (Q_F) and an experimentally derived transmittance coefficient (Tr), such that:

$$Tr = S\,(1 - K_D/Q_B) \tag{4}$$

where S is the solute sieving coefficient. Thus, Tr for a particular solute is dependent on the efficiency of diffusive removal. At very low values of K_D/Q_B, diffusion has a very small impact on blood compartment concentrations and the convective component of clearance closely approximates the quantity $S \cdot Q_F$. However, with increasing efficiency of diffusive removal (i.e. increasing K_D/Q_B), blood compartment concentrations are significantly influenced. The result is a decrease in Tr and, consequently, in the convective contribution to total clearance.

Blood Water and Plasma Clearance

An implicit assumption in the determination of whole-blood clearance is that the volume from which the solute is cleared is the actual volume of blood transiting through the dialyzer at a certain time. This assumption is incorrect for two reasons. First, in both the erythron and plasma components of blood, a certain volume is comprised of solids (proteins or lipids) rather than water. Second, for solutes like creatinine and phosphate which are distributed in both the erythron and plasma water, slow mass transfer from the intracellular space to the plasma space (relative to mass transfer across the dialyzer) results in relative sequestration (compartmentalization) in the former compartment [22]. This reduces the *effective* volume of distribution from which these solutes can be cleared *in the dialyzer*. As such, whole-blood dialyzer clearances derived by using plasma water concentrations in conjunction with blood flow rates, a common practice in dialyzer evaluations, results in a significant overestimation of actual solute removal. The more appropriate approach is to employ blood water clearances, which account for the above Hct-dependent effects on effective intradialyzer solute distribution volume [23]:

$$Q_{BW} = 0.93 \cdot Q_B[1 - Hct + K(1 - e^{-\alpha t})Hct] \tag{5}$$

where Q_{BW} is blood water flow rate. In this equation, for a given solute, K is the red blood cell (RBC) water/plasma water partition coefficient for a given solute, α is the transcellular rate constant (units: $time^{-1}$), and t is the characteristic dialyzer residence time. Estimates for these parameters have been provided by numerous prior studies and have been summarized by Shinaberger et al. [24]. (The factor 0.93 in equation 2 corrects for the volume of plasma occupied by plasma proteins and lipids.) Finally, K_{BW} can be calculated by substituting Q_{BW} for Q_B in equation 1.

Although the distribution volume of many uremic solutes approximates total body water, it is much more limited for other toxins, particularly those of larger molecular weight. For example, the distribution space of β_2-microglobulin and many other low-molecular-weight proteins is the plasma volume. Consequently, when using equation 2 to determine β_2-microglobulin clearance, plasma flow rates (inlet and outlet) should replace blood flow rates in the first term of the right-hand side of the equation.

The distinction between whole-blood, blood water and dialysate-side clearances is very important when interpreting clinical data. However, clearances provided by dialyzer manufacturers are typically in vitro data generated from experiments in which the blood compartment fluid is an aqueous solution. Although these data provide useful information to the clinician, they overestimate actual dialyzer performance that can be achieved clinically (under the same conditions). This overestimation is related to the inability of aqueous-based experiments to capture the effects of RBCs (see above) and plasma proteins on solute mass transfer.

Clearance versus Mass Removal Rate

It is important to recognize that clearance is *not* a measure of actual dialytic mass removal of a particular solute. As equation 1 indicates, clearance is the ratio of mass removal rate to blood concentration for a given solute. In HD, the mass removal rate of small solutes like urea is very high during the early stage of an intermittent HD treatment due to a favorable transmembrane concentration gradient for diffusion at this time. As the treatment proceeds, a proportional decrease in the blood urea nitrogen and the urea mass removal rate, which is determined by the instantaneous blood urea nitrogen, occurs [19]. Equation 1 predicts that a proportional decrease in these parameters results in a constant dialyzer clearance during the treatment (provided that dialyzer function is preserved; fig. 2). Despite not being a measure of actual dialytic solute removal, clearance remains a very reasonable parameter to assess dialyzer function. The discordance between solute clearance and mass removal rate described above is a much more relevant consideration when a whole-body (rather than dialyzer) clearance approach is used (see below).

Determinants of Diffusive Solute Clearance

Diffusion is the dominant mass transfer mechanism mediating small solute removal in HD. Diffusive solute removal involves sequential mass transfer from the dialyzer blood compartment, through the membrane, and into the dialysate compartment. To quantify a dialyzer's diffusive capabilities, the concept of mass transfer resistance is frequently employed [25]:

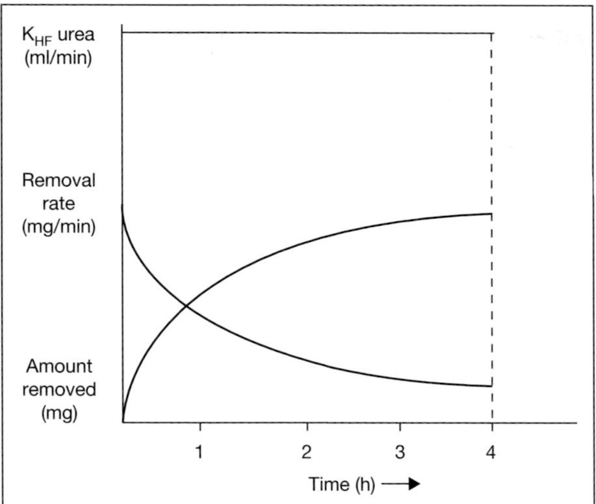

Fig. 2. Relationship between solute clearance (K_{HF}), mass removal rate and cumulative removal during a 4-hour HD treatment. Even with constant dialyzer clearance, the mass removal rate falls during the treatment due to a reduced concentration gradient. Reprinted with permission from Clark and Henderson [19].

$$R_O = R_B + R_M + R_D \tag{7}$$

In the above equation, the overall resistance to diffusive mass transfer of a particular solute (R_O) by a dialyzer has three components: blood compartment resistance (R_B), resistance due to the membrane itself (R_M) and dialysate compartment resistance (R_D). In turn, R_O is the inverse of the overall mass transfer coefficient (K_O), which is a component of the overall mass transfer-area coefficient (K_OA) discussed below. After a discussion of membrane properties above, the blood and dialysate compartments are discussed below.

Blood Compartment

A fundamental relationship exists between diffusive clearance and blood flow rate for all solutes. For a given solute, a graph of clearance versus Q_B has two domains [26]. In the relatively low Q_B regime, an effectively linear relationship exists between these two parameters. For all solutes, the line defined by this relationship falls below the line of identity, thus indicating that dialyzer clearance can never exceed the blood flow rate. For a given dialyzer, the slope of the line defining this flow-limited regime is inversely related to solute size. Beyond a certain Q_B, the curve defining the clearance versus Q_B relationship for a given solute/dialyzer combination demonstrates a plateau. This plateau defines the K_OA-limited region. For a given solute/dialyzer combination, the

K_OA parameter can be regarded as the maximal clearance attainable under a given set of flow conditions. Both the Q_B at which the transition from the blood-flow-limited to the K_OA-limited region occurs and the plateau clearance value are specific for a given solute/dialyzer combination [26]. For a given solute, an increase in either membrane diffusivity (K_O) or area (A) has the effect of increasing both the transition Q_B and the plateau clearance value.

Minimizing the mass transfer resistance in the blood compartment is achieved primarily by the use of relatively high flow rates (i.e. shear rates) that minimize effects related to boundary (unstirred) layers. A boundary layer can be conceptualized as a stagnant film of fluid residing on the membrane surface. However, another important factor influencing blood compartment resistance is Hct. Blood is a complex fluid in which RBCs are suspended in plasma. Plasma is an aqueous-based solution but does have a solid component (approx. 7% by volume) consisting of proteins and lipids. The erythron is also primarily aqueous, with water constituting approximately 70% of the total erythron and the remaining solid component being comprised primarily of cellular membranes. Although many uremic solutes are distributed in the aqueous phase of both the RBC and plasma fractions of blood, solute removal during HD can occur only from plasma water. Before actual dialytic removal of solutes with this type of distribution can be achieved, mass transfer from the RBC water to the plasma water must occur. In turn, the rate at which this latter process occurs is solute specific. Prior data [27] indicate that urea movement across the RBC membrane is relatively fast. Therefore, during HD, urea in the plasma water leaving the dialyzer is in equilibrium with urea in the RBC water, with the ratio of these concentrations (approx. 0.76) being determined by the ratio of the water fractions of the aqueous and RBC compartments. On the other hand, the transcellular rate of movement for other uremic solutes, such as creatinine and phosphate, is small (or negligible) relative to the rate of dialytic removal [28]. For a given unit volume of whole blood, an increase in Hct causes a relative increase in the distribution of solute in the RBC water, resulting in a relative sequestration of solutes with low RBC membrane diffusivity.

The application of rheological principles to the flow of blood in a dialyzer also raises concerns that blood compartment mass transfer may be impaired by increasing Hct. For a given solute, diffusive mass transfer resistance in the blood compartment of a dialyzer is the ratio of effective diffusive path length to effective solute diffusivity, both of which may be influenced by Hct [28]. As the volume comprised by the RBC mass per unit volume of blood increases with increasing Hct, solutes diffusing to the membrane surface are relatively more likely to encounter an RBC, causing an effective lengthening of the diffusion distance. In addition, solute diffusivity may decrease as a function of increasing Hct due to the latter's effect on viscosity, itself a determinant of mass transfer resistance.

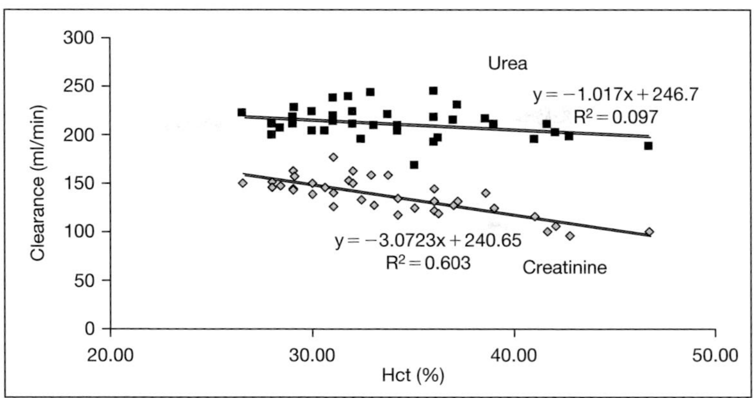

Fig. 3. Small-solute clearance as a function of Hct in HD. Reprinted with permission from Ronco et al. [28].

Lim et al. [23] studied 5 patients in whom pre-HD Hct was raised from a mean of 22.9 to 37.8% with the use of erythropoietin. Whole-blood (K_B) and dialysate-side (K_D) clearances of urea, creatinine and phosphate were measured under the following (prescribed) conditions: Q_B, 400 ml/min; dialysate flow rate (Q_D), 500 ml/min; treatment time, 180 min. Dialysate-side clearance was used as the truer ('gold standard') estimate of mass removal. The ratio K_D/K_B, an estimate of the degree to which whole-blood clearance overestimates mass removal, was observed to decrease significantly for both creatinine and phosphate but not for urea. In urea kinetic analyses (based on the direct dialysate quantification method), both Kt/V (1.21 vs. 1.17) and percent urea reduction (64.2 vs. 61.6%) decreased but not significantly. Interestingly, in a separate group of 7 patients in whom Hct was raised from 19.1 to 29.5% with RBC transfusions, both Kt/V (1.32 vs. 1.19) and percent reduction (66.4 vs. 62.7%) decreased significantly.

Data from Ronco et al. [28] suggest that Hct may also influence flow distribution within the blood compartment of a dialyzer. These investigators employed a computerized-tomography-based technique to measure fiber bundle perfusion of blood with varying Hct (25–40%). A centralized distribution of flow was observed. Moreover, the extent of this maldistribution was proportional to Hct. In fact, at Hct = 40%, the flow velocity and wall shear rate were 2- to 3-fold higher in the central region of the bundle than in its peripheral region. For clinical correlation, these investigators also measured dialyzer urea and creatinine clearances as a function of Hct. As shown in figure 3, this study corroborated the differential effect of increasing Hct on urea and creatinine clearance reported by Lim et al. [23].

Dialysate Compartment

In recent years, enhanced blood compartment and transmembrane small-solute mass transfer efficiency has been attained by the use of high blood flow rates and improved membrane designs, respectively. Consequently, most recent efforts have focused on dialysate-side mass transfer. Based on the K_OA concept introduced above, both the dialysate-side mass transfer coefficient and membrane surface area may influence mass transfer. The dialysate-side mass transfer coefficent is determined largely by boundary layer phenomena, as in the blood compartment. As discussed below, effective mass transfer area is not necessarily equal to the manufacturer-reported (nominal) value.

Dialyzer characteristics which influence dialysate-side mass transfer include packing density, fiber undulation (also known as crimping), and the presence or absence of spacer yarns. Packing density is defined as the ratio of the area comprised of hollow fibers to the area of the dialyzer housing, based on a cross-sectional cut through the dialyzer. Recent magnetic resonance imaging and computed tomography studies [28, 29] suggest that nonoptimized packing density may be the cause of channeling of dialysate at standard flow rates. These investigations demonstrate that a large proportion of the dialysate stream may flow peripherally to the fiber bundle in dialyzers that are not optimally configured. From a physical perspective, the interior of a fiber bundle packed too tightly represents a path of relatively large resistance while the peripheral pathway is the path of least resistance. Obviously, an inwardly situated hollow fiber cannot participate in diffusive mass exchange if it is not perfused with dialysate. Packing density values beyond the optimum may account for the recent finding that dialyzers with a large surface area (i.e. greater than $1.7\,m^2$) are generally associated with less efficient dialysate small-solute mass transfer, relative to dialyzers of smaller surface area [30].

Another dialyzer characteristic that influences hollow-fiber perfusion with dialysate is fiber bundle spacing. Dialysate may not be able to perfuse the area between adjacent fibers that are spatially too close. As is the case for nonoptimized packing density, this reduces the effective membrane surface area available for mass exchange. Two recently developed approaches to address this fiber spacing problem are spacer yarns and a specific fiber undulation pattern. Spacer yarns are multifilament, linear structures interspersed longitudinally in a specific spatial distribution within the fiber bundle [28]. With respect to undulation, all hollow fibers are manufactured with a relatively specific periodicity (amplitude and frequency). However, as discussed below, recent evidence suggests that specific fiber undulation approaches improve dialysate flow distribution and small-solute mass transfer.

In a recent clinical evaluation, Ronco et al. [28] measured the effect of ‘microcrimping’ and spacer yarns on both small-solute removal and dialysate

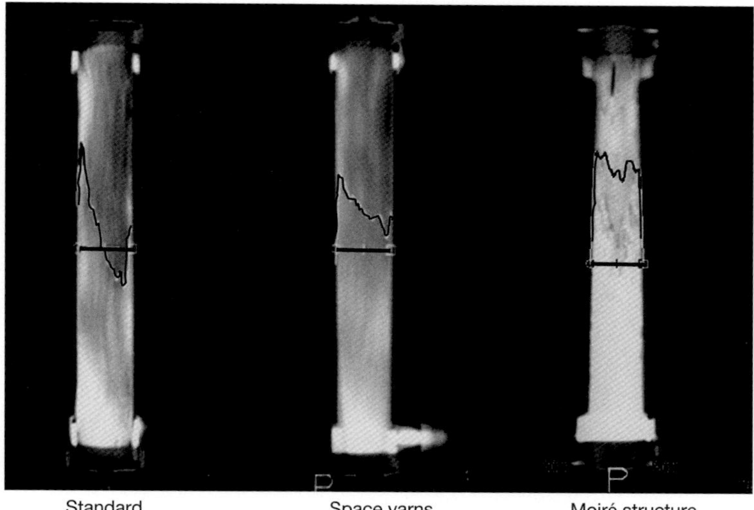

Fig. 4. Dialysate flow distribution in dialyzers having different structures. (Moiré structure corresponds to microcrimped fibers.) Reprinted with permission from Ronco et al. [28].

flow distribution. The microcrimped fibers contained in the dialyzers used in this study have a relatively low amplitude and high frequency. In comparison to conventional dialyzers (i.e. fibers with standard undulation and no spacer yarns), urea clearances were found to be significantly higher for dialyzers with both microcrimped fibers and spacer yarns. Based on a computerized-tomography-based technique, these investigators also found that dialysate flow distribution was most homogeneous in dialyzers with microcrimped fibers and least homogeneous in conventional dialyzers, with dialyzers having spacer yarn technology in an intermediate range (fig. 4). These data suggest that both of these newer approaches improve dialysate flow distribution and, thus, increase effective membrane surface area.

In addition to this influence on effective surface area, microcrimping may also reduce dialysate-side mass transfer resistance essentially by disrupting ('agitating') the boundary layer. Another way in which boundary layer effects may be attenuated is through creation of a turbulent flow regime with a relatively high Q_D. At a relatively common Q_B and Q_D combination of 300 and 500 ml/min, respectively, it is possible that dialysate-side mass transfer is rate limiting under certain conditions. For several high-efficiency and high-flux dialyzers, Leypoldt et al. [30] reported a mean increase of 14% in in vitro urea K_OA when Q_D was increased from 500 to 800 ml/min at a constant Q_B of 450 ml/min. These laboratory data have been corroborated clinically [31, 32].

Two important points about Q_D-related effects on small-solute mass transfer require comment. First, for Q_D to have a significant effect on K_OA, a minimal Q_B must be achieved. Specifically, if the Q_B is much less than 50% of the Q_D at baseline, an increase in the latter is not expected to derive much benefit [33]. Second, it is important to note that the beneficial effect of increasing Q_D on small-solute mass transfer may also be due to a reduction in channeling with improved perfusion of the inner fiber bundle. Thus, the mass transfer benefit of both microcrimping and increased dialysate flow mechanisms may be due to dissipation of boundary layer effects, an increase in effective membrane surface area or both.

References

1 Lysaght MJ: Evolution of hemodialysis membranes; in Bonimini V, Berland Y (eds): Dialysis Membranes: Structure and Predictions. Contrib Nephrol. Basel, Karger, 1995, vol 113, pp 1–10.

2 Lysaght MJ: Hemodialysis membranes in transition; in Colasanti G, D'Amico G (eds): Nephrology and Dialysis Updated. Contrib Nephrol. Basel, Karger, 1988, vol 61, pp 1–17.

3 Hoenich N, Woffindin C, Cox P, Goldfinch M, Roberts S: Clinical characterization of Dicea, a new cellulose membrane for haemodialysis. Clin Nephrol 1997;48:253–259.

4 Ronco C, Brendolan A, Everard P, et al: Cellulose triacetate: another membrane for continuous renal replacement therapy. J Nephrol 1999;12:241–247.

5 Funck-Bretano J, Sausse A, Man NK, Granger A, Rondon-Nucete M, Zingraff J, Jungers P: A new hemodialysis treatment associating a membrane highly permeable to middle molecules with a closed circuit dialysate system. Proc EDTA 1972;9:55–66.

6 Streicher E, Schneider H: The development of a polysulfone membrane: a new perspective in dialysis? In Streicher E, Seyffart G (eds): Highly Permeable Membranes. Contrib Nephrol. Basel, Karger, 1985, vol 46, pp 1–13.

7 Gohl H, Buck R, Strathmann H: Basic features of polyamide membranes; in Shaldon S, Koch KM (eds): Polyamide – The Evolution of a Synthetic Membrane for Renal Therapy. Contrib Nephrol. Basel, Karger, 1992, vol 96, pp 1–25.

8 Bonomini M, Fiederling B, Bucciarelli T, Manfrini V, Di Ilio C, Albertazzi A: A new polymethylmethacrylate membrane for hemodialysis. Int J Artif Organs 1996;19:232–239.

9 Jaber BL, Gonski JA, Cendoroglo M, Balakrishnan VS, Razeghi P, Dinarello C, Pereira BJG: New polyethersulfone dialyzers attenuate passage of cytokine-inducing substances from Pseudomonas aeruginosa contaminated dialysate. Blood Purif 1998;16:210–219.

10 Ronco C, Crepaldi C, Brendolan A, et al: Evolution of synthetic membranes for blood purification: the case of the Polyflux family. Nephrol Dial Transplant 2003;18(suppl 7):vii10–vii20.

11 Rockel A, Hertel J, Fiegel P, Abdelhamid S, Panitz N, Walb D: Permeability and secondary membrane formation of a high flux polysulfone hemofilter. Kidney Int 1986;30:429–432.

12 Ledebo I: Principles and practice of hemofiltration and hemodiafiltration. Artif Organs 1998;22: 20–25.

13 Clark WR, Hamburger RJ, Lysaght MJ: Effect of membrane composition and structure on performance and biocompatibility in hemodialysis. Kidney Int 1999;56:2005–2015.

14 Ronco C, Ballestri M, Gappelli G: Dialysis membranes in convective treatments. Nephrol Dial Transplant 2000;15(suppl 2):31–36.

15 Ronco C: Backfiltration: a controversial issue in modern dialysis. Int J Artif Organs 1988;11: 69–74.

16 Ronco C, Brendolan A, Lupi A, Metry G, Levin N: Effects of a reduced inner diameter of hollow fibers in hemodialyzers. Kidney Int 2000;58:809–817.

17 Clark WR, Macias WL, Molitoris BA, Wang NHL: β2-Microglobulin membrane adsorption: equilibrium and kinetic characterization. Kidney Int 1994;46:1140–1146.
18 Clark WR, Macias WL, Molitoris A, Wang NHL: Plasma protein adsorption to highly permeable hemodialysis membranes. Kidney Int 1995;48:481–488.
19 Clark WR, Henderson LW: Renal versus continuous versus intermittent therapies for removal of uremic toxins. Kidney Int 2001;59(suppl 78):S298–S303.
20 Clark WR, Shinaberger JH: Clinical evaluation of a new high-efficiency hemodialyzer: polysynthane (PSNn). ASAIO J 2000;46:288–292.
21 Jaffrin MY: Convective mass transfer in hemodialysis. Artif Organs 1995;19:1162–1171.
22 Slatsky M, Schindhelm K, Farrell P: Creatinine transfer between red blood cells and plasma: a comparison between normal and uremic subjects. Nephron 1978;22:514–521.
23 Lim V, Flanigan M, Fangman J: Effect of hematocrit on solute removal during high efficiency hemodialysis. Kidney Int 1990;37:1557–1562.
24 Shinaberger J, Miller J, Gardner P: Erythropoietin alert: risks of high hematocrit hemodialysis. Trans Am Soc Artif Intern Organs 1988;34:179–184.w
25 Huang Z, Clark WR, Gao D: Determinants of small solute clearance in hemodialysis. Semin Dial 2005;18:30–35.
26 Leypoldt JK, Cheung AK: Optimal use of hemodialyzers; in Ronco C, La Greca G (eds): Hemodialysis Technology. Contrib Nephrol. Basel, Karger, 2002, vol 137, pp 129–137.
27 Cheung A, Alford M, Wilson M, Leypoldt JK, Henderson LW: Urea movement across erythrocyte membrane. Kidney Int 1983;23:866–869.
28 Ronco C, Brendolan A, Crepaldi C, Rodighiero M, Scabardi M, Ghezzi PM: Blood and dialysate flow distributions in hollow fiber hemodialyzers analyzed by computerized helical scanning technique. J Am Soc Nephrol 2002;13(suppl 1):S53–S61.
29 Poh CK, Hardy PA, Liao Z, Huang Z, Clark WR, Gao DY: Effect of flow baffles on the dialysate flow distribution in hollow-fiber hemodialyzers: a non-intrusive experimental study using MRI. J Biomech Eng 2003;125:481–489.
30 Leypoldt JK, Cheung AK, Agodoa LY, Daugirdas JT, Greene T, Keshaviah PR: Hemodialyzer mass transfer-area coefficients for urea increase at high dialysate flow rates. Kidney Int 1997;51:2013–2017.
31 Ouseph R, Ward RA: Increasing dialysate flow rate increases dialyzer urea mass transfer-area coefficients during clinical use. Am J Kidney Dis 2001;37:316–320.
32 Hauk M, Kuhlmann M, Riegel W, Kohler H: In vivo effects of dialysate flow rate on Kt/V in maintenance hemodialysis patients. Am J Kidney Dis 2000;35:105–111.
33 Sigdell J, Tersteegen B: Clearance of a dialyzer under varying operating conditions. Artif Organs 1986;10:219–225.

William R. Clark, MD
Gambro Renal Products
4322 Wythe Lane
Indianapolis, IN 46250 (USA)
Tel. +1 317 691 1438, Fax +1 317 849 4599, E-Mail william.clark@us.gambro.com

Ronco C, Canaud B, Aljama P (eds): Hemodiafiltration.
Contrib Nephrol. Basel, Karger, 2007, vol 158, pp 34–49

Fluid Mechanics and Crossfiltration in Hollow-Fiber Hemodialyzers

Claudio Ronco

Department of Nephrology, St. Bortolo Hospital, Vicenza, Italy

Abstract

The efficiency of a hemodialyzer is largely dependent on its ability to facilitate diffusion between blood and dialysis solution. The diffusion process can be impaired if there is a mismatch between blood and dialysate flow distribution in the dialyzer. For this reason it is important that average and regional blood and dialysate flow velocities do not differ significantly. Single-fiber flow velocity should be similar in the center and the periphery of the bundle. Similarly, dialysate flow in the central region of the dialyzer and in the peripheral areas should be similar. In this way the best blood-to-dialysate flow countercurrent configuration is obtained, and the diffusive process is optimized. Unfortunately this optimal situation is hard to achieve, and frequently a significant blood-to-dialysate flow mismatch may occur in hollow-fiber hemodialyzers either due to uneven blood flow distribution or to a dialysate channeling phenomenon external to the fiber bundle. Attempts to optimize flows has been made in the blood compartment designing specific blood ports while, in the dialysate, different options have been proposed such as space yarns (spacing filaments preventing contact between fibers) or the moiré structure (waved shape of fibers to prevent contact between adjacent fibers). Furthermore, the process of transmembrane crossfiltration along the length of the dialyzer can be very different in quantity and direction, thus interfering significantly with the diffusion process. In particular, maximal rates of direct filtration (blood to dialysate) are achieved in the proximal part of the dialyzer, while in the distal part ultrafiltration is minimal and it can also change direction producing significant amounts of backfiltration.

Small-solute removal is obtained primarily by diffusion [1–5]. Convection represents an additional mechanism mostly important for larger molecules. The efficiency of a hemodialyzer is therefore dependent on its ability to facilitate the diffusion process and optimize its interaction with convection [6–9]. Diffusion is affected by blood and dialysate flow rates, temperature, surface area of the dialyzer and thickness of the membrane. Assuming that all other factors are constant, the diffusion process is basically dependent on the concentration gradient between blood and dialysate [10, 11]. This is strongly affected by the blood and dialysate flow rates and by the distribution of the countercurrent flows in their relative compartments. It is evident that any possible mismatch between blood and dialysate flow distributions can create a significant reduction in the efficiency of the filter [10]. In some cases blood flow distribution may be less than optimal due to blood viscosity properties or to a poor distribution of the flow at the blood inlet port [11, 12]. In this case, the external fibers of the bundle may be penalized by a lower flow velocity compared to the fibers located in the central region of the bundle. On the other hand, fiber packing density may be higher in the central region of the bundle, and dialysate flow may be limited in that region by an increased resistance. Under these circumstances, dialysate tends to flow at higher speed in those regions of the filter where blood flow velocity is minimal and vice versa [13]. This effect may be the cause of inconsistent performances of the hemodialyzer, and clearance values may be lower than those expected from theoretical calculations [14].

When convection is taken into account, the regional flux across the membrane becomes an important factor affecting solute transport. This is due to the solvent drag effect but also to the potential negative interference of the filtration fluxes with the diffusion process. Thus, as far as hydraulics is concerned, three fundamental aspects should be considered to analyze the solute transport processes inside hollow-fiber hemodialyzers: (a) the fluid mechanics in the blood compartment, (b) the fluid mechanics in the dialysate compartment, (c) the transmembrane crossfiltration flux with its direct and reverse components.

Fluid Mechanics in the Blood Compartment

The uremic syndrome is characterized by the retention of a host of solutes that interfere with various biochemical functions. Over the past decade, much clinical research has been carried out on the adequacy of dialysis, mainly focusing on the clearance of the small-molecular-weight substances like urea, with much less consideration for the middle-molecular-weight substances, such as β_2-microglobulin [15]. Moreover, treatment of renal anemia by recombinant human erythropoietin has increased dramatically the average hematocrit (Hct) in the dialysis population. Although positive effects were expected on cardiovascular function, there has been increasing concern that increasing Hct values beyond a certain level will adversely affect dialyzer clearance necessitating a modification in dialysis therapy. Besarab et al. [16] reported that changes in dialyzer clearances after erythropoietin treatment were not significant. Other authors [17, 18] found that in patients receiving either high-flux or conventional dialysis during treatment with erythropoietin, there was only a slight decrease in clearances of creatinine, potassium and phosphate in the presence of higher Hcts. However, in other studies [19, 20], creatinine and phosphate clearances significantly decreased in the presence of high Hct values, while urea clearance was minimally affected. Burr and Martin [21] noted that dialysis efficiency for creatinine decreased by approximately 10% in patients with high Hct.

In a specifically designed study we showed that creatinine and phosphate clearances negatively correlated with the levels of Hct, whilst urea clearance only displayed a negative trend [22]. This is a finding which is in agreement with previous studies [19, 20]. Urea is a highly diffusible molecule, freely mobile between the extracellular and intracellular compartments. As a consequence, urea should not be significantly affected by changes in plasma volume/red cell volume ratio. On the other hand, creatinine and phosphate are slowly moving across the red cell membrane, and for dialytic purposes they can be considered confined to plasma water. Relative plasma volume is reduced when Hct increases, and this may decrease the delivery of creatinine and phosphate to the hemodialyzers due to a decrease in effective plasma flow.

Although this appears the most logical explanation, our in vitro results seem to suggest a further possible effect played by an impaired blood flow distribution in the dialyzer occurring when Hct increases.

Blood is a concentrated suspension of red cells in an aqueous electrolyte-protein solution, which shows a viscoelastic property [23]. The viscoelasticity of the blood is traceable to the elastic red cells. When the red cells are at rest, they tend to aggregate and stick together (fig. 1). In order to flow freely, the aggregates must disintegrate and the cells must undergo elastic deformation and orientation to each other. This process depends upon several factors including Hct, plasma proteins and fibrinogen [24]. The blood flow in a narrow vessel with an inner diameter $<300\,\mu m$ is determined by how the cells glide past each other and how interaction between cells and vessel walls takes place [25]. Therefore an insight into the blood flow mechanics within the dialyzer is needed to understand the complicated effects of increasing Hct levels.

One should consider the important function of the arterial blood port of the hemodialyzer. This component is crucial to ensure a good distribution of blood into the fibers. The presence of turbulence, dead spaces or preferential pathways might interfere with a good distribution, and peripheral fibers may be penalized in terms of flow delivery.

Assuming a physiological difference in flow delivery between the central (higher) and the peripheral (lower) regions of the bundle, there may be an additional effect inducing a further reduction of flow velocity in the peripheral fibers

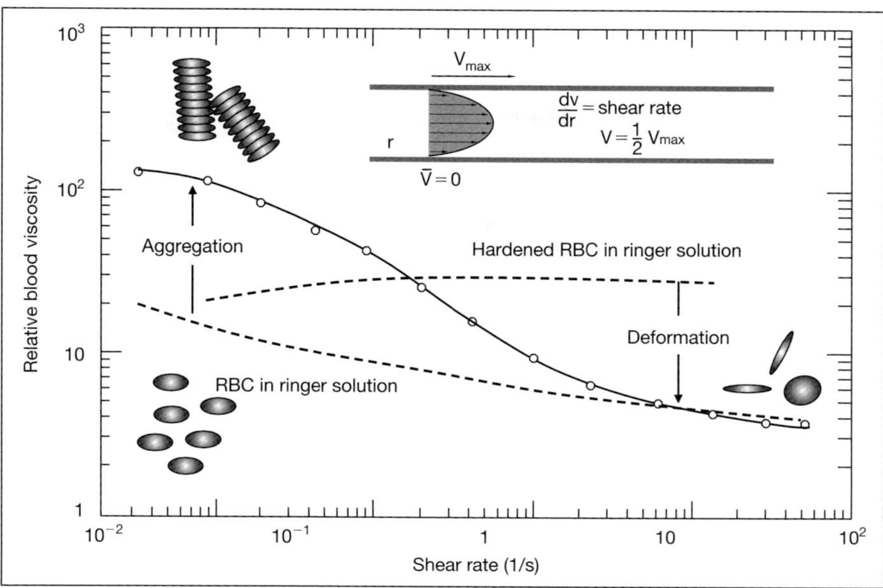

Fig. 1. Characteristics of blood as a non-Newtonian viscoelastic fluid and behavior of red cells suspended in different media.

(fig. 2) [14]. Due to the hydraulic design of the hemodialyzer, a transmembrane pressure (TMP) gradient will be equally applied to all fibers of the bundle. If the single-fiber blood flow is slightly lower from the beginning in the peripheral regions of the bundle, these fibers will experience a slightly higher filtration fraction. In fact, for the same permeability coefficient and the same TMP gradient, equal amounts of ultrafiltration will be produced in all fibers. However, since peripheral fibers tend to have a lower blood flow per fiber, this will result in a higher single-fiber filtration fraction and higher hemoconcentration in the fiber. This in turn will result in an increase in blood viscosity and a possible increase in the resistance to flow in those specific fibers. This phenomenon may contribute to a further reduction in flow velocity and a new steady-state profile. The phenomenon only leads to a new steady-state profile, and not to a progressive obstruction of the peripheral fibers for two reasons. One is due to the lower wall shear rates present in these fibers and the consequent formation of a boundary layer that limits ultrafiltration. The second is linked to a progressive increase in the oncotic pressure generated by plasma proteins that acts against ultrafiltration. Assuming that these considerations are true, one could expect a different flow distribution profile within the hemodialyzer, in the presence of constant Hct and blood flow but variable levels of ultrafiltration.

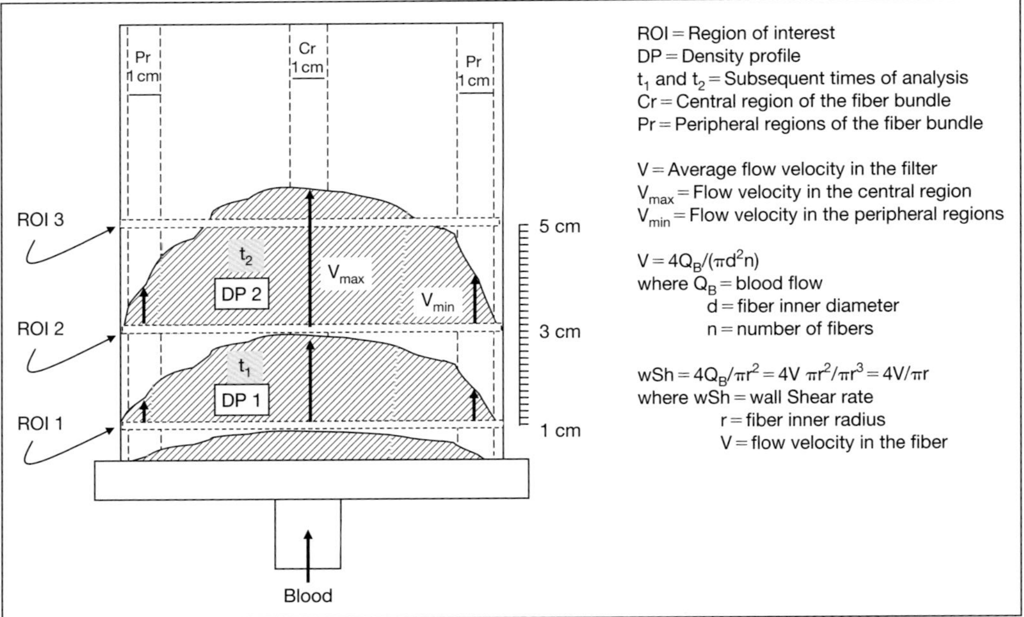

Fig. 2. Flow distribution in the blood compartment and effects of local ultrafiltration on viscosity and concentration polarization. Two flow distribution profiles describing two subsequent times (t_1 and t_2) are presented. Analysis of distribution profiles is carried out in different regions of interest (ROI 1, ROI 2 and ROI 3) with a specific radiographic method. Once the blood enters the blood port of the hemodialyzer, a flow distribution curve starts to build up. Regional velocities are different at different moments and in different regions of the bundle.

Considering the rheological properties of blood and its typically non-Newtonian behavior, alternative hypotheses can be formulated. Blood is a fluidized suspension of red blood cells, which has viscoelastic properties reflecting the cumulative effects of plasma viscosity and Hct. Since the smaller the velocity and the shear rate applied to blood, the higher its viscosity, one can speculate that the lower flow velocity observed in the peripheral fibers further aggravates the flow-dynamic conditions because of a relative increase in blood viscosity in those fibers.

In summary, blood is distributed nonproportionally in the hemodialyzer. This uneven distribution is strongly affected by the level of Hct. The final effect is reflected on efficiency and solute clearances. We assume that this effect can be individualized to the patients, since it can be affected by several factors, e.g. the degree of ultrafiltration, the presence of stiff erythrocytes and the blood flow rate.

As far as the blood compartment is concerned, hemodialyzer design has been quite constant over the last 20 years. The average Hct of patients has however increased significantly. Therefore, a careful evaluation of dialysis adequacy parameters is strongly advisable when dealing with patients in which Hct levels progressively increase.

These considerations apply even more when treatments with high convective components are involved. In fact, hemodiafiltration (HDF) may induce a significant hemoconcentration in the blood compartment, and increased viscosity can be experienced along the length of the hollow fibers. This effect is mostly observed in postdilution modalities, while in predilution or middilution this effect is mitigated and an improved performance of the fiber is observed. Nevertheless, a general recommendation should be made to increase blood flows as much as possible when convective therapies are utilized.

Fluid Mechanics in the Dialysate Compartment

Some studies have demonstrated that the flow distribution in the dialysate compartment might be less than optimal due to channeling phenomena [26]. Under such circumstances, the hypothesis of a blood-to-dialysate flow mismatch as a major cause of dialyzer malfunction or impaired efficiency becomes realistic.

The flow distribution in the dialysate compartment can be theoretically modeled using equations of physical chemistry and transport [27, 28] and can be assimilated to the flow distribution in packed beds [29].

As in packed beds, the packing structure of the hollow fibers is usually quite complex, and the resulting flow pattern external to the fibers is extremely complicated. In well-packed columns, the diversity of channel diameters and of velocities in the individual channels is small. In this case the packed bed can be approximated to a bundle of tortuous capillary tubes. In the case of the dialysate compartment of a hollow-fiber hemodialyzer, some wide-diameter channels and gaps in the packing structure may be present resulting in wide variations of local flow velocity. This may cause the undesirable phenomenon of so-called channeling of the flow. As discussed in detail in a recent publication [29], the fundamental principle governing the flow of fluids through packed beds is Darcy's law. The free cross-section of the dialysate compartment bed (total internal area of the case – total area occupied by the fibers) is constituted by the interfiber gaps (interparticle porosity) and constitutes the fluid pathway external to the fibers. The dimension of the specific permeability of the compartment is square centimeters but it could be given in Darcy units (1 darcy = 10^{-8} cm^2). Unfortunately, the bundle can be concentrated and packed in the central region of the dialyzer,

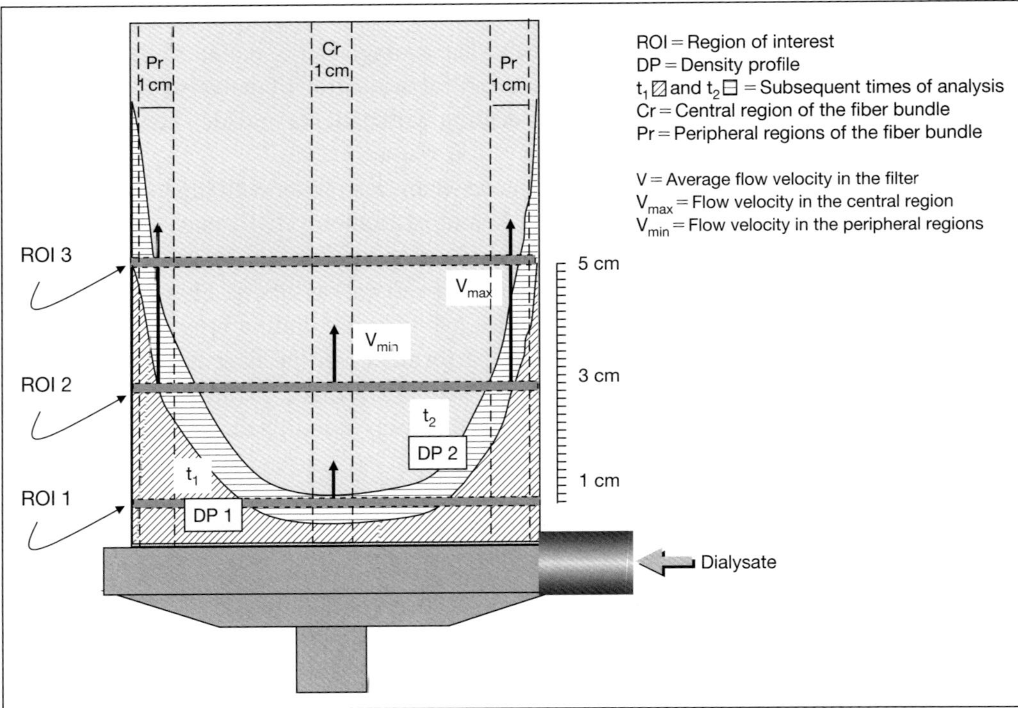

Fig. 3. Flow distribution in the dialysate compartment. Two flow distribution profiles (describing two subsequent times t_1 and t_2) are presented. Analysis of distribution profiles is carried out in different regions of interest (ROI 1, ROI 2 and ROI 3) with a specific radiographic method. Once the dialysate enters the Hansen connector of the hemodialyzer, a flow distribution curve starts to build up. Regional velocities are different at different moments and in different regions of the bundle.

and low-resistance pathways can be created in the more peripheral regions of the compartment. This results in a greater flow velocity in the peripheral regions while a significant stagnation can be observed in the central region. In this case, the specific permeability of the interfiber space of the bundle in the central region becomes much smaller than that observed in the peripheral regions and the efficacy of the countercurrent flow is impaired (fig. 3).

The most uniform flow profile in packed beds can be obtained when beds are packed tightly with spherical particles of equal size. If the ratio of the tube diameter to the particle diameter is less than 100, this may have a significantly positive effect on the flow distribution profile.

In hollow-fiber dialyzers, the fibers and their external surface substitute the particles of a porous bed. Since the fibers are not tightly packed, preferential fluid pathways may be generated. This explains why the packing density of hollow fibers is an important parameter in the design of a hemodialyzer. Further, it seems that special configurations designed to prevent a close contact of adjacent fibers may induce a significant improvement on the flow distribution. Studies have permitted the evaluation of the possible impact of new solutions oriented to the improvement of the dialysate pathway configuration. In particular, the use of space yarns external to hollow fibers may help in reducing the negative effects due to dialysate channeling. A more homogeneous distribution of the dialysate has been however obtained by the waved configuration of the hollow fibers in the bundle, creating the so-called moiré structure [14].

The optimization of dialysate distribution in the modified hemodialyzers is also confirmed by an improved performance in terms of urea clearance. This suggests a definite improvement of the diffusion processes inside the dialyzer due to an optimization of the countercurrent effect on blood-to-dialysate solute gradients [11, 30].

Crossfiltration in Hollow-Fiber Hemodialyzers

Water flux across the dialysis membrane in each axial segment (dl) of the dialyzer may occur in two directions: from blood to dialysate, which is termed filtration, or from dialysate to blood, which is termed backfiltration.

Backfiltration may occur inside any kind of filter, and during any kind of treatment, when the TMP gradient at a given point becomes negative – that is when the hydraulic pressure of dialysate (P_D) together with the oncotic pressure exerted by plasma proteins (π) exceeds the hydraulic pressure of the blood inside the fiber (P_B). This condition may happen occasionally during the treatment or for the entire duration of the session affecting solute fluxes [31–33]. TMP is generally expressed in average values with the simplified equation 1:

$$TMP = (P_{Bi} + P_{Bo})/2 + (P_{Di} + P_{Do})/2 + (\pi_i + \pi_o)/2 \quad (1)$$

where i and o represent the inlet and the outlet of the filter for blood and dialysate, respectively. However, this representation only describes an average phenomenon and it does not define the actual profile of local pressures along the length of the filter. Although TMP is positive, the local pressure gradient ΔP is not necessarily positive at every point along the length of the filter. Equation 1 also assumes that the pressure drop inside the blood and dialysate compartment is linear which according to the Hagen-Poiseuille law is only true under certain circumstances. The pressure drop is linear only when blood viscosity remains constant along the fibers, and this would only occur if no crossfiltration is present. Crossfiltration in fact either increases blood viscosity when it is direct or reduces viscosity when it is reverse. Thus, since crossfiltration cannot be null, viscosity is subject to change, and pressure drop cannot be linear.

The local water flux in a single surface element (ds) of the dialyzer is described by the equation $Q_F = K_M \times \Delta P$ (K_M being the hydraulic permeability coefficient of the membrane and ΔP the algebraic sum of hydraulic and oncotic pressures). Expanding this concept to the whole dialyzer, the overall water flux in a given dialyzer will be expressed by the formula described in equation 2:

$$Q_F = \int\int_o^l \Delta P \times K_M \times ds \quad (2)$$

where ds is a single surface element of the dialyzer and s is the surface of the dialyzer, o is the initial segment of the dialyzer and l is the most distal segment of the dialyzer after n segments of dimension dl.

Arbitrarily assuming K_M to be a constant on the whole surface area s, and ΔP to be identical in any point of a cross-sectional segment of the dialyzer, equation 2 can be simplified as follows:

$$Q_F = K_M \int_o^l \Delta P \times dl \quad (3)$$

where l is the length of the dialyzer and ΔP is the local TMP gradient in a cross-sectional segment of the dialyzer (dl). For simple calculation we can use the formula:

$$Q_F = K_D \int_o^l \Delta P \times dl/l \quad (4)$$

where $\int_o^l \Delta P \times dl/l$ is the average TMP gradient (avTMP) and K_D is the dialyzer ultrafiltration coefficient. Thus, the overall net water flux will be

$$Q_F = K_D \times avTMP. \quad (5)$$

While this is a commonly used equation to simplify the phenomena inside the dialyzer, a more complex crossfiltration and pressure profiles have been experimentally determined by nuclear scintigraphic methods [34] (fig. 4). Linear models are in fact not accurate to predict filtration and backfiltration fluxes empirically measured by the changes in concentration of a nondiffusible marker molecule along the length of the fibers.

The water flux inside the dialyzer is then the result of two opposing fluxes:

$$Q_F = Q_{F1} - Q_{F2} = (K_{M1} \times \int_0^x \Delta P \times dl) - (K_{M2} \times \int_x^l \Delta P \times dl) \quad (6)$$

where Q_F = net ultrafiltration; Q_{F1} = filtration; Q_{F2} = backfiltration; K_{M1} = membrane direct ultrafiltration coefficient; K_{M2} = membrane reverse ultrafiltration coefficient; x = point of inversion of pressure gradient and water flux.

Most of the effects observed along the length of the filter are related to variations in blood viscosity and plasma protein concentration. In fact, in highly permeable hollow-fiber hemodialyzers, although with higher filtration rates

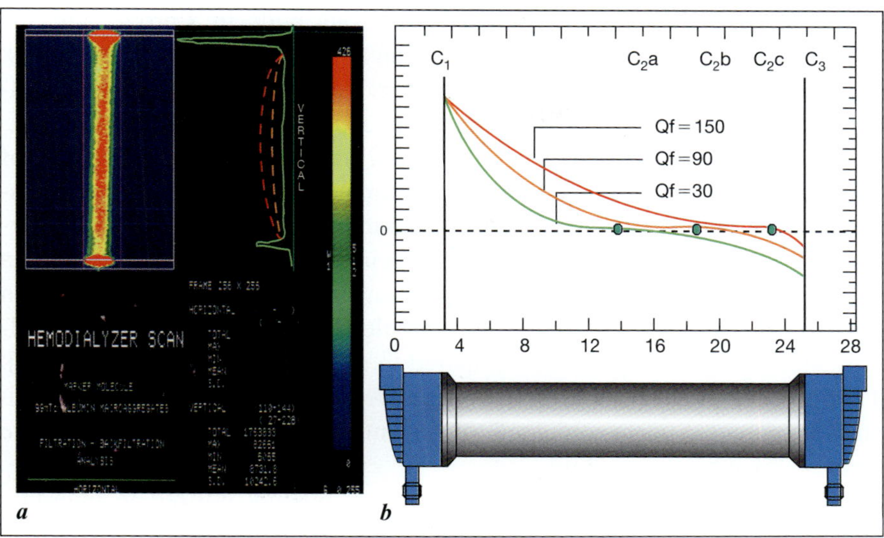

Fig. 4. Examples of local crossfiltration fluxes along the length of the dialyzer at different net filtration rates. a The scintigraphic curves of the nondiffusible marker molecule generated by the gamma camera are reported. b Filtration fluxes are positive in the proximal part of the dialyzer while backfiltration occurs distally. Even at very high filtration rates, backfiltration cannot be avoided.

backfiltration is minimized, the flux of reverse filtration cannot be avoided since plasma proteins operate small but significant amounts of oncotic-pressure-driven backfiltration. Thus, while the linear model suggests to identify three possible conditions, i.e. (a) spontaneous filtration, (b) critical filtration (the minimal amount of filtration necessary to avoid backfiltration) and (c) zero net filtration (the flux of filtration equals that of backfiltration), the experimental findings clarify that even at high filtration rates, small amounts of backfiltration are always present.

Several lines of evidence demonstrate the importance of middle-molecule removal in hemodialysis [35]. The use of high-flux membranes and the increased use of convective techniques have permitted to improve the efficiency of hemodialysis leading to better removal of solutes in the middle-molecular-weight range [36, 37].

The improvement achieved with synthetic membranes is mainly due to their higher hydraulic permeability and their increased sieving capacity compared to classic cellulose membranes. These properties result in higher middle-molecule clearance. This clearance improvement is due to larger amounts of ultrafiltration per treatment and a more important contribution of convection to the overall transport process [38].

Synthetic high-flux membranes are used both in Europe and the USA, with different modes of application [35, 36]. In Europe, high-flux dialysis and HDF are used as treatment modalities for chronic renal failure. Conventional HDF utilizes large convective transport with ultrafiltration rates above 70 ml/min. Since the ultrafiltration rate exceeds the rate of desired weight loss in the patient, sterile replacement fluid must be administered. The net ultrafiltration rate in the patient will be equal to the difference between total ultrafiltration rate and reinfusion rate. Total ultrafiltration varies between 12 and 15 l/session. The enhanced convective transport in HDF permits an increased removal of middle- to high-molecular-weight solutes such as β_2-microglobulin compared to standard hemodialysis [35–39]. The major drawbacks of this treatment are the complexity of the system and the increased costs compared to conventional hemodialysis due to large amounts of substitution fluid.

In the USA, high-flux membranes are commonly utilized in high-flux dialysis in which net filtration rates are volumetrically controlled. This results in a complex fluid balance within the dialyzer where true filtration rates are counterbalanced by significant amounts of backfiltration. In this setting, convective transport is partially maintained and the clearance of large molecules is improved compared to conventional hemodialysis, although not as much as in HDF. The magnitude of net filtration in high-flux dialysis is controlled by the dialysis machine. In contrast, the amounts of true filtration and backfiltration are determined by the hydraulic permeability and surface of the membrane, by the geometry of the dialyzer and by the hydrostatic and oncotic forces acting on the dialysis membrane. In previous studies, we measured the internal water fluxes in high-flux dialyzers using an experimental dialysis circuit at zero net filtration [34]. In such conditions, the rate of filtration and concomitantly of backfiltration could be precisely determined.

Convective transport and the rates of filtration-backfiltration can be increased in high-flux dialyzers, by modifying the geometry of the filter but also of the hollow fiber. The rates of filtration-backfiltration at a given blood flow are directly correlated with the resistance of the filter, i.e. with the pressure drop in the blood compartment and that in the dialysate compartment. Filtration-backfiltration rates can be increased experimentally by the application of a fixed O ring external to the fiber bundle to alter the dialysate end-to-end pressure drop [40]. In the blood compartment this effect could be achieved by modifying the length of the filter and/or its cross-sectional area. The cross-sectional area of a dialyzer can be modified by changing the number of hollow fibers in the bundle or by using hollow fibers with a different inner diameter. A reduced inner diameter is in fact expected to increase proximal filtration and distal backfiltration, by increasing the resistance to flow in the blood compartment. In all cases, improved convective removal of large solutes is expected because of the increased internal filtration [41].

Internal crossfiltration is governed by the hydraulic and oncotic forces acting along the length of the dialyzer on each side of the membrane. In each point of the dialyzer, the local pressure differential is termed TMP. When the TMP is positive, the water flux is from the blood compartment to the dialysate compartment. When the TMP is negative, backfiltration occurs. The removal of middle molecules can be enhanced by increasing the positive pressure differential in the proximal part of the dialyzer, thus increasing internal filtration. Adequate net filtration is maintained by the ultrafiltration control system by a parallel increase in the negative pressure differential in the distal part of the dialyzer. This would result in increased rates of proximal filtration and distal backfiltration without affecting the 'net' filtration rate.

The relationship of TMP, ultrafiltration (UF) and membrane ultrafiltration coefficient (K_M) is expressed in the equation:

$$K_M = UF/TMP. \quad (7)$$

High-flux membranes have a K_{UF} >20 ml/h/mm Hg. Therefore, these membranes can have UF rates of 4,000 ml/h with a TMP = 300 mm Hg. The clearance of middle molecules at this UF rate would be ideal, but the patient cannot tolerate these rates. HDF, as carried out in Europe, operates in conditions of high filtration rates, but significant amounts of replacement fluid are required to maintain the patient's fluid balance.

In high-flux dialysis, volumetric control regulates the net ultrafiltration; however as stated previously, the convective transport is limited by the rate of internal filtration. Modification of the dialyzer structure could increase the peaks of positive and negative TMP along the length of the dialyzer, thereby increasing filtration and backfiltration [34].

When high rates of backfiltration are utilized, a high quality of dialysate is needed to prevent any inconvenient or side effect related to pyrogen transfer into the patient's circulation [42, 43]. For this treatment the use of last-generation hemodialysis machines is strongly suggested. New machines are equipped with a built-in pyrogen filter to prepare ultrapure dialysate. The reinfusion via backfiltration is providing an extra step of safety since the fluid is filtered again across the hemodialysis membrane prior to reaching the blood compartment.

The modification of the inner diameter of the fiber may become an interesting approach to increasing the TMP without introducing major changes in the dialyzer design. In previous experiments, this approach resulted in a positive increase in the TMP in the proximal portion of the dialyzer and a negative increase in the distal portion of the dialyzer [41]. The difference in pressure drop when the inner diameter is even marginally reduced becomes significant as it is predicted by the Hagen-Poiseuille formula

$$\Delta P = Q_B \times (8\eta l/\pi r^4) \quad (8)$$

where ΔP = end-to-end pressure drop, Q_B = blood flow, η = blood viscosity.

Since the pressure drop in a fiber correlates with the internal radius of the fiber to the fourth power, it seems logical to attempt solutions that involve modifications of the fiber geometry. One may speculate that a reduction of the inner diameter of the hollow fiber will also result in an increase in the average blood flow velocity per fiber and a consequent increase in wall shear rates. This additional factor may in fact result in a 'cleaning' effect at the blood-membrane interface. Higher shear rates lead in fact to a reduction of the thickness of the protein boundary layer and improve membrane permeability counterbalancing the concentration polarization phenomenon. This will certainly help not only to obtain a better performance of the membrane in terms of filtration rates at a given local TMP gradient, but also an optimal utilization of the sieving capacities of the membrane.

From this observation the importance of the blood flow rate as a major determinant of convective clearance becomes evident. In fact, at a given blood flow, the viscosity of blood and the cross-sectional area of the conduct govern the end-to-end pressure drop in the blood compartment. If blood flow is increased, the end-to-end pressure drop will increase according to the Hagen-Poiseuille law and so will the TMP gradient in the proximal and distal parts of the hemodialyzer. For this reason, the same amount of convective transport in specifically modified dialyzers was obtained at lower blood flow rates compared to standard dialyzers [40, 41]. This is in fact a good chance to achieve a remarkable convective clearance during high-flux dialysis without reaching dangerously high filtration fractions and an increased risk of clotting in patients who cannot be treated with traditional convective therapies such as hemofiltration or HDF because of insufficient blood flow.

The final consideration concerns the better performance of the hollow fibers in the filtration-backfiltration mode, as compared to the filtration-postdilution mode. In the latter mode in fact, a greater impact of protein concentration polarization is expected and the boundary layer at the blood-membrane interface will be thicker resulting in a significant decrease in membrane permeability.

In conclusion, two directions will probably be undertaken in the near future: one consists in modifications of the design of hollow fibers leading to simplified HDF techniques without the need for replacement solutions, but simply utilizing internal filtration as a main way to increase convective transport; in contrast, the second consists in the maximization of the convective transport utilizing replacement solutions produced online (and therefore cheaply and in large amounts) possibly infused in predilution mode to improve performance of the fibers [43].

Conclusions

After the accurate analysis of the mechanics of fluid in the blood and dialysate compartments together with the profiles of crossfiltration along the length of the dialyzer, we can conclude that diffusion and convection are two membrane separation processes that continuously interfere making it impossible to clearly distinguish the separate contribution of each phenomenon to the final solute removal. We may say that while in hemodialysis diffusion is the prevalent mechanism, in HDF convection may become the prevalent mechanism, and in high-flux dialysis a really mixed form of transport is observed inside the filter without a prevalent mechanism of removal.

References

1 Kill F: Development of a parallel flow artificial kidney in plastics. Acta Chir Scand Suppl 1960; 253:S142–146.
2 Malchesky PS, Mrava GI, Nose Y: A totally disposable presterilized dialyzer. Arch Intern Med 1971;127:278–283.
3 Kolff VJ, Watshinger B: Further development of a coil kidney. J Lab Clin Med 1956;47:969–974.
4 Haas G: Dialysieren des strömenden Blutes am Lebenden. Klin Wochenschr 1923;2:1888–1894.
5 Nakagawa S, Koshikawa S, Ishida Y, Uematsu M, Ishibashi K: Development of flat type hollow fibre dialyzer (NF-01) achievement of better performance than cylinder type with same membrane area; in Frost TH (ed): Technical Aspects of Renal Dialysis. Tunbridge Wells, Petman Medical, 1977, pp 29–37.
6 Sigdell JE: Hollow fiber dialyzers on the market. Artif Organs 1988;12:4–11.
7 Sigdell JE: Comparison of the hollow dialyzers. Artif Organs 1981;5:4–9.
8 Sakai K: Technical determination of optimal dimension of hollow fibre membranes for clinical dialysis. Nephrol Dial Transplant 1989;4(suppl):S73–S77.
9 Ronco C, Ballestri M: New developments in hemodialyzers. Blood Purif 2000;18:267–275.
10 Vander Velde C, Leonard EF: Theoretical assessment of the effect of flow maldistributions on the mass transfer efficiency of artificial organs. Med Biol Eng Comput 1985;23:224–229.
11 Hoenich N, Ronco C: Dialyzer evaluation; in Winchester J, Koch K, Jacobs C, Kjiellestrand C (eds): Replacement of Renal Function by Dialysis. Dordrecht, Kluwer Academic Publishers, 1996, pp 256–270.
12 Leypoldt JK, Cheung AK, Agodoa LY, Daugirdas JT, Greene T, Keshaviah PR: Hemodialyzer mass transfer-area coefficients for urea increase at high dialysate flow rates. The Hemodialysis (HEMO) Study. Kidney Int 1997;51:2013–2017.
13 Ronco C, Ghezzi PM, Metry G, Spittle M, Brendolan A, Rodighiero M, Milan M, Zanella M, La Greca G, Levin N.W: Effects of hematocrit and blood flow distribution on solute clearance in hollow-fiber hemodialyzers. Nephron 2001;89:243–250.
14 Ronco C, Brendolan A, Crepaldi C, Rodighiero MP, Scabardi M: Blood and dialysate flow distributions in hollow-fiber hemodialyzers analyzed by computerized helical scanning technique. J Am Soc Nephrol 2002;13:S53–S61.

15 Skroder N, Jacobson S, Holmquist B, Kjellstrand P, Kjellstrand C: β2-Microglobulin generation and removal in long slow and short fast hemodialysis. Am J Kidney Dis 1993,21:519–526.

16 Besarab A, Girone J, Erslev A, et al: Recent developments in the anemia of chronic renal failure. Semin Dial 1989;2:87–97.

17 Acchiardo S, Quinn B, Burk L, et al: Are high flux dialysis and erythropoietin treatment in a collision course? ASAIO Trans 1989;14:19–25.

18 Paganini E, Latham D, Abdulhadi M: Practical considerations of recombinant human erythropoietin therapy. Am J Kidney Dis 1989; 14(suppl 1):19–25.

19 Zehnter E, Pollock M, Longere F, Bramsiepe P, Ziegenhagen D, Baldamus C: Urea kinetics in patients on RDT treated with recombinant erythropoietin (abstract). Kidney Int 1988;33:242.

20 Shinaberger J, Miller J, Gardner P: Erythropoietin alert: risks of high hematocrit hemodialysis. ASAIO Trans 1988;34:179–184.

21 Burr T, Martin L: Secondary effects of erythropoietin on metabolism and dialysis efficiency in stable hemodialysis patients. Clin Nephrol 1990;34:230–335.

22 Chiou W, Lee H: Effect of change in blood flow on hemodialysis clearance studied by a simple unified organ clearance approach. Res Commun Chem Pathol Pharmacol 1989;65:393–396.

23 Thurston G: Viscoelasticity of human blood. Biophys J 1972;12:1205–1217.

24 Schweiger B, Pohl I, Driessen G, Heidtmann H, Schmid-Schönbein H: Influence of fibrinogen concentration on flow velocity of RBCs in rat mesentery; in Gaehtgens P (ed): Recent Advances in Microcirculatory Research. Bibl Anat. Basel, Karger, 1981, vol 20, pp 220–233.

25 Secomb T: Red blood cell mechanics and capillary blood rheology. Cell Biophys 1991;18: 231–251.

26 Ronco C, Scabardi M, Goldoni M, Brendolan A, Crepaldi C, La Greca G: Impact of spacing filaments external to hollow fibers on dialysate flow distribution and dialyzer performance. Int J Artif Organs 1997;5:261–266.

27 Jost W: Diffusion in Solids, Liquids, Gases. New York, Academic Press, 1965.

28 Scheidegger AE: The Physics of Flow through Porous Media. New York, McMillan, 1960.

29 Ronco C, Ghezzi PM, Morris A, Rosales L, Wang E, Zhu F, Metry G, De Simone L, Rahmati S, Adhikarla R, Bashir A, Manzoni C, Spittle M, Levin NW: Blood flow distribution in sorbent beds: analysis of a new sorbent device for hemoperfusion. Int J Artif Organs 2000;23:125–130.

30 Ronco C: Dialysis delivery versus dialysis prescription. Int J Artif Organs 1993;16:628–635.

31 Ronco C: Hemofiltration and hemodiafiltration; in Bosch JP (ed): Hemodialysis: High Efficiency Treatments. New York, Churchill Livingstone, 1993, pp 119–133.

32 Ronco C, Brendolan A, Bragantini L, Chiaramonte S, Feriani M, La Greca G: Technical and clinical evaluation of four different highly efficient short dialysis techniques; in Colasanti G, D'Amico G (eds): Nephrology and Dialysis Updated. Contrib Nephrol. Basel, Karger, 1988, vol 61, pp 46–53.

33 Ronco C: Backfiltration: a controversial issue in modern dialysis. Int J Artif Organs 1988;11: 69–74.

34 Ronco C, Brendolan A, Feriani M, Milan M, Conz P, Lupi A, Berto P, Bettini MC, La Greca G: A new scintigraphic method to characterize ultrafiltration in hollow fiber dialyzers. Kidney Int 1992; 41:1383–1393.

35 Ohmi T, Muto C, Nishibori F: Investigation on plasma clearance of beta-2-microglobulin in hemodialysis with PMMA membrane. Jpn J Artif Organs 1991;20:116–121.

36 Lee CjHsiong CH, Chang YL, Cheng CH, Lian JD: Statistical and parameteric analysis of beta-2 microglobulin removal from uremic patients in high flux hemodialysis. ASAIO J 1994;40:62–66.

37 Floege J, Granolleras C, Deschodt G, Heck M, Baudin G, Branger B, Tournier O, Reinhard B, Eisenbach GM, Smeby LC: High flux synthetic versus cellulosic membranes for beta-2 microglobulin removal during hemodialysis, hemodiafiltration and hemofiltration. Nephrol Dial Transplant 1989;4:653–657.

38 Locatelli F, Mastrangelo F, Redaelli B, Ronco C, Marcelli D, La Greca G, Orlandini G: Effects of different membranes and dialysis technologies on patient treatment tolerance and nutritional parameters. Kidney Int 1996;50:1293–1302.

39 Miller Jh, von Albertini B, Gardner PW, Shinaberger JH: Technical aspects of high flux hemodiafiltration for adequate short (under 2 hours) treatment. Trans Am Soc Artif Intern Organs 1984; 30:377–380.
40 Ronco C, Brendolan A, Lupi A, Bettini MC, La Greca G: Enhancement of convective transport by internal filtration in a modified experimental hemodialyzer. Kidney Int 1998;54:979–985.
41 Ronco C, Brendolan A, Lupi A, Metry G: Effects of a reduced inner diameter of hollow fibers in hemodialyzers. Kidney Int 2000;58:809–817.
42 Ronco C, Cappelli G, Ballestri M, Lusvarghi E, Frisone P, Milan M, Dell'Aquila R, Crepaldi C, Dissegna D, Gastaldon F, La Greca G: On-line filtration of dialysate: structural and functional features of an asymmetric polysulfone hollow fiber ultrafilter (Diaclean). Int J Artif Organs 1994; 10:515–520.
43 Canaud B, Bosc JY, Leray-Moragues H, et al: On-line haemodiafiltration: safety and efficacy in long-term clinical practice. Nephrol Dial Transplant 2000;5(suppl 1):S60–S67.

Dr. Claudio Ronco
Department of Nephrology, St. Bortolo Hospital
Viale Rodolfi 16
IT–36100 Vicenza (Italy)
Tel. +39 0444753650, Fax +39 0444753949, E-Mail cronco@goldnet.it

Ronco C, Canaud B, Aljama P (eds): Hemodiafiltration.
Contrib Nephrol. Basel, Karger, 2007, vol 158, pp 50–56

Mechanisms of Solute and Fluid Removal in Hemodiafiltration

Akihiro C. Yamashita

Department of Materials Science and Engineering, College of Engineering, Shonan Institute of Technology, Fujisawa, Japan

Abstract

Background: Prescribing therapeutic conditions for online predilution hemodiafiltration (HDF) with fixed total dialysate flow rate Q_{Dtotal} is not straightforward, since the increase in the substitution flow rate Q_S is compensated by the decrease in the net dialysate flow rate Q_{Dnet}. **Methods:** Clearances of various solutes under online predilution HDF were clinically evaluated with fixed Q_{Dtotal} (=520 ml/min) divided into Q_{Dnet} and Q_S. Three polysulfone membrane dialyzers and 5 polyester polymer alloy membrane dialyzers were chosen to measure sieving coefficients (SC) for albumin in vitro at 37°C to predict when the albumin loss is greatest during clinical treatment. **Results:** Clearances of small solutes such as urea and creatinine increased in vivo with the increase in blood flow. These values, however, slightly but steadily decreased with the increase in Q_S because the increase in Q_S decreased Q_{Dnet}. Clearances of β_2-microglobulin and α_1-microglobuin increased with the increase in Q_S and decreased with the increase in Q_{Dnet}, because clearances of larger solutes were more strongly dependent on ultrafiltration than on diffusion. The SC for albumin in vitro showed a peak at the beginning of the experiment in those membranes with large proportions of polyvinylpyrroridone (PVP), which may lead to large amounts of albumin loss at the beginning of the treatment. **Conclusions:** Dialysis prescription in online predilution HDF in terms of maximizing clearance for the solute of interest may be different for each target solute. The amount of albumin loss may be closely related to the amount of PVP included in the membrane.

Hemodiafiltration (HDF) is accepted as one of the intermittent blood purification modalities for treating end-stage renal disease (ESRD) patients, since it removes toxins over a wide molecular-weight range [1–3]. In HDF treatments, however, since molecular diffusion and considerable amount of ultrafiltration occur at the same time in one dialyzer, the solute and fluid transport mechanisms are much more complicated than other treatment modalities in which either diffusion or convection is used with a limited effect of the other mechanism. Many factors affect the fluid and mass transport in HDF, and the following 2 factors need to be considered before starting discussion. The first concerns the mode of dilution. Postdilution has been the preferred form of treatment, owing to its optimal cost-effectiveness. However, the use of online prepared dialysate as the substitution fluid has solved the economic problem of predilution. Moreover, since it may be easier to control the amount of albumin loss with predilution HDF, this mode is preferred when dialyzers with larger pore sizes are used. Secondly, in recent years, many petroleum-based synthetic polymers have been used as dialysis membranes; however, these materials are too hydrophobic in nature to use for blood purification treatment. A hydrophilic agent is therefore often added to these materials to improve their compatibility with blood, more specifically to prevent thrombosis. The most common is polyvinylpyrrolidone (PVP), which has been used with many polymers, including polysulfone, polyether sulfone, polyamide and polyester polymer alloy (PEPA). However, PVP affects not only biocompatibility, but also solute transport, including the amount of albumin loss. Then we will consider online predilution HDF with fixed total dialysate flow rate, which is sometimes difficult for prescribing therapeutic conditions, since an increase in the substitution flow rate is compensated by a decrease in the net dialysate flow rate. Mechanisms of albumin loss in HDF with high-flux dialyzers using PVP are also discussed in this section.

Materials and Methods

The amount of PVP used in the membrane is semiquantitatively scaled in the following 4 categories based on the membrane casting procedure: PVP− = no PVP, PVP+ = a small amount, PVP++ = an increased amount, and PVP+++ = a large amount.

Clearances for urea [molecular weight (MW) = 60], creatinine (MW = 113), β_2-microglobulin (β_2-MG, MW = 11,800) and α_1-microglobulin (α_1-MG, MW = 33,000) were clinically measured in hemodialysis (HD) and in online predilution HDF mode with various substitution flow rates (Q_S) from 180 to 260 ml/min. Blood flow rates (Q_B) ranged from 200 to 230 ml/min while the total dialysate flow rate (Q_{Dtotal}) was fixed at 520 ml/min, which was divided into Q_S and net dialysate flow rate (Q_{Dnet}) in all clinical studies.

The sieving coefficients (SC) for albumin were measured in vitro with 6 commercial dialyzers (table 1), the membranes of which included various amounts of PVP. Measurements were done at 37°C with 2 liters of phosphate buffer solution (pH = 7.4) with bovine albumin (Wako Pure Chemical Ind. Co., Osaka, Japan) in a glass container. The flow rate of the test solution (pseudo-blood) was 200 ml/min, and the ultrafiltration rate (Q_F) was fixed at 10 ml/min. The ultrafiltrate and the test solutions were returned to the glass container during the course of the experiment for 630 min. Samples were taken at various times, and concentrations were analyzed by either spectrophotometry or HPLC.

Table 1. Technical specifications of investigated ultrafilters

Name	Abbreviated name	Surface area, m^2	Membrane materials	Hydrophilic agent	Pore size	Manufacturer
PS-1.6UW	PS	1.6	PS	PVP+++	NA	Fresenius-Kawasumi, Tokyo, Japan
FLX-15GW	FLX	1.5	PEPA	PVP−	standard	
FDX-15GW	FDX	1.5	PEPA	PVP+	standard	
FDY-15GW	FDY	1.5	PEPA	PVP+	larger	Nikkiso Co., Tokyo, Japan
FDX-150GW	new FDX	1.5	PEPA	PVP++	standard	
FDY-150GW	new FDY	1.5	PEPA	PVP++	larger	

PS = Polysulfone; − = no PVP; + = small amount; ++ = increased amount; +++ = large amount.

Theoretical Background

Dialyzer clearances (C_L) were calculated for various solutes (urea, creatinine, β_2-MG, α_1-MG) using the following equation:

$$C_L = \frac{C_{Bi} - C_{Bo}}{C_{Bi}} Q_{Bo} + Q_F \quad (1)$$

where C_{Bi}, C_{Bo} are concentrations in the test solution at the inlet and outlet of the dialyzer, respectively, and Q_{Bo} is the blood flow rate at the outlet of the dialyzer.

The definition of the *SC* is the ratio between the concentration in the downstream to that in the upstream, and the definitive equations may be found elsewhere. We used the following semiquantitative definition SC_4, proposed by the authors [4, 5]:

$$SC_4 = \frac{C_F}{\sqrt{C_{Bi} C_{Bo}}} \quad (2)$$

where C_F is the solute concentration in the ultrafiltrate.

Results and Discussion

Although Q_F was changed within a certain range (20–280 ml/min), clearances for urea and creatinine in vivo increased sharply with Q_B, implying that clearances for these solutes were strongly dependent on Q_B. The clearance for α_1-MG, however, never showed a sharp increase with Q_B but showed a relatively large deviation, caused by the change in Q_F. This implied that the transport of large solutes cannot be controlled only by Q_B.

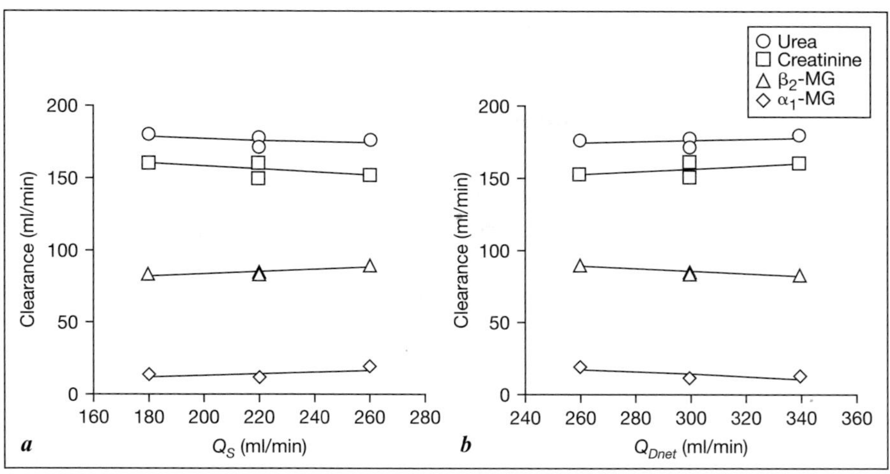

Fig. 1. Clearances for various solutes in online predilution HDF. $Q_B = 200$ ml/min, $Q_{Dtotal} = 520$ ml/min.

Figure 1a shows another clinical relationship between solute clearances and Q_S in online predilution HDF treatments with a fixed blood flow rate $Q_B = 200$ ml/min. With the increase in Q_S, clearances for small solutes such as urea and creatinine decreased slightly but steadily, while clearances for β_2-MG and α_1-MG increased. In online treatments in general, since Q_{Dtotal} is usually fixed at some value and was fixed at 520 ml/min in these treatments, an increase in Q_S will decrease Q_{Dnet} ($Q_{Dnet} = Q_{Dtotal} - Q_S$). Then the abscissa of figure 1a is replaced by Q_{Dnet} to yield figure 1b, which is a mirror image of figure 1a. Since urea and creatinine transport is a diffusion-limited process, a decrease in Q_{Dnet} has a more crucial negative effect on clearances of these solutes than an increase in Q_S (or Q_F), which should have a positive effect on clearances. However, since transport of β_2-MG-and α_1-MG is a bulk flow-limited (convection-limited) process, for clearances of these solutes an increase in Q_S (or Q_F) is much more effective than a decrease in Q_{Dnet}, which should have an adverse effect. Since transport phenomena of this kind never happen in postdilution HDF (neither online nor off-line) [6], great attention should be paid to the target solutes that should be removed by the treatment in online predilution HDF. There is still some debate on dilution modes because in terms of solute removal it is in general better to treat patients with postdilution HDF. Canaud et al. [7], however, showed that solute removal performance in predilution can match that in postdilution. Moreover, Ahrenholz et al. [8] showed that the rate of albumin loss can exceed 7,000 mg/session in postdilution HDF; in that case, it is safer to perform HDF in predilution mode. Since recent dialyzers have high hydraulic permeability as well as high solute permeability, ultrafiltration from the blood compartment to the dialysate and reverse filtration from the dialysate to the blood are induced in one dialyzer at the same time, which is termed the internal filtration [9]. There are several commercial dialyzers that are designed to increase the internal filtration rate. With an increased internal filtration similar (on a limited scale) to postdilution HDF, albumin loss may also be increased, and this should therefore be monitored. The internal filtration is suppressed by increasing Q_F; therefore, it is minimized in predilution HDF that induces by far the largest Q_F. Consequently, the reduced albumin loss in predilution HDF is caused not only by the low albumin concentration due to diluted blood but also by the suppressed internal filtration due to extremely high Q_F. Reducing albumin loss without changing clearances for other solutes may in many cases fit clinical requirements.

The time courses of SC_4 for albumin, using a PS-1.6UW dialyzer (PS, Fresenius-Kawasumi Co., Tokyo, Japan) in aqueous solution with various albumin concentrations, showed strong time-dependent patterns with peak values approximately 10 min after start of the experiments. The lower the albumin concentration, the higher the values and the longer the time required for achieving steady state. Moreover, Ahrenholz et al. [8] pointed out that as much as 50% of albumin loss occurred within the first 30 min of the treatment. From these facts, large albumin losses may be expected at the beginning of each treatment with such membranes that take the peak SC values [10, 11].

The SC_4 for albumin of 3 PEPA dialyzers, FLX, FDX and FDY gradually increased with time and never reached peak values. The membranes used in the FLX and FDX had the same pore size, the only difference being that the latter contained a small amount of PVP on the inner surface of the membrane. The fact that the FDX showed much lower SC_4 values than the FLX can be explained in the following way. The membrane used in the FDX soon reached the adsorption saturation of albumin due to reduced hydrophobic interaction. In contrast, since the FLX had higher adsorption characteristics to albumin, the albumin concentration in the test solution (C_{Bi} and C_{Bo}) drastically decreased, which decreased the value of the denominator of the SC_4, while the numerator did not change much because adsorbed albumin molecules may have been slowly released from the membrane. The membrane material used in the FDX is the same as the one used in the FDY, which had a 5% larger pore diameter analyzed by the classic pore theory [12]. By enlarging the pore diameter in the FDY, the SC_4 increased in accordance with the enlargement.

The time courses of SC_4 for albumin of the latest models of PEPA dialyzers (new FDX and new FDY with PVP++) showed peak values at 6 min after starting the experiments. The peaks found with the new PEPA membranes were quite similar to the one found with the PS (PVP+++) dialyzer, which may be because of the increased amount of PVP. We have already reported that an increase in PVP may induce larger changes in C3a concentration in vivo [11]. Then the peak SC_4 values for albumin and the blood compatibility of the membrane may be related to the amount of PVP or hydrophilicity of the membrane.

Since the albumin concentrations of the test solutions were lower by a factor of 1/30–1/10 than the standard albumin concentration in human blood (3.6–4.0 g/dl), the SC_4 values for albumin shown above do not correspond directly to the clinical results. One should, however, consider the membrane separation characteristics that depend on the membrane materials, including both the main material and hydrophilic agents, as well as the experimental conditions.

Conclusions

Solute removal characteristics in online predilution HDF were demonstrated with a fixed total dialysate flow rate. Clearances for small solutes decreased with increasing Q_F, and clearances for β_2-MG-and α_1-MG increased with increasing Q_F.

Since the SC for albumin reached a peak value at the beginning of the experiment with those membranes containing relatively large amounts of PVP (less adsorption), a large amount of albumin loss may be expected at the beginning of the treatment.

The amount of PVP used in the membrane may be closely related to biocompatibility as well as the solute removal characteristics.

References

1 Sprenger KB: Haemodiafiltration. Life Support Syst 1983;1:127–136.
2 Ofsthum NJ, Leypoldt JK: Ultrafiltration and backfiltration during hemodialysis. Artif Organs 1995;19:1143–1161.
3 Leypoldt JK: Solute fluxes in different treatment modalities. Nephrol Dial Transplant 2000;1:3–9.
4 Yamashita AC, Sakiyama R, Hamada H, Tojo K: Two new definitive equations of the sieving coefficient. Kidney Dial (Jin To Toseki) 1998;45:S36–S38.
5 Yamashita AC: New dialysis membrane for removal of middle molecule uremic toxins. Am J Kidney Dis 2001;38(suppl 1):S217–S219.
6 Masakane M: Selection of dilutional method for on-line HDF, pre- or post-dilution. Blood Purif 2004;22(suppl 2):49–54.
7 Canaud B, Levesque R, Krieter D, Desmeules S, Chalabi L, Moragues H, Morena M, Cristol JP: On-line hemodiafiltration as routine treatment of end-stage renal failure: why pre- or mixed dilution mode is necessary in on-line hemodiafiltration today? Blood Purif 2004;22(suppl 2):40–48.
8 Ahrenholz PG, Winkler RE, Michelsen A, Lang DA, Bowry SK: Dialysis membrane-dependent removal of middle molecules during hemodiafiltration: the b2-microglobulin/albumin ratio. Clin Nephrol 2004;62:21–28.

9 Dellana F, Baldamus CA: Does internal-filtration have a benefit? Abstr Meet 'Quality care for haemodialysis patients', Wiesbaden, May 11–13, 1995, p 51.
10 Yamashita AC, Tomisawa N, Takezawa A, Sato Y: Separation characteristics of newly developed polymer alloy membrane. Proc 8th Jpn Int SAMPE Symp, Tokyo, 2003, pp 415–418.
11 Yamashita AC, Tomisawa N, Takesawa A, Sakurai K, Sakai T: Blood compatibility and filtration characteristics of newly developed polyester polymer alloy (PEPA) membrane. Hemodial Int 2004;8:373–337.
12 Pappenheimer JR, Renkin EM, Borrero LM: Filtration, diffusion and molecular sieving through peripheral capillary membranes – a contribution to the pore theory of capillary permeability. Am J Physiol 1951;167:13–46.

Prof. Akihiro C. Yamashita, PhD
Department of Materials Science and Engineering
College of Engineering, Shonan Institute of Technology
1–1–25 Tsujido-Nishikaigan
Fujisawa, Kanagawa 251-8511 (Japan)
Tel./Fax +81 466 30 0234, E-Mail yama@la.shonan-it.ac.jp

Ronco C, Canaud B, Aljama P (eds): Hemodiafiltration.
Contrib Nephrol. Basel, Karger, 2007, vol 158, pp 57–67

Membranes and Filters for Haemodiafiltration

Nicholas A. Hoenich

School of Clinical Medical Sciences, Faculty of Medical Sciences,
Newcastle University, Newcastle upon Tyne, UK

Abstract

Online haemodiafiltration is an extracorporeal technique, utilizing highly permeable and highly biocompatible membranes, which permits the combination of convective and diffusive solute removal from the blood and offers increased removal of medium-weight uraemic solutes, compared to the more frequently used low- and high-flux haemodialysis. The objective of this chapter is to review the membranes and filters available for haemodiafiltration and to discuss factors that influence their performance during clinical use.

The treatment of patients with chronic kidney disease in the absence of a suitable kidney for transplantation relies upon the use of artificial support to sustain life. The most widely used support modality is haemodialysis, a treatment in which non-protein-bound solutes from the blood are removed by diffusion into an electrolyte solution (dialysis fluid) across a semi-permeable membrane. This treatment modality is highly efficient in removing small-molecular-weight uraemic toxins, but offers only a limited clearance of larger-molecular-weight substances, some of which, e.g. β_2-microglobulin, are associated with the development of long-term treatment complications. Improved removal of such compounds can be achieved by convective therapies such as haemofiltration, a treatment modality introduced into clinical practice in the mid-1970s, using hollow-fibre devices containing highly permeable membranes.

During haemofiltration, plasma water is filtered across a highly permeable membrane at a rate far beyond that needed to normalize intertreatment fluid gain. The excess fluid removed is replaced with a sterile replacement fluid infused into the extracorporeal circuit either before (pre-dilution) or after (postdilution) the filter, with early treatments using prepared sterile replacement fluid. Owing to cost considerations, the volume of the fluid used was typically 5–10 litres, up to a maximum of 15 litres.

As a result of water movement, solutes able to pass through the pores of the membrane are dragged across the membrane independently of their molecular size, provided this size is less than the size of the membrane pores. Consequently, this treatment offered a higher rate of medium- and large-molecular removal than conventional haemodialysis, but removal of small-molecular compounds was inferior. Leber et al. [1], in the late 1970s, proposed combining haemodialysis and haemofiltration into a single treatment (haemodiafiltration). As in haemofiltration, early applications relied on the use of prepared sterile infusate. Today, technological advances permit the online production of fluid derived from bicarbonate-buffered dialysis fluid to be used for the infusate, allowing safe use of high-exchange volumes (online haemodiafiltration) [2].

In this chapter, the membranes and filters used in haemodiafiltration will be reviewed, together with their functional performance, and the factors influencing performance during clinical use will be discussed.

Membrane Materials

In the early 1970s, membrane requirements focused on small-molecular clearance and hydraulic permeability or ultrafiltration; since the 1980s, the emphasis has shifted to the clearance of larger molecules and flux. Today, major manufacturers produce families of membranes or devices suitable for conventional haemodialysis, high-flux dialysis, haemofiltration or haemodiafiltration. Classification of the membranes may be according to their hydraulic permeability or their chemical composition (fig. 1).

In contrast to membranes intended for use in conventional low-flux haemodialysis, which have a permeability to water of 5–6 ml/h · mm Hg · m^2, membranes intended for use in haemodiafiltration have higher permeabilities (30–40 ml/h · mm Hg · m^2), and additionally exhibit a high removal rate for β_2-microglobulin, a compound implicated in the evolution of long-term complications associated with haemodialysis treatment, and which has become an important surrogate parameter of dialysis efficiency regarding medium-molecule removal. High-permeability membranes in current clinical use are not selective, and whilst a certain degree of selectivity can be achieved by the manipulation of the membrane structure during manufacture [3], such selectivity is not optimal and is associated with some albumin loss. Short-term clinical experience with such membranes suggests improved anaemia correction, decreased total plasma homocysteine concentrations and reduced plasma

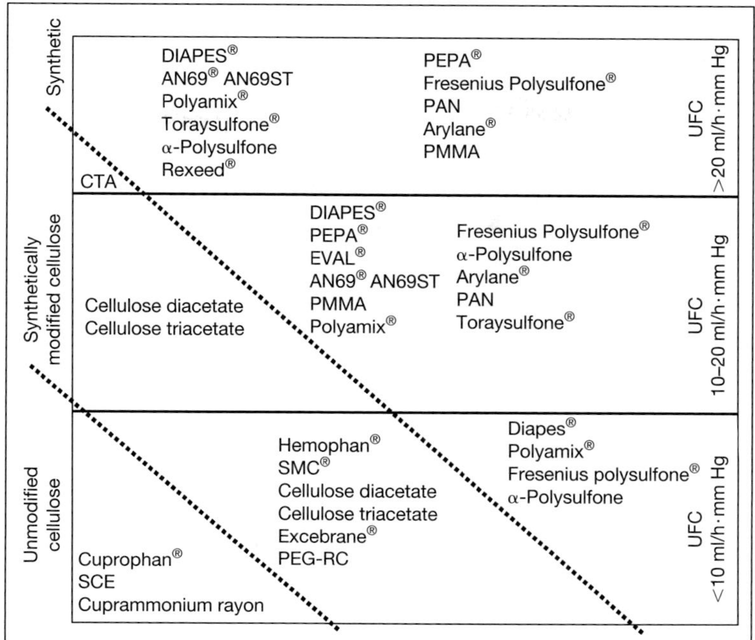

Fig. 1. Membranes suitable for haemodiafiltration classified according to their chemical composition and hydraulic permeability. UFC = Ultrafiltration coefficient.

concentrations of glycosylated and oxidized proteins, but it is not yet clear whether the routine use of such membranes is warranted [4]. Furthermore, whilst it can be speculated that a considerable albumin loss across the membrane may lead to hypo-albuminaemia and malnutrition, at least in those patients who are unable to supply a sufficient protein intake, it remains impossible to quantify an acceptable upper limit for albumin loss for extracorporeal renal replacement therapies or to define the optimum membrane permeability.

Haemodiafilter Design

Today, the most commonly used haemodialyser is the hollow-fibre or capillary design. Such a design can be subject to limitations in respect of an even flow through and around the fibres [5]. Nevertheless, it offers considerable manufacturing flexibility, enabling devices of a range of sizes to be manufactured for use in a range of clinical applications merely by altering the number, length or type of fibre, and all major manufacturers of haemodialysers produce

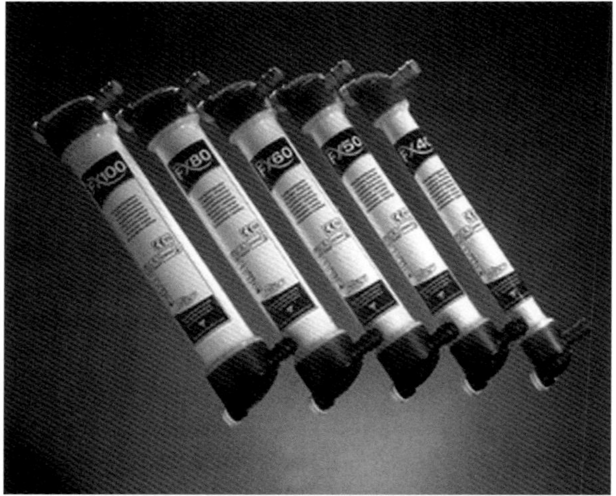

a

Fig. 2. ***a*** Modern hollow-fibre devices, suitable for use as haemodiafilters, utilizing fibres with a three-dimensional microwave structure, incorporated into a specifically designed housing for optimized flow distribution in both the blood and dialysate pathways (photograph courtesy of Fresenius Medical Care AG, Bad Homburg, Germany).

hollow-fibre devices suitable for haemodiafiltration in either pre- or postfilter dilution mode (fig. 2a).

A deviation from this approach is the Olpur MD 190H mid-dilution filter (Nephros Inc., New York, N.Y., USA). This has a circular groove incorporated into the fibre bundle tube at one end, such that when the header cap is added, two discrete but serially connected paths for blood are formed: an outer or annular path, and an inner or core path. The header cap splits the fibre bundle and also functions as a mixing chamber for the infused substitution fluid. The other end of the device uses a dual port header which acts as an inlet and outlet manifold for the blood. The dialysis fluid enters and leaves the device in the conventional manner (fig. 2b).

Fundamentals of Performance

Solute Transport

Solute transport across the membrane can occur via diffusion or convection. Diffusive solute transport is the transport in the presence of a concentration

Fig. 2. ***b*** The Olpur 190 Mid-dilution filter for haemodiafiltration (photographs courtesy of Nephros Inc., New York, N.Y., USA).

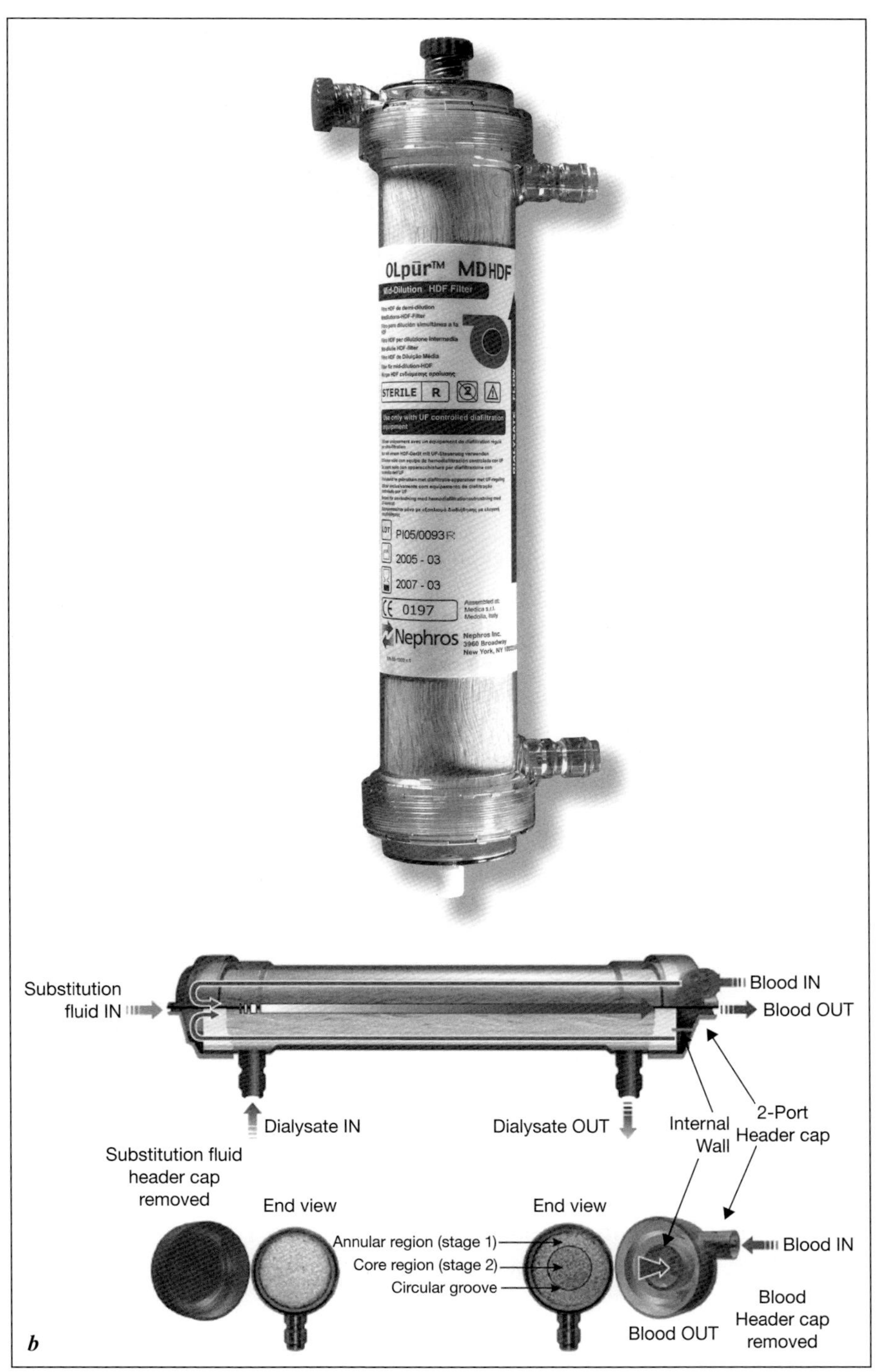
OLpūr™ MD HDF
Mid-Dilution HDF Filter
STERILE R
PI05/0093R
2005 - 03
2007 - 03
0197
Nephros
Substitution fluid IN
Blood IN
Blood OUT
Dialysate IN
Dialysate OUT
Internal Wall
2-Port Header cap
Substitution fluid header cap removed
End view
End view
Annular region (stage 1)
Core region (stage 2)
Circular groove
Blood IN
Blood OUT
Blood Header cap removed
b

gradient. It is governed by Fick's law, which can be expressed mathematically as

$$J_D = -D\,A\,\frac{dC}{dx}$$

Where J_D is the diffusive flux, D is the solute diffusion coefficient, A the area available for transport, and dC/dx the concentration gradient.

Convective solute transport is a consequence of filtration of fluid through the membrane. All solutes that can pass through the pores of the membrane, i.e. which are sieved by the membrane, are carried along by the filtered fluid. Thus, the sieving properties of the membrane determine what is removed. In contrast to diffusive transport, convective transport remains constant over a wide range of molecular sizes but decreases as the molecular size approaches that of the pores. Mathematically, it can be expressed as

$$J_C = Q_F\,C\,S$$

Where J_C is the convective flux, Q_F the rate of fluid transfer across the membrane, C the solute concentration in the fluid, and S the sieving coefficient, a parameter that represents the magnitude of restriction of the pore size relative to the molecular size and varies between 0 for a freely permeable molecule and 1 for a completely impermeable molecule.

Solute transport in haemodiafiltration occurs as a consequence of both diffusion and convection. Early theoretical approaches assumed that the diffusive and convective mass transfer took place sequentially, and this approach remains applicable to the paired filtration dialysis system, a variant of online haemodiafiltration [6].

In the presence of simultaneous convective and diffusive mass transport, the combined solute transport is not the sum of the individual components, because of an interaction between the convective and diffusive components. Several models have been proposed to explain this mathematically, of which the simplest is

$$K_{HDF} = K_0 + Q_F T$$

where K_0 is the clearance at zero ultrafiltration, Q_F the ultrafiltration rate and T the transmittance coefficient, a parameter which is a function of the flow conditions and membrane properties.

An expression for the transmittance coefficient that is universal for all solutes has been proposed by Jaffrin et al. [7], namely

$$K_{HDF} = K_0 + 0.46 Q_F$$

for ultrafiltration rates below 70 ml/min, which is modified to

$$K_{HDF} = K_0 + 0.43Q_F + 0.00083Q_F^2$$

for ultrafiltration rates above 70 ml/min.

Hydraulic Permeability

The hydraulic permeability (L_p) of the membrane is a parameter which reflects the relationship between the volumetric flux and the transmembrane pressure difference (ΔP). In the absence of an osmotic pressure difference the volumetric flux (J_V) can be expressed mathematically as

$$J_V = L_p \Delta P$$

which in the presence of an osmotic pressure difference becomes

$$J_V = L_p \Delta P - L_p \Delta \pi_s$$

where $\Delta\pi_s$ is the osmotic pressure difference across the membrane and σ the Staverman or osmotic reflection coefficient, whereby a value of 0 applies to a non-selective membrane, and a value of 1 applies to an impermeable membrane.

Biocompatibility

Extracorporeal circulatory procedures involve repeated exposure of the patient's blood to foreign materials, of which the membrane represents the largest contact surface. Such exposure is associated with a number of biological sequelae, the magnitude of which is determined to a large extent by the membrane's surface characteristics; however, in the case of high-flux membranes, transmembrane transport of activated components also contributes [8, 9].

Considerable uncertainty exists as to the long-term clinical impact of membrane biocompatibility; however, what is beyond doubt is that clinical application of haemodiafiltration exposes patients to highly biocompatible membranes which are used in conjunction with ultrapure dialysis fluid and infusion solutions, offering the highest possible treatment-associated biocompatibility [10].

Performance of Haemodiafilters

The laboratory performance of haemodiafilters is generally measured by manufacturers in accordance with an internationally recognized standard: ISO 8637:2004 – Cardiovascular implants and artificial organs – Haemodialysers, haemodiafilters, haemofilters and haemoconcentrators. Table 1 summarizes comparative data for currently produced devices in terms of urea clearance and β_2-microglobulin and protein sieving coefficients.

Table 1. Comparative performance characteristics of hollow-fibre devices suitable for haemodiafiltration

Device	Area m^2	Membrane	Clearance performance ml/min[a]			UFC ml/h · mm Hg[b]	Sieving coefficient	
			urea	creatinine	PO_4		β_2-microglobulin	albumin
PolyfluxS	1.7	Polyamix	254 280[c]	229 262[c]	223 258[c]	71	0.63	<0.01
PF-170H	1.7	Purema	274	259	240	74	0.8	NA
FX80	1.8	Helixone	276	250	239	59	0.8	0.001
Rexeed 18A	1.8	Rexbrane	280	265	250	71	0.85	0.002
Olpur MD 190H	1.9	Polyethersulfone	276	264	257	90	0.8	0.005
PolyfluxS	2.1	Polyamix	267 280[c]	245 262[c]	240 258[c]	83	0.63	<0.01
PF-210H	2.1	Purema	285	272	253	80	0.8	NA
Rexeed 21A	2.1	Rexbrane	284	272	257	74	0.85	0.002
FX100	2.2	Helixone	278	261	248	73	0.8	0.001

Data shown extracted from manufacturers' product specification sheets and measured in accordance with ISO 8637. NA = Not given in product sheet; UFC = ultrafiltration capacity.

[a] At a blood flow rate of 300 ml/min, dialysis fluid flow rate 500 ml/min, ultrafiltration rate 0 ml/min.

[b] Measured using bovine blood.

[c] At a blood flow rate of 300 ml/min, dialysis fluid flow rate 500 ml/min, ultrafiltration rate 60 ml/min.

Operational Factors Influencing Efficiency

Solute Transport

The efficiency of haemodiafiltration is influenced, as for conventional haemodialysis, by the blood and dialysate flow rates and the red cell concentration. In addition, solute transport efficiency is also influenced by the site of the infusion fluid.

In postdilution, the clearance of both small and medium molecules is increased compared to conventional haemodialysis, and can be considered as the most efficient method of haemodiafiltration. In this modality, however, as the infusion fluid is added after the filter, the blood flowing through the filter is subject to haemoconcentration. Therefore, to mimimize the risk of compromising the extracorporeal circuit through clotting, the total ultrafiltration rate (i.e. the sum of the substitution fluid replacement rate and the net ultrafiltration) should not exceed 30% of the blood flow rate to ensure that the postfilter haematocrit does not exceed 50%.

In predilution HDF, where the substitution fluid is added to the blood before the filter, a dilution of the blood entering the filter occurs. This ensures better rheological conditions, and higher convective or large-molecular clearances, but this advantage is offset by the dilution of the concentration available for diffusion, resulting in reduced small-molecular clearance, to a level below that achieved in conventional haemodialysis [11]. In an online setting, this approach, however, permits infusion rates of up to 10–12 l/h to be used, which can prove useful when treating patients with high haemoglobin levels or when high exchange volumes are required.

Simultaneous pre- and postfilter dilution has also been proposed, but has not been used clinically. Instead, the mid-dilution approach with its specially designed filter appears to combine the high clearance of small-molecular-weight toxins (such as urea) associated with postdilution haemodiafiltration with the high clearance of medium-weight molecules (such as β_2-microglobulin) associated with predilution haemodiafiltration [12].

Irrespective of the strategy used, an important contributing element to the removal of large-molecular-weight compounds such as β_2-microglobulin is adsorption to the membrane, a characteristic which differs between membranes [13]. Therefore, the future development of membrane materials with a greater affinity for adsorption of β_2-microglobulin could theoretically result in higher removal rates than achieved by the combination of convection and diffusion. A logical extension of this is the future immobilization of proteins on the surface of the membrane to act as immunoadsorptive devices for this and other compounds.

Hydraulic Permeability

Membrane permeability is a key determinant of performance; in vivo, the hydraulic permeability is affected by the formation of a protein layer on the membrane surface, reducing ultrafiltration, and convective fluxes influencing the exchange volumes are possible as well as the convective solute removal.

Adequacy of Treatment when Using Haemodiafiltration

In haemodiafiltration, the additional flux compared to low- or high-flux haemodialysis treatments increases removal of small-molecular-weight compounds and facilitates the attainment of a high Kt/V. Additionally, removal of medium-molecular-weight compounds such as β_2-microglobulin is also increased, with the increase influenced by the volume of the substitution fluid used [14]. Thus, with a typical treatment duration of 240 min, and a blood flow rate of 300 ml/min, postfilter substitution volumes of 22 litres are potentially possible when maintaining the ultrafiltration rate of 30% of the blood flow rate, rising to 29 litres at a blood flow rate of 400 ml/min. Whilst theoretically it would be possible to use higher exchange volumes with the use of prefilter infusion, this would require a longer treatment period to compensate for the reduction of small-molecular clearance. Increasing the clearance of molecules such as β_2-microglobulin is subject to physiological constraints as a recent study by Ward et al. [15] indicated. Consequently, higher removal may require alternative strategies such as increased treatment times or frequency of treatment, to further reduce plasma β_2-microglobulin concentrations.

References

1 Leber HW, Wizemann V, Goubeaud G, Rawer P, Schutterle G: Hemodiafiltration: a new alternative to hemofiltration and conventional hemodialysis. Artif Organs 1978;2:150–153.

2 Aires I, Matias P, Gil C, Jorge C, Ferreira A: On-line haemodiafiltration with high volume substitution fluid: long-term efficacy and security. Nephrol Dial Transplant 2007;22:286–287.

3 Ronco C, Bowry S: Nanoscale modulation of dimensions, size distribution and structure of a new polysulfone-based high-flux dialysis membrane. Int J Artif Organs 2001;24:726–735.

4 Ward RA: Protein-leaking membranes for hemodialysis: a new class of membranes in search of an application? J Am Soc Nephrol 2005;16:2421–2430.

5 Ronco C, Levin N, Brendolan A, Nalesso F, Cruz D, Ocampo C, Kuang D, Bonello M, De Cal M, Corradi V, Ricci Z: Flow distribution analysis by helical scanning in polysulfone hemodialyzers: effects of fiber structure and design on flow patterns and solute clearances. Hemodial Int 2006;10: 380–388.

6 Ghezzi PM, Dutto A, Gervasio R, Botella J: Hemodiafiltration with separate convection and diffusion: paired filtration dialysis; in D'Amico G, Colasanti G (eds): Clinical Nephrology: Immunologic Considerations, Invasive Techniques and Dialytic Strategies. Contrib Nephrol. Basel, Karger, 1989, vol 69, pp 141–161.

7 Jaffrin MY, Ding LH, Laurent JM: Simultaneous convective and diffusive mass transfers in a hemodialyser. J Biomech Eng 1990;112:212–219.

8 Kaiser JP, Oppermann M, Gotze O, Deppisch R, Gohl H, Asmus G, Rohrich B, von Herrath D, Schaefer K: Significant reduction of factor D and immunosuppressive complement fragment Ba by hemofiltration. Blood Purif 1995;13:314–321.

9 Gasche Y, Pascual M, Suter PM, Favre H, Chevrolet JC, Schifferli JA: Complement depletion during haemofiltration with polyacrilonitrile membranes. Nephrol Dial Transplant 1996;11:117–119.

10 Macleod AM, Campbell M, Cody JD, Daly C, Donaldson C, Grant A, Khan I, Rabindranath KS, Vale L, Wallace S: Cellulose, modified cellulose and synthetic membranes in the haemodialysis of patients with end-stage renal disease. Cochrane Database Syst Rev. 2005;3:CD003234.

11 Wizemann V, Kulz M, Techert F, Nederlof B: Efficacy of haemodiafiltration. Nephrol Dial Transplant 2001;16(suppl 4):27–30.

12 Santoro A, Conz PA, De Cristofaro V, Acquistapace I, Gaggi R, Ferramosca E, Renaux JL, Rizzioli E, Wratten ML: Mid-dilution: the perfect balance between convection and diffusion; in Ronco C, Brendolan A, Levin NW (eds): Cardiovascular Disorders in Hemodialysis. Contrib Nephrol. Basel, Karger, 2005, vol 149, pp107–114.

13 Padrini R, Canova C, Conz P, Mancini E, Rizzioli E, Santoro A: Convective and adsorptive removal of β_2-microglobulin during predilutional and postdilutional hemofiltration. Kidney Int 2005;68:2331–2337.
14 Lornoy W, Becaus I, Billiouw JM, Sierens L, Van Malderen P, D'Haenens PR: On-line haemodiafiltration. Remarkable removal of β_2-microglobulin. Long-term clinical observations. Nephrol Dial Transplant 2000;15(suppl 1):49–54.
15 Ward RA, Greene T, Hartmann B, Samtleben W: Resistance to intercompartmental mass transfer limits β_2-microglobulin removal by post-dilution hemodiafiltration. Kidney Int 2006;69:1431–1437.

Nicholas A. Hoenich
School of Clinical Medical Sciences
Faculty of Medical Sciences, Newcastle University
Newcastle upon Tyne NE2 4HH (UK)
Tel. +44 191 222 6998, Fax +44 191 222 0723, E-Mail nicholas.hoenich@ncl.ac.uk

Ronco C, Canaud B, Aljama P (eds): Hemodiafiltration.
Contrib Nephrol. Basel, Karger, 2007, vol 158, pp 68–79

Technical Aspects of Online Hemodiafiltration

Hans-Dietrich Polaschegg[a], *Thomas Roy*[b]

[a]Medical Devices Consultant, Köstenberg, Austria; [b]Research and Development, Fresenius Medical Care Deutschland GmbH, Bad Homburg, Germany

Abstract

The chapter describes and analyzes the most commonly used systems for online substitution fluid production in hemofiltration and hemodiafiltration, covering in detail systems comprising 2 multiuse filters, or 2 multiuse filters in combination with 1 disposable filter. A generally applicable risk analysis for the process of online substitution fluid preparation is provided. It is concluded that both system variants discussed perform in a safe manner, provided the operator fully complies with the manufacturer's instructions for use.

Many scientists, clinicians and technologists in Japan, the USA and Europe have contributed to the development of hemofiltration (HF) and hemodiafiltration (HDF) with online-produced substitution fluid. Today's most widely used commercial systems were developed by the companies Gambro and Fresenius Medical Care using various technologies. These systems formed the basis upon which other companies designed their systems. For this reason these most common systems will be described in detail, while the later developed systems will be discussed only briefly, using the basic systems as a reference.

Over the years, various systems for online HDF from various manufacturers have been used clinically. However, the routine application of online HDF is technically dominated by equipment from Fresenius Medical Care (FME), Germany, and Gambro AB, Sweden. Both companies entered the field of online fluid preparation before others, and provided online HDF equipment first on request from enthusiastic doctors and later as a regular option for all their mainstream hemodialysis (HD) machines (Gambro: AK series; FME: 2008 and 4008 series).

The trend to use online HDF as a cost-efficient, highly effective treatment mode for end-stage renal disease was low before the 1990s owing to uncertainties regarding the regulatory situation of these systems. However, with the so-called Medical Devices Directive [1], coming into effect in 1993, and subsequent interpretations of this directive [2], online HDF equipment including consumables were classified as medical devices and – in consequence – could be CE marked and distributed in the European Community, leading to increased application of this modality. For the FME 5008, the most current FME HD machine, online HDF is part of the standard device configuration.

Gambro and FME online HDF equipment, exemplified in the following paragraphs, underwent various modifications since the mid-1980s on the way from prototype-like experimental devices to the current state of professionally made medical equipment, but still represent the 2 most common approaches to solve the problem of safe and efficient online preparation of intravenously injectable substitution fluid.

Both systems are adapted to the specific properties of the underlying HD machines, in particular to the design of the respective dialysate circuits. Other online HDF machines that were developed later employ principles used by either the FME or the Gambro system or both.

In general it can be said that both systems, to the authors' knowledge, have a clean safety record. According to FME internal reports, between the years 2000 and 2006 approximately 15 million single online HDF treatments were performed with the current technical system (brand name Online plus™) without any report of patient injury due to failures of the specific online fluid preparation components of the device.

Gambro HD machines are traditionally characterized by an ultrafiltration control system comprising 2 electromagnetic flow meters before and behind the dialyzer (fig. 1). Fluid balance is regulated by means of 2 flow restrictors and 2 pumps installed before and behind the flow cell unit.

Incoming process water is filtered through an ultrafilter (type U8000S, surface area 2.1 m^2, membrane material polyamide S). The water filter is operated in cross-flow mode, in which a small amount of fluid is continuously drained off to prevent accumulation of possible contaminants on the inlet side of the filter. In the next step the 2 concentrate components for bicarbonate dialysate are added. In the context of 'intended use', the manufacturer requires for the device that the incoming water complies with at least the Association for the Advancement of Medical Instrumentation standard for HD water quality [3], and that the bicarbonate concentrate is generated in situ by the machine from powder to avoid the hazards of liquid bicarbonate concentrate, which easily develops major bacterial contamination.

After passing the flow cell, the now ready-to-use dialysate is filtered through another U8000S ultrafilter, this one running in dead-end mode. A valve

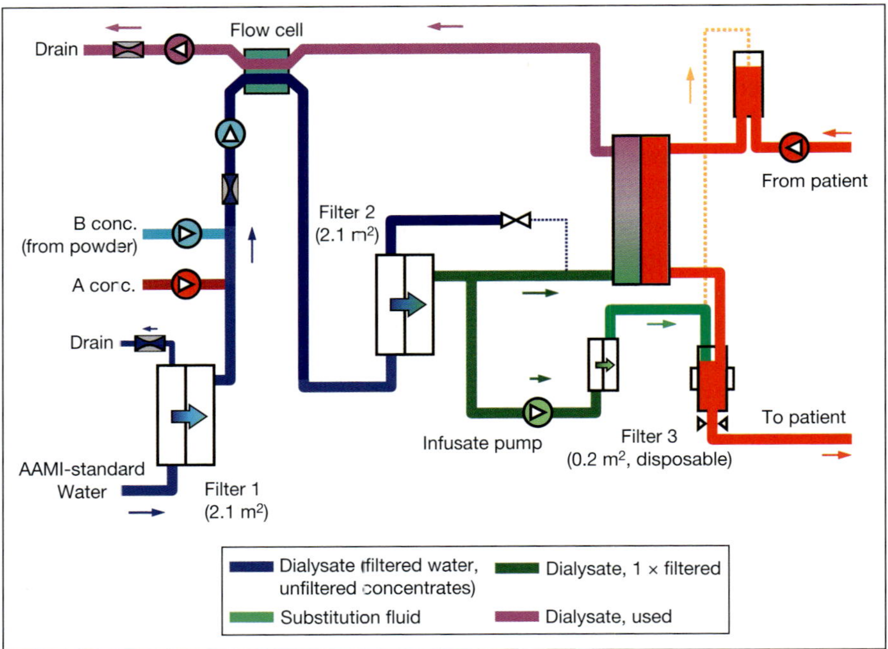

Fig. 1. Gambro 3-filter hemodialysis system. Online HDF-related components and simplified flow scheme for Gambro AK 200 S Ultra. Components not required for online HDF are not shown. AAMI = Association for the Advancement of Medical Instrumentation; conc. = concentrate. Redrawn from HCEN9291: AK 200 Ultra S Service Manual, with kind permission of Gambro Corporate R&D, Lund, Sweden.

in the cross-flow path of the filter is operated only during the cleaning and disinfection cycle of the machine. Both U8000S filters are multiple-use components, are included in the cleaning and disinfection cycles of the machine, and are routinely used for 1 month. However, depending on the microbiological test results of the fluid quality at the end of the routine filter lifetime, this period may be extended [4].

Injectable substitution fluid is generated from this purified dialysate stream by means of further filtration across a low-surface-area polyamide filter (0.2 m^2). This filter is an integral part of a sterile disposable set consisting of the filter, the connection lines to the machine and to the extracorporeal circuit, and a roller pump segment. Depending on the desired dilution mode, this fluid is injected into the bloodstream before or after the dialyzer.

The safe operation of online HDF systems depends on ultrafilter integrity during its entire lifetime. In the case of the system described here, the U8000S filters are exposed to a pressure test procedure at the end of the manufacturing

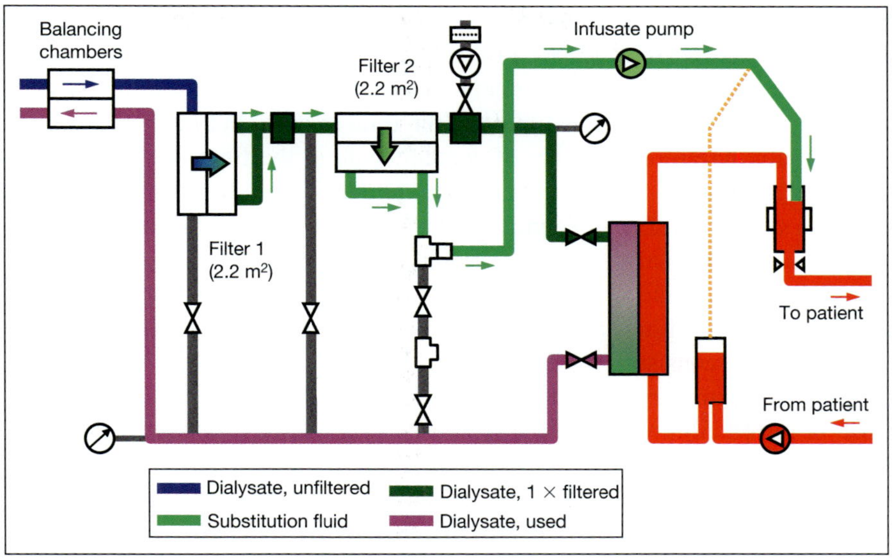

Fig. 2. FME 2-filter hemodialysis system. Online HDF-related components and simplified flow scheme for FME Online plus systems. Redrawn from Fresenius Medical Care Online plus 7/07.03 (OP), Fresenius Medical Care, Bad Homburg, Germany.

process. Filters showing a pressure drop exceeding a certain limit over time (>0.3 bar at a test pressure of 1.6 bar) are discarded [5]. The third disposable filter undergoes a similar test procedure during manufacturing and is guaranteed by the manufacturer.

Instead of using 3 filters for substitution fluid preparation as described above, it is possible to design systems with equal safety and performance on the basis of 2 large-surface, multiple-use filters. The FME system (fig. 2) takes advantage of the design of the volumetric dialysate circuit, which is common to nearly all HD machines of this manufacturer. The fluid space behind the so-called balancing chamber represents a precisely constant volume. In modern HD machines, using extensive microprocessor control, it is possible to activate all hydraulic components such as valves or pumps in an independent and highly flexible manner to run a variety of procedures and tests. These test capabilities in particular are essential for the design and operation of a cost-efficient 2-filter system.

The FME system comprises 2 identical large-surface ultrafilters (type Diasafe® plus, surface area 2.2 m^2, membrane material Fresenius Polysulfone®). The filter housing and connector technology were specifically developed for online fluid preparation. In the context of 'intended use' the manufacturer defines minimum quality requirements for process water, concentrates and ready-to-use dialysate (water: <100 CFU/ml and <0.25 EU/ml endotoxin; ready-to-use dialysate: <1,000 CFU/ml, <1 EU/ml endotoxin).

The input to the first filter is ready-to-use dialysate. For reasons of dialysate economy this filter is operated most of the time in dead-end mode. To prevent a potentially hazardous buildup of contaminants in the filter, the inlet side is frequently flushed to the drain via a valve. The fluid from this first filter passes the inlet side of the second, identical filter, operated in cross-flow mode, and is used to supply the dialyzer with the required flow.

Substitution fluid is generated by drawing the required amount of fluid across the second filter using a standard roller pump on a simple disposable tubing section consisting of 2 connectors, a pump segment and the required tubing to the extracorporeal blood circuit for the desired mode of dilution (pre-, post- or mixed dilution).

It must be emphasized here, and this is true for all systems used for online substitution fluid preparation, that connector technology is crucial for all components in contact with the potentially intravenously injectable fluid. Since it has been known for many years that the standard dialysate connectors (Hansen type) are prone to contamination and nearly impossible to clean and disinfect, these connectors should not be found together with online HDF or online HF systems. Instead, special types of connector and sealings have been developed, mostly using the existing experience from peritoneal-dialysis connectors regarding safety against touch contamination.

The nominal lifetime of the 2 filters is 12 weeks or 100 online HF/HDF treatments. A filter must be changed when the predialysis filter integrity test fails. The filters may be cleaned with sodium hypochlorite according to a defined procedure. The HD machine monitors these procedures together with filter lifetime and, for safety reasons, blocks all online specific functions apart from standard dialysis in the case of deviations from the specified regimen.

The design of a safe 2-filter system requires that the 2 filters are truly redundant, which means that 1 filter alone has sufficient retention capability to protect the patient from any hazards by contamination, at least for a limited period of time. This property must be validated during the approval procedure for a given design.

Furthermore, it is essential for a safe 2-filter system that every treatment starts with 2 functioning ultrafilters. To verify this, the device must be able to run a filter integrity test procedure before every treatment. For reasons of comfort and reliability this procedure should be automated.

Figure 3 demonstrates such an integrity test routine for the FME 2-filter system [6]. The test makes use of the property of the filter membrane to let fluid pass but to block air. For test purposes the system is pressurized with filtered air which displaces the fluid from both filters. Once the respective

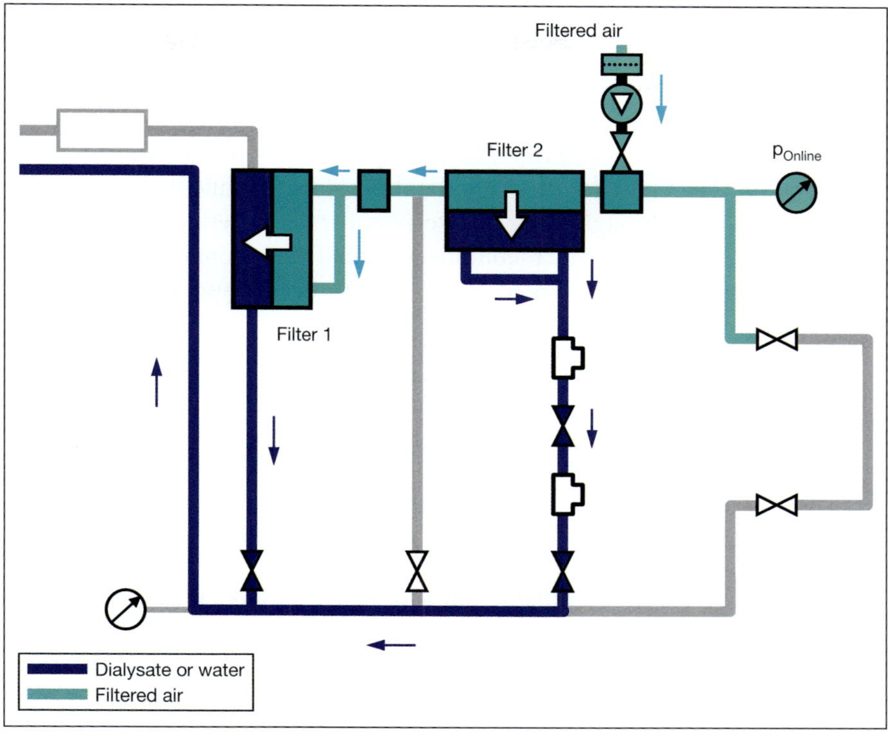

Fig. 3. Filter integrity test procedure and related components for FME Online plus systems. p = Pressure. Redrawn from Fresenius Medical Care Online plus 07/07.03 (OP), Fresenius Medical Care, Bad Homburg, Germany.

filter compartments have been completely filled with air, the system builds up pressure across the membrane, which is measured by a suitable pressure transducer. After reaching the required test pressure of approximately 1 bar the system is hermetically closed. In the case of an intact membrane, the pressure drop is small or zero. A hazardous filter leak is shown by a pressure drop above a certain design-specific limit. This test procedure is very similar to the process used in manufacture to ensure dialyzer integrity. The test pressure is sufficient to detect filter leaks at levels which can represent a safety hazard for the patient (see below).

After a successful test the air is removed from the system, which is then ready for treatment. In the case of repeated negative test results the device must not be used for treatments with online fluid preparation, but can be operated in standard dialysis mode. A negative test is not able to differentiate which of the 2 filters is faulty; this must be done later during the required servicing of the HD machine.

Other Machines

The B. Braun system uses the principles pioneered by FME. Like the FME machines, the B. Braun Dialog HDF Online comprises a volumetric balancing system for ultrafiltration control. The 2 dialysate filters are used in the same configuration: The first filter can be periodically flushed while the second filter is operated in flow-through mode. These filters are also periodically checked. Unlike the FME system, which comprises special filter connectors excluding the use of noncompatible filters by design, the B. Braun system uses standard connectors.

The Nikkiso system uses a single dialysate filter that is regularly tested by a pressure-holding test (like the FME system) in combination with a single-use filter (like the Gambro system). The system was originally equipped with a dialysate filter with conventional connectors, which makes this system compatible to the B. Braun filter and vice versa. The later version comprises a special filter housing and a dedicated filter, which improves filter handling and eliminates the risk of touch contamination.

Nephros is a small company that originally embarked on the development of an integrated HDF system comprising several novel features. This development is well documented by patents. Eventually, however, the company decided to offer a 2-stage dialyzer for mid-dilution HDF which is marketed in Europe. In a next stage the company developed an add-on device for online HDF in combination with conventional HD machines. This device [7] is aimed at the US market where online HDF is not yet available. It incorporates an integrated 2-stage dialysate filter [8], each with a surface area of $0.5\,m^2$, which can be disinfected and tested by the device. This device was recently cleared for clinical trials by the US Food and Drug Administration (FDA).

Bellco, building upon its well-established paired-filtration dialysis method, developed a device for the regeneration of filtrate removed from the ultrafiltration stage. The regenerated filtrate is reinfused into the bloodstream. This principle builds upon decades of experience with dialysate regeneration by adsorption and ion exchange. The double filter can be operated with the filtrate stage first, followed by the dialysis stage, or vice versa.

Safety Aspects

Safety is the freedom from unacceptable risk [9]. Because risk cannot be avoided entirely, 'absolute safety', a term not only used by marketing departments but also by the European Best Practice Guidelines (EBPG) [10], does not exist. Complying with safety regulations and safety standards means that the manufacturer has weighed risks and benefits and has come to the conclusion that the benefits outweigh the risks. This process is checked by notified bodies (e.g. TÜV) in the European Union, by the FDA in the USA and by other national bodies in other countries.

The level of accepted risk depends on the application. For medical devices it is assumed that prevention of a hazard to the patient or user after a single fault is sufficient (safety under single-fault condition). Because single systems produced under normal quality conditions have failure rates of around 10^{-4}, redundant systems reduce the likelihood of a hazard to around 10^{-8}, which is equivalent to one accident in 10^8 treatments [11]. In Europe the manufacturer is obliged to set up a risk management system which includes risk analysis, risk mitigation and market surveillance. The authors have asked the major companies to lay open their risk analysis data, but received the uniform answer that these documents contain proprietary information and will not be published.

For this reason, the risks of online HDF and HF and possible methods for risk mitigation will be discussed using general knowledge and related to the various methods employed by the manufacturers.

The primary risk of online HDF and HF is related to the infusion into the bloodstream of dialysate that may be contaminated with particulate matter, bacteria and/or endotoxin. Secondary risks are the possible infusion of air into the extracorporeal circuit and ultrafiltration errors. These secondary risks do not differ qualitatively from risks in regular HD with high-flux dialyzers. In terms of numbers the additional risk is small and can be neglected, provided that the alarm limits of the dialysis machine are set correctly. Unfortunately, often this is not the case with the venous pressure monitor. Incorrect settings of this monitor may not only cause undetected blood loss to the environment but also undetected weight loss in the case of a leak in the infusion line for the online-produced substitution fluid.

The primary risk is mitigated by filtering contaminated dialysate through a filter capable of preventing the passage of particulates, bacteria and endotoxin. For the purpose of this discussion, the term endotoxin includes all Limulus-amebocyte-lysate-reactive substances. The filters used today have membranes similar to high-flux dialyzers. This means that particulate matter and bacteria are held back by size exclusion. Endotoxin fractions and other potentially hazardous debris from bacteria are not filtered because of the low molecular weight. Membrane materials used for dialysate filtration are capable of adsorbing this potentially hazardous debris on the membrane surface, including the inner surface of the membrane pores. Tests have shown that the rejection fraction of these membranes for bacteria exceeds 10^6–10^9 (detection limit) and for endotoxin around 10^3 [12, 13].

The EBPG (rule IV.4.3) [10] demand an endotoxin concentration for ultrapure dialysate below the detection limit. The detection limit is defined by these guidelines at better than 0.03 EU/ml. With a rejection fraction of around 300 the endotoxin concentration of the incoming dialysate must not exceed 10 EU/ml, which exceeds the limits set for regular dialysate by rule IV.4.2 EBPG of 0.25 EU/ml. Clinical improvements have been reported with lower endotoxin concentrations (0.001 IU/ml) apparently measured with a more sensitive test [14]. This limit can still be achieved with a typical 1-stage dialysate filter. This means that a single filter is sufficient if faults can be excluded.

Fault exclusion for a dialysate filter is not possible – any filter may fail. Potential failure modes are: a gross leak either in the potting material that separates the inside and outside of the filter capillaries at the filter ends or a broken fiber, a leak in the fiber caused by wear or exposure to unsuitable disinfection fluids (e.g. bleach for polysulfone membranes), and saturation of the membrane by endotoxin.

The worst-case scenario for a gross leak is that large amounts of contaminated dialysate are infused into the bloodstream. The hazard is primarily related to bacterial contamination. The endotoxin content of dialysate complying with the EBPG is low compared to previous years when membranes permeable to endotoxin (e.g. cuprophane) were used. Infusion of this endotoxin in the case of an isolated event may be regarded as less severe.

Gross leaks can in principle be detected by measuring filtrate pressures or by pressure holding tests. FME employs an automatic pressure holding filter test [15, 16]. The filter is filled with air on one side while the pores and the other side remain filled with fluid. A pressure difference is generated between the air and the fluid side with the higher pressure on the air side. Because filters employ hydrophilic membranes, air cannot penetrate the filters in physical form in the absence of a gross leak. If the air side is closed, a gross leak will be detected by a rapid pressure drop. If the air side is open, air bubbles can be detected on the fluid side. This test is called the bubble point test. The sensitivity of such tests can be estimated. For the typical test conditions employed by HD machines the diameters of leaks that can be detected is around 5 μm, which would allow the passage of bacteria. Leaks of this kind are discussed below.

Membrane leaks caused by wear or unsuitable disinfection fluids cannot be detected by mechanical tests that would be applicable inside a dialysis machine. The effect of such leaks will be the passage of bacteria and endotoxin. The upper limit for the bypass flow caused by a single pore leak with a 5-μm diameter can be estimated with the Bernoulli equation. For a dialysate filter with an ultrafiltration coefficient of 5 ml/min · mm Hg, the pressure drop at 500 ml/min dialysate flow is 100 mm Hg. This results in a flow of around 0.025 ml/min, which is $5 \cdot 10^{-5}$ of the actual flow through a single leak not detectable by the usual pressure holding test. The actual value will be less and we can use 10^{-6} (1 : 1 million) for the further estimate. Assuming 1,000 CFU/ml in the unfiltered dialysate, the filtered dialysate will still comply with the requirement for ultrapure dialysate (0.01 CFU/ml). The same applies for endotoxin. If, however, 10 or more such pores develop simultaneously, ultrapure dialysate is no longer guaranteed. Similar calculations can be done for smaller pores but larger numbers.

The failure mode assumes that the diameter of existing pores is increased, which means that the flow resistance will decrease, but also that the effective surface area for diffusion of air during the pressure holding test will increase, causing a faster drop in pressure. In principle it may be possible to detect this fault by a sensitive pressure test, taking historical data into account. Technically this is feasible with existing dialysis machines. It is unknown whether this possibility has been investigated by companies.

In the absence of a sensitive test, these leaks can only be avoided by strict process control, including regular changing of the filter, and limiting the exposure time to aggressive disinfectants according to the instructions for use. Modern machines make use of microprocessors to remind the user about the need to change the filter and may also be able to detect the use of unsuitable disinfection fluids.

The adsorption capacity of filters depends on the capillary surface area. It also depends on the membrane material and on the physical structure of the membrane which influences the total surface area of the pores. This means that quantitative test results achieved for one type of filter cannot be used for other filters, even if the same membrane raw material is used.

Weber et al. [13] measured the passage and adsorption capacity for synthetic lipid A and lipopolysaccharide (LPS) from *Pseudomonas aeruginosa*. While no passage was detected, the membranes used for dialysate filters typically adsorbed around 50 μg of lipid A (approx. 5,200 EU) per square meter of nominal capillary surface area, or around 500 ng/m^2 of LPS (approx. 6,000 EU). In both cases this corresponded to around 50% of the total challenging dose. Because only half of the material was adsorbed, it is assumed that the rest was size excluded. With this data the 'adsorption' lifetime can be estimated, assuming that LPS remains adsorbed on the surface. A 2-m^2 filter would be able to adsorb around 12,000 EU and reject approximately the same amount by size exclusion. The sum is then estimated at around 25,000 EU. With the incoming dialysate concentration limited to 0.25 EU/ml, 100,000 ml or 100 liters of dialysate could be filtered, which corresponds approximately to the dialysate consumption of 1 treatment.

Because filters are used for up to 100 treatments, it can be concluded that LPS and lipid A are desorbed during the cleaning cycle or that the challenging test mentioned above was insufficient to reveal the true adsorption capacity of the membranes.

The likelihood of a filter to fail because of a gross leak has not been published or made available by the manufacturers. An estimate can be made based on the claim that no serious adverse events related to dialysate fluid filters for HF/HDF have become known so far. Assuming 15 million treatments and with 2 filters in series, the likelihood of both filters failing during a treatment can be estimated to be less than 10^{-6} to 10^{-8} (both filters having been tested before the start of the treatment). The likelihood of a single filter failing is then 10^{-3} to 10^{-4} per treatment. This estimate is applicable for the FME system.

The Gambro system comprises two filters that are changed each month, but not tested before treatment, and a single disposable filter. Estimating the likelihood of failure is more difficult for this system, because the probability of contamination between filters 1 and 2 must be estimated. Since manipulations involving connectors take place when the system is being set up, contamination cannot be entirely excluded. The integer single disposable filter will still be able to prevent the infusion of bacteria into the bloodstream. No published information is known to the authors whether this single small-surface-area filter is capable of adsorbing the majority of endotoxin in the case of both dialysate filters failing. If not, such failures may go undetected for several treatments, and exposure to endotoxin may go on for several weeks.

In summary it can be concluded that the application of risk analysis to the existing systems using published data is consistent with the assumption that these systems are safe, although 'absolute safety' does not exist. The limitation of the number of treatments between filter changes seems to be based on clinical experience rather than quantitative knowledge about the processes involved. As long as sound research results about membrane destruction and membrane adsorption capacity are lacking, users are strongly advised to comply fully with the instructions given by the manufacturers.

Declaration of Conflict of Interest

Hans-Dietrich Polaschegg is an independent scientific consultant for medical devices. He has no financial interest in any of the companies mentioned and no consulting project for on-line hemodiafiltration. Thomas Roy is an employee of Fresenius Medical Care Deutschland GmbH, Bad Homburg, Germany.

References

1 Community Directive 93/42/EEC on Medical Devices. Official Journal of the European Communities No L169, 12 July 1993.

2 Pirovano D: Regulatory issues for on-line haemodiafiltration. Nephrol Dial Transplant 1998;13(suppl 5):21–23.

3 Association for the Advancement of Medical Instrumentation: Water Treatment Equipment for Hemodialysis Applications (ANSI/AAMI RD62:2001). American National Standard. Arlington, AAMI, 2001.

4 AK 200 ULTRA S – Operator's manual. HCEN9752 Revision.12.2003, Lund, Gambro AB, 2003.

5 Ledebo I: On-line preparation of solutions for dialysis: practical aspects versus safety and regulations. J Am Soc Nephrol 2002;13:S78–S83.

6 Online plus™ Operating Instructions, part No 676 894 1, Revision: 7/07.03, Bad Homburg, Fresenius Medical Care, 2003.

7 Collins GR, Summerton J, Spence E (inventors), Nephros Inc (assignee): Method and apparatus for a hemodiafiltration delivery module. US patent 6916424. 07/12/2005.

8 Summerton J, Collins G (inventors), Nephros Inc (assignee): Sterile fluid filtration cartridge and method for using same. US patent 6635179. 10/21/2003.

9 ISO 14971 1, 2007-02-28: Medical devices – Application of risk management to medical devices.

10 EBPG Expert Group on Haemodialysis: European best practice guidelines for haemodialysis (part 1), section IV: dialysis fluid purity – IV.4 haemodialysis-proportioning machine. Nephrol Dial Transplant 2002;17:1–111.

11 Polaschegg HD, Levin N: Hemodialysis machines and monitors; in Winchester J, Koch R, Lindsay R, Ronco C, Horl W (eds): Replacement of Renal Function by Dialysis, ed 5. New York, Kluwer Academic Publishers, 2004, pp 323–447.

12 Frinak S, Polaschegg HD, Levin NW, Pohlod DJ, Dumler F, Saravolatz LD: Filtration of dialysate using an on-line dialysate filter. Int J Artif Organs 1991;14:691–697.

13 Weber C, Linsberger I, Rafiee-Tehrani M, Falkenhagen D: Permeability and adsorption capacity of dialysis membranes to lipid A. Int J Artif Organs 1997;20:144–152.

14 Arizono K, Nomura K, Motoyama T, Matsushita Y, Matsuoka K, Miyazu R, Takeshita H, Fukui H: Use of ultrapure dialysate in reduction of chronic inflammation during hemodialysis. Blood Purif 2004;22:26–29.

15 Polaschegg HD, Mathieu B (inventors), Fresenius AG (assignee): Verfahren zum Prüfen von Sterilfiltern eines Hämofiltrationsgeräts. DE patent 3448262. 06/21/1990.

16 Wamsiedler R, Matheiu B (inventors), Fresenius AG (assignee): Verfahren zur Überprüfung von mindestens einem im Dialysierflüssigkeitssystem einer Vorrichtung zur extrakorporalen Blutbehandlung angeordneten Filter. DE patent 19534417. 03/20/1997.

Hans-Dietrich Polaschegg
Scientific Consultant
A-9231 Koestenberg (Austria)
Tel. +43 4274 4045, Fax +43 4274 4096, E-Mail hdp@aon.at

Ronco C, Canaud B, Aljama P (eds): Hemodiafiltration.
Contrib Nephrol. Basel, Karger, 2007, vol 158, pp 80–86

Quality of Water, Dialysate and Infusate

Gianni Cappelli, Marco Ricardi, Decenzio Bonucchi, Sara De Amicis

Nephrology Dialysis and Renal Transplantation Unit, University Hospital of Modena, Modena, Italy

Abstract

Great improvements in water treatment technology and the spread of ultrafiltration for cold sterilization have been the basic support for the development and diffusion of on-line dialysis treatments. Some 20 years ago, nephrologists recognized that the official standards for dialysis fluids were insufficient with respect to these new treatment modalities, and ultrapure water (bacteria <0.1 CFU/ml; endotoxin <0.03 EU/ml) was proposed as a reference. Today, ultrapure water is included in most guidelines and recommended standards, but there remains a need for harmonization between standards. To achieve and ensure these levels of purity, technology must be supported by commitment of resources to an active quality assurance programme with adequate maintenance, monitoring, cleaning, sanitizing and problem analysis procedures.

Background

Several lines of evidence have accumulated in the last 10–15 years which show that optimizing water purity in dialysis, in terms of bacterial contamination, is a fundamental issue for preventing inflammation in most dialysis-related pathologies in end-stage renal disease patients [1–7]. Until the mid-80s, the concern regarding water quality was mostly concentrated on chemical contaminants but after the relationship between the bacterial burden in dialysate and pyrogenic reactions had been established [8–10], the emphasis moved to microbiological contamination. Ultrafiltration was at that time in the phase of preliminary experimentation, but several groups were already reporting its use with consistent results in obtaining sterile bacteria- and endotoxin-free solutions to be used as dialysate or infusate in haemo(dia)filtration [11–15].

The Search for Harmonization of Standards

The pressure to redefine adequate microbiological standards became urgent in the early 90s, due to the spreading use of highly permeable membranes, the spread of online treatments and the feasibility offered by dialysis technology in obtaining sterile fluids. Now, at the beginning of the 21st century, while there is a worldwide general agreement on maximum levels of most chemical contaminants, some differences between countries still remain regarding permitted levels of microbiological contaminants.

The lack of harmonization is due to both scientific and economic reasons. For the first part, the clinical evidence for using ultrapure fluids is still under discussion, since (i) most data are from different groups with no controlled clinical trials, (ii) endotoxin evaluation does not cover all microbially derived products (including bacterial DNA) that have been demonstrated to cross the dialysis membrane, and (iii) the purity of dialysis fluids is part of a multifactorial aetiology for chronic inflammatory response in end-stage renal disease patients, which also includes vascular access, dental infection and membrane biocompatibility.

As to the economic question, the main points are: (i) capital investments have to be made in water systems and monitors, (ii) resources must also be committed to quality assurance and monitoring, and (iii) in some countries where reimbursements from government organizations are linked to adherence to water quality standards, new limits must be implemented gradually.

A recent review [16] discusses the opportunity of harmonization to achieve a widely applicable set of standards, taking into consideration all these aspects and, most of all, best practice for patient safety.

Table 1 lists recommended maximum concentrations of chemical contaminants in water for haemodialysis, comparing the Association for the Advancement of Medical Instrumentation (AAMI) with the European Pharmacopoeia [17, 19]. In table 2 are the maximum levels of bacterial contaminants for water for dilution and standard dialysate, recently issued as recommendations or national standards of some professional associations or organizations for standardization.

From these tables it is clear that, in spite of a large production of standards, the ideal purity of dialysis fluid is still under development. In recent papers and reviews, ultrapure fluids, as originally defined (<0.1 CFU/ml, <0.03 EU/ml) [25], are indicated as new 'gold standards' for both dialysis water and dialysate, and according to European Renal Association/European Dialysis and Transplant Association (ERA-EDTA) guidelines they are suggested for all dialysis treatment modalities [26].

Table 1. Recommended levels of chemical contaminants in water for haemodialysis

Contaminant	Maximum contaminant concentration mg/l	
	ANSI/AAMI RD62-2001 [17]	European Pharmacopoeia ed. 5 [18]
Calcium	2 (0.1 mEq/l)	2
Magnesium	4 (0.3 mEq/l)	2
Potassium	8 (0.2 mEq/l)	2
Sodium	70 (3.0 mEq/l)	50
Ammonia	–	0.2
Antimony	0.006	–
Arsenic	0.005	–
Barium	0.10	–
Beryllium	0.0004	–
Cadmium	0.001	–
Chromium	0.014	–
Chloride	–	50
Lead	0.005	–
Mercury	0.0002	0.001
Selenium	0.09	–
Silver	0.005	–
Aluminium	0.01	0.01
Chloramine	0.10	–
Free chlorine	0.50	–
Total available chlorine	–	0.1
Copper	0.10	–
Fluoride	0.20	0.20
Nitrate (as N)	2.00	2.00
Sulphate	100	50
Thallium	0.002	–
Total heavy metals	–	0.10
Zinc	0.10	0.10

Technology to Obtain Ultrapure Fluids

Producing ultrapure fluids is not a trivial task, as it requires appropriate technology and most of all a commitment of resources and a quality control programme to put it on a routine basis. Current water treatment techniques offer optimal results and can be adapted to most situations. Only general indications can be proposed for a new system, since detailed suggestions must be based on

Table 2. Recommended levels of microbiological contaminants in solutions for haemodialysis

	AAMI (USA) [17, 19]	Eur. Pharma. ed. 5 [18]	ESBP ERA-EDTA [20]	CSA (Canada) [21]	Renal Association (UK) [22]	CARI (Australia) [23]	JSDT (Japan) [24]
Water for dialysis							
Bacteria, CFU/ml	200[a]	100	100	100	100	100	–
Endotoxin, EU/ml	2[a]	0.25	0.25	2	0.25	0.25	0.05
Standard dialysate							
Bacteria, CFU/ml	200[a]	–	100	100	100	100	–
Endotoxin, EU/ml	2[a]	–	0.25	2	0.25	0.25	0.05
Ultrapure dialysate							
Bacteria, CFU/ml	0.1	–	0.1	–	0	0.1	–
Endotoxin, EU/ml	0.03	–	0.03	–	0.015	0.03	0.01
Infusate for haemo(dia)filtration							
Bacteria, CFU/ml	10^{-6}	10^{-6}	10^{-6}	–	0	10^{-6}	–
Endotoxin, EU/ml	0.03	0.25	0.03	–	0.015	0.03	0.01

CARI = Caring for Australasians with Renal Impairment; CSA = Canadian Standards Association; ESBP = European Best Practice Guidelines; JSDT = Japanese Society for Dialysis Therapy.

[a] Defined an action level at 50 CFU/ml for bacteria and 1 EU/ml for endotoxins.

local water quality, taking into account also seasonal variability and disinfection methodology [27].

The optimal water purification system is the result of a 2-stage procedure: pretreatment and final treatment (fig. 1). Pretreatment technology is dictated by raw water quality and is usually based on softeners and carbon tanks containing granulated activated charcoal. Pretreatment includes a depth filter, sometimes added to remove particulate matter from feeding water, and a 5-μm cartridge filter used to protect the reverse osmosis (RO) membrane from leached carbon particles. Final treatment with RO provides an excellent barrier to most chemicals and microbiological contaminants, and the use of a double RO in series improves performance. When a deionizer is used as a supplement to RO installation, an ultrafilter after the deionizer is mandatory to achieve consistent microbiological results. Distribution of the purified water to individual dialysis machines is a key point, as bacterial growth in the distribution pipes is the most common source of contamination. New piping materials have been proposed, featuring no leaching of contaminants, smoother surfaces and low adherence to bacterial cells in order to prevent biofilm formation, but frequent and periodical disinfections remain the best strategy to assure a high microbiological level. A continuous loop design is the recommended circuit to minimize biofilm formation and to assure a pure water

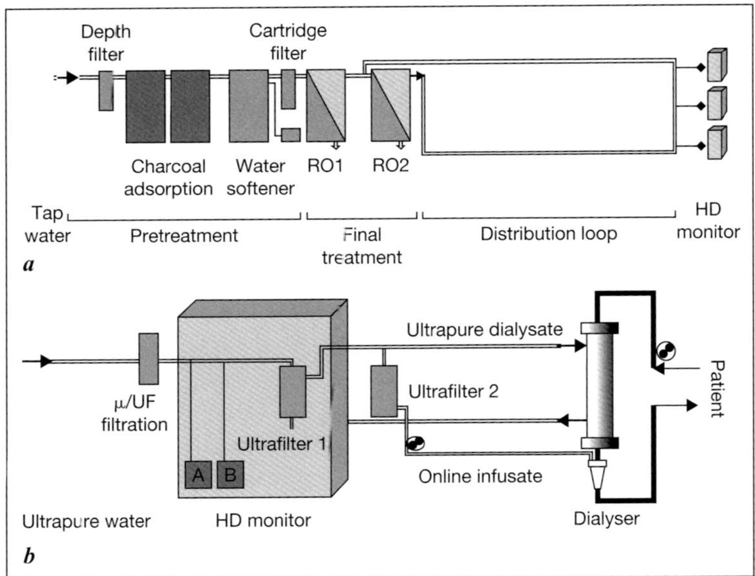

Fig. 1. Water treatment system and dialysis apparatus to obtain fluids for online treatments. ***a*** Water plant with pretreatment and final treatment based on a double RO in series. ***b*** Water from distribution loop enters the dialysis monitor and, after a first ultrafiltration to obtain ultrapure dialysate, is passed through a second ultrafilter to obtain substitution fluid. HD = Haemodialysis; µ/UF filtration = micro- or ultrafiltration.

transfer according to ultrapure dialysate prescription. As to the regulatory aspects of components of water treatment and distribution systems, producers of water purification systems are regulated by the Food and Drug Administration (FDA) in the USA or by Directive 93/42/EEC for medical devices in the European Union. Water systems, dialysis machines and high-permeability dialysers are mandated as class II medical devices by the FDA and as class II-b by the European Union and require diligent tracking of critical components and a complaint investigation system in place. The quality level of ultrapure dialysate technology should be user-friendly and budget-compatible, but nephrology professionals, including nurses and technicians, should be aware that monitors and ultrafilters must be used according to manufacturers' instructions, and adequate disinfection as suggested by each manufacturer must be periodically performed. The choice of disinfectant is based on compatibility with the materials used in the water system, on manufacturers' suggestions and on results from monitoring the dialysis fluid production process. Disinfectants are also regulated as class II medical devices, being accessories to the devices that they are intended to disinfect, and therefore dialysis staff must strictly adhere to manufacturers' instructions.

Quality Assurance

The experience accumulated in past years with online treatments of thousands of patients has overcome the problem of safety. At each stage, ultrafiltration is able to reduce bacteria and endotoxin by factors of at least 10^7 and 10^3, respectively, providing a 'cold sterilization' device [28]. To stay within operational limits the lowest possible bacterial and endotoxin mass must be presented to the ultrafiltration point and redundancy in terms of surface area must be provided by the device to optimize filtration and absorption processes. The impossibility of online monitoring of results is therefore balanced by the assurance of maintaining a high absorption capacity.

Staff should be aware of the importance of the hygiene of the entire fluid path, from tap water to the distribution loop, including the hydraulic dialysis-monitoring circuit. To avoid failure of the most critical component of the water treatment system, the human one, a quality assurance procedure has to be instituted, based on appropriate maintenance, monitoring, cleaning and sanitizing procedures for the whole production chain. It includes acceptance or redefinition of limit values for each part of the system, depending on local needs, as well as definition of laboratory methods and tests to check the process. Auditing for analysis of operational problems should be part of the quality assurance system.

References

1 Baz M, Durand C, Ragon A, Jaber K, Andrieu D, Merzouk T, Purgus R, Olmer M, Reynier JP, Berland Y: Using ultrapure water in hemodialysis delays carpal tunnel syndrome. Int J Artif Organs 1991;14:681–685.

2 Sitter T, Bergner A, Schiffl H: Dialysate related cytokine induction and response to recombinant human erythropoietin in haemodialysis patients. Nephrol Dial Transplant 2000;15:1207–1211.

3 Schiffl H, Lang SM, Stratakis D, Fischer R: Effects of ultrapure dialysis fluid on nutritional status and inflammatory parameters. Nephrol Dial Transplant 2001;16:1863–1869.

4 Matsuhashi N, Yoshioka T: Endotoxin-free dialysate improves response to erythropoietin in hemodialysis patients. Nephron 2002;92:601–604.

5 Schiffl H, Wendinger H, Lang SM: Ultrapure dialysis fluid and responsiveness to hepatitis B vaccine. Nephron 2002;91:530–531.

6 Matsuhashi N, Yoshioka T: Endotoxin-free dialysate improves response to erythropoietin in hemodialysis patients. Nephron 2002;92:601–604.

7 Blagg C, Twardowski Z, Bower J, Kjellstrand C: Cardiovascular instability and dialysate purity. ASAIO J 2003;49:190.

8 Favero MS, Carson LA, Bond WW, Petersen NJ: Factors that influence microbial contamination of fluids associated with hemodialysis machines. Appl Microbiol 1974;28:822–830.

9 Gordon SM, Oettinger CW, Bland LA, Oliver JC, Arduino MJ, Aguero SM, McAllister SK, Favero MS, Jarvis WR: Pyrogenic reactions in patients receiving conventional, high-efficiency, or high-flux hemodialysis treatments with bicarbonate dialysate containing high concentrations of bacteria and endotoxin. J Am Soc Nephrol 1992;2:1436–1444.

10 Mion CM, Canaud B, Garred LJ, Stec F, Nguyen QV: Sterile and pyrogen-free bicarbonate dialysate: a necessity for hemodialysis today. Adv Nephrol Necker Hosp 1990;19:275-314.

11 Henderson LW, Beans E: Successful production of sterile pyrogen-free electrolyte solution by ultrafiltration. Kidney Int 1978;14:522–525.
12 Henderson LW, Sanfelippo ML, Beans E: 'On line' preparation of sterile pyrogen-free electrolyte solution. Trans Am Soc Artif Intern Organs 1978;24:465–467.
13 Shaldon S, Beau MC, Deschodt G, Flavier JL, Nilsson L, Ramperez P, Mion C: Three years of experience with on-line preparation of sterile pyrogen free infusate for hemofiltration. Int J Artif Organs 1983;6:25–26.
14 Canaud B, N'Guyen QV, Lagarde C, Stec F, Polaschegg HD, Mion C: Clinical evaluation of a multipurpose dialysis system adequate for hemodialysis or for postdilution hemofiltration/hemodiafiltration with on-line preparation of substitution fluid from dialysate; in Streicher E, Seyffart G (eds): Highly Permeable Membranes. Contrib Nephrol. Basel, Karger, 1985, vol 46, pp 184–186.
15 Erley CM, von Herrath D, Hartenstein-Koch K, Kutschera D, Amir-Moazami B, Schaefer K: Easy production of sterile, pyrogen-free dialysate. ASAIO Trans 1988;34:205–207.
16 Ward RA: Worldwide water standards for hemodialysis. Hemodial Int 2007;11:S18–S25.
17 Association for the Advancement of Medical Instrumentation: Water Treatment Equipment for Hemodialysis Applications. ANSI/AAMI RD62:2001. Arlington, Association for the Advancement of Medical Instrumentation, 2001.
18 European Pharmacopoeia Commission: Monograph 01/2005:1167 Haemodialysis Solutions, Concentrated, Water for Diluting. European Pharmacopoiea, ed 5. Strasbourg, European Pharmacopoeia Commission, 2006.
19 Association for the Advancement of Medical Instrumentation: Dialysate for hemodialysis. ANSI/AAMI RD52:2004. Arlington, Association for the Advancement of Medical Instrumentation, 2004.
20 European Renal Association-European Dialysis and Transplant Association: European best practice guidelines for haemodialysis (part I), section IV: dialysis fluid purity. Nephrol Dial Transplant 2002;17(suppl 7):45–62.
21 Canadian Standards Association: Water Treatment Equipment and Water Quality Requirements for Hemodialysis. CSA Standard Z364.2.2–03. Mississauga, Canadian Standards Association, 2003.
22 The Renal Association and the Royal College of Physicians of London: Treatment of Adults and Children with Renal Failure: Standards and Audit Measures, ed 3. London, Lavenham Press, 2002.
23 CARI Guidelines: Dialysis adequacy guidelines – water quality for hemodialysis. Nephrology 2005;10:S61–S80.
24 Masakane I: Review: clinical usefulness of ultrapure dialysate – recent evidence and perspectives. Ther Apher Dial 2006;10:348–354.
25 Ledebo I, Nystrand R: Defining the microbiological quality of dialysis fluid. Artif Organs 1999;23:37–43.
26 Kjellstrand CM, Kjellstrand P: Beyond ultrapure hemodialysis: a necessary and achievable goal. Hemodial Int 2007;11:S39-S48.
27 Cappelli G, Perrone S, Ciuffreda A: Water quality for on-line haemodiafiltration. Nephrol Dial Transplant 1998;13(suppl 5):12–16.
28 Canaud B, Bosc JY, Leray H, Stec F: Microbiological purity of dialysate for on-line substitution fluid preparation. Nephrol Dial Transpl 2000;15(suppl 2):21–30.

Prof. Gianni Cappelli
Nephrology Dialysis and Renal Transplantation Unit
Department of Medicine and Medical Specialties
University Hospital of Modena
Via Del Pozzo, 71
IT–41100 Modena (Italy)
Tel. +39 059 422 5220, Fax +39 059 422 2167, E-Mail cappelli@unimo.it

Ronco C, Canaud B, Aljama P (eds): Hemodiafiltration.
Contrib Nephrol. Basel, Karger, 2007, vol 158, pp 87–93

Fluids in Bags for Hemodiafiltration

Ingrid Ledebo

Gambro Research, Lund, Sweden

Abstract

The objective of hemodiafiltration (HDF) is to increase the convective transport of solutes poorly removed by diffusion, and therefore ultrafiltration (UF) beyond the desired weight loss is prescribed. The excess UF is compensated for by infusion of a physiological solution which should be sterile and nonpyrogenic. This replacement solution can be provided either in bags containing commercially prepared infusion solution, i.e. so-called classic HDF, or by an integrated stepwise filtration of the dialysis fluid, i.e. so-called online HDF. In both cases the composition of the replacement solution should mirror that of plasma water. When the fluid is provided in bags, practical handling is a limiting factor, and the amount of convection that can be delivered is most often restricted to 10–12 l/session. Results from clinical studies show that the degree of convective transport obtained in classic HDF corresponds to what can be achieved in contemporary high-flux dialysis, where uncontrolled UF and backfiltration take place inside the dialyzer. Classic HDF with replacement fluid in bags offers the possibility of delivering an HDF treatment with controlled convective dose and fluid quality, albeit with a limited amount of convection.

Definitions and Terminology

The difference between hemodialysis (HD) and hemodiafiltration (HDF) is that in the latter therapy, ultrafiltration (UF) exceeds the desired weight loss, and the difference is made up with a replacement solution, according to common definitions [1]. The original definition states that the replacement solution should come from an external source. However, with our increased understanding of the transport processes that take place in blood purification therapies, it is now acknowledged that so-called internal replacement of excess UF can produce a similar result, and therapies comprising this feature should also be regarded as HDF [2].

The objective of excessive UF is to increase the removal of solutes that are poorly transported by diffusion. UF is accompanied by convective transport of all those solutes that can pass the membrane, and the amount of convection is determined by the UF volume and the membrane permeability. Thus, in low-flux HD convective transport is negligible, because the UF corresponds only to the weight loss and the membrane has a low solute permeability. Modern high-flux membranes are highly permeable to water as well as to solutes up to a molecular weight of 20–30 kDa, and thus have the potential to provide considerable convective clearance. These membranes are used in HDF as well as in high-flux dialysis. When used in HD with modern equipment providing volume control, the net UF corresponds to the desired weight loss, but significant fluid flux takes place inside the dialyzer in both directions across the membrane and generates convective solute transport [3]. Blood is ultrafiltered at the arterial end of the dialyzer, and the excess is replaced by dialysis fluid backfiltered across the membrane at the venous end. Under conditions of countercurrent flow, the backfiltered fluid is relatively fresh and can be regarded as replacement fluid, although not quite of the same composition and quality. The result is convective solute transport and fluid replacement, both of which occur automatically and are uncontrolled.

With the use of externally provided replacement fluid, the amount of convection can be prescribed and controlled by settings on the machine. The total convective volume corresponds to the volume of UF, which is a product of the UF rate and the treatment time. The blood flow rate is a limiting factor, and UF rates corresponding to 30% of the blood flow rate can usually be achieved in postdilution HDF. The amount of replacement fluid required is the total UF volume corrected for the desired weight loss. To avoid symptoms of under- and overhydration, it is vital that the control mechanism for fluid removal and fluid replacement be accurate. The flow rates should be matched so that the difference corresponds to the desired weight loss rate for the specific patient and treatment, just as in an HD treatment. The replacement solution is most commonly continuously provided through an integrated online preparation that consists of stepwise UF of dialysis fluid under controlled conditions [4]. However, the replacement fluid can also be provided as an intravenous solution in bags, which is the focus of this chapter. An overview of the characteristics of the replacement fluids used for the various forms of HDF is given in table 1.

Composition of Replacement Fluid

The replacement fluid as well as the dialysis fluid should be physiological, and the composition should mirror that of plasma water. With stable

Table 1. Replacement fluid characteristics for various forms of HDF

	High-flux dialysis	Classic HDF	Online HDF
Source of fluid	internal, dialysis fluid	external, bags	external, online
Mode of preparation	backfiltration	autoclaving	stepwise filtration
Fluid composition	as dialysis fluid	choice between available fluids	as dialysis fluid
Fluid quality	variable, not likely to be sterile	sterile and nonpyrogenic according to *Pharmacopoeia*	sterile and nonpyrogenic
Prescription of convective volume	not possible	limited by fluid volume in bags	not limited by access to fluid
Infusion mode	only postdilution	only postdilution	pre- or postdilution
Extra work compared to HD	simple, automatic	handling of bags	hygiene of system
Cost compared to HD	similar	+ cost of fluid in bags	+ cost of ultrafilters
Risk to patient	use of unsterile fluid	low, if fluid quality OK	low, if system operated according to manuals

HD patients who are transferred to HDF, it is recommended to start with the same composition of the replacement fluid as has been used for the dialysis fluid. This may not always be possible when using fluid in bags, since the choice of available compositions is limited. When alternative compositions have to be used, it is wise to aim for more physiological solutions, since the replacement fluid needs no concentration gradient for transport across a membrane.

In the early days of HDF the buffer source was a limiting factor. When acetate was used in the dialysis fluid, lactate was the obvious choice in the replacement fluid. However, when acetate was replaced with bicarbonate, the drawbacks of using unphysiological buffer sources became obvious, and bicarbonate-containing fluid in bags was developed. The use of bicarbonate in fluids prepared, sterilized and stored in bags makes particular demands on the packaging. To avoid precipitation, the bicarbonate ions must be separated from the divalent cations until the moment of mixing. Therefore, separate bags or 2-compartment bags must be used. The benefits of using bicarbonate as the sole buffer source in dialysis therapy were clearly illustrated in a trial which tested 4 different buffer combinations, and which demonstrated that acid-base correction as well as patient tolerance were superior when bicarbonate was used as the buffer source in both fluids [5]. Today, the majority of fluid in bags for HDF contains bicarbonate at a concentration of 32–35 mmol/l, which corresponds to the buffer concentration most commonly used in dialysis fluid.

When discussing the composition of replacement solution, it should also be mentioned that certain forms of HDF therapy require special solutions, e.g. acetate-free biofiltration. This is HDF with buffer-free dialysis fluid and an external replacement fluid consisting of sodium bicarbonate at a concentration of 145 mmol/l, provided in bags and used in volumes of 8–10 l/session [6]. Several studies have documented the benefits of optimal acid-base correction and hemodynamic stability, but comparisons have generally been made with HD rather than HDF. For further information about acetate-free biofiltration, readers are referred to the chapter by Santoro et al. (pp. 138–152) in this book.

Quality of Replacement Fluid

Replacement fluid is classified as a drug, an infusion solution, which must be sterile and which must contain less than 0.25 endotoxin units/ml (EU/ml) according to the *European Pharmacopoeia* [7].

However, if fluid of such quality were to be used in convective therapies, the maximum recommended endotoxin exposure for healthy individuals (5 EU/kg body weight and hour) would be exceeded already at moderate infusion rates and body weights. It is therefore important that the replacement solution for HDF is of considerably higher microbiological quality than just meeting the limit prescribed by current regulations.

Example: $70\,\text{kg} \times 5\,\text{EU/(kg} \cdot \text{h)} = 0.25\,\text{EU/ml} \times 1{,}400\,\text{ml/h}$

Experience from the early days of using replacement fluid in bags for convective therapies, at that time mainly hemofiltration, shows a number of serious, even fatal, incidences of contamination from these fluids, either from handling of the fluid or from the fluid itself [8]. Quellhorst et al. [9] measured the endotoxin concentration in various fluids and found that the mean concentration in 721 samples of commercially prepared substitution solution was 17.5 ± 6.8 pg/ml, well below the target recommended by the *Pharmacopoeia*, but still 4 times higher than the average in the 1,364 samples of online prepared fluid (4.1 ± 0.6 pg/ml). However, the quality of the dialysis fluid is also important because fluid flux across the dialysis membrane may occur. Panichi et al. [10] found that HDF using replacement fluid in bags was associated with production of proinflammatory cytokines during periods when backfiltration of standard-quality dialysis fluid was known to take place, but not when backfiltration was avoided.

Volume of Replacement Fluid

With the use of replacement fluid in bags, mainly practical but also economical considerations pose serious limitations on the volume used and thus the dose of convection delivered. Large volumes of fluid are heavy and difficult to handle, and modern bicarbonate-containing fluids are costly. Most users of HDF with fluid in bags therefore limit the amount of replacement fluid to 9 liters, which translates into two 4.5-liter bags. Adding the UF that corresponds to the weight loss gives a total convective volume of 10–12 liters. This limitation in fluid volume also means that administration in postdilution mode is the only realistic alternative.

From a therapeutic point of view the volume of convective transport should be maximized. To justify the additional cost when switching patients from high-flux dialysis to HDF, the convective transport should be considerably increased. However, the degree of convection already achieved in contemporary high-flux HD appears to correspond to HDF treatments with approximately 10 liters of convective transport, i.e. classic HDF sessions. This is shown by studies comparing the clearance and plasma levels of convectively removed marker molecules, such as β_2-microglobulin. Similar levels of β_2-microglobulin were achieved with high-flux dialysis and classic HDF in the Italian Cooperative Dialysis Study [11], and similar β_2-microglobulin clearance and reduction ratios were observed in high-flux dialysis and HDF when infusion rates of 40 ml/min were used [12]. Thus, the major benefit of switching from high-flux dialysis to HDF with fluid in bags appears to be the improved control of convective volume and assurance of fluid quality.

To be able to achieve considerably increased convective volumes there must be no limitation in access to fluid, and online fluid preparation is the only realistic alternative. An average online HDF session, performed at a blood flow rate of 300–400 ml/min, would generate a UF rate of 90–120 ml/min, assuming that 30% of the blood flow can be ultrafiltered. In 4 h, 22–29 liters of ultrafiltrate would be generated and would require some 20–26 liters of replacement solution. The convective transport would be at least twice that achieved with high-flux dialysis or classic HDF, with 9 liters of replacement fluid in bags.

Use of HDF with Fluid in Bags

If the purpose of a therapy prescription is to achieve as high a convective clearance as possible in combination with a certain amount of diffusive clearance, HDF with unlimited access to replacement fluid, i.e. online HDF, is the obvious choice. However, in situations when this is not possible due to unavailability of equipment or regulatory obstacles, the use of classic HDF, i.e. with the replacement fluid provided in bags, is a good alternative. This will allow the user to prescribe a certain, although limited, amount of convection and administer it under conditions of controlled fluid quality. High-flux dialysis, on the other hand, may provide similar amounts of convective clearance, but unless the quality of the dialysis fluid and the characteristics of the dialysis membrane are such that endotoxin transfer is reduced to safe levels, the risk to the patient is considerable. It may be claimed that high-flux dialysis is widely used and even associated with superior survival, thus indicating that it is beneficial rather than risky [13]. Still, the biologic response to chronic exposure to bacterial products may be subtle, only evident as a microinflammation or even blunted by the benefit of enhanced convective solute removal. Finally, the use of HDF with fluid in bags is also justified when the composition of the fluid has a purpose beyond mere physiological replacement, such as in acetate-free biofiltration. Thus, there are special cases when HDF with replacement fluid in bags is the better choice, but in general online fluid preparation is an essential prerequisite for optimal HDF therapy [14].

References

1 Gurland HJ, Davison AM, Bonomini V, et al: Definitions and terminology in biocompatibility. Nephrol Dial Transplant 1994;9(suppl 2):4–10.

2 von Albertini B, Miller JH, Gardner PW, et al: High-flux hemodiafiltration: under six hours/week treatment. Trans Am Soc Artif Intern Organs 1984;30:227–231.

3 Ronco C: Backfiltration: a controversial issue in modern dialysis. Int J Artif Organs 1988;11: 69–74.

4 Ledebo I: On-line preparation of solutions for dialysis: practical aspects versus safety and regulations. J Am Soc Nephrol 2002;13:S78–S83.

5 Biasiolo S, Feriani M, Chiaramonte S, et al: Different buffers for hemodiafiltration. a controlled study. Int J Artif Organs 1989;12:25–30.

6 Galli G, Panzetta G: Acetate free biofiltration (AFB): from theory to clinical results. Clin Nephrol 1998;50:28–37.

7 European Pharmacopoeia, ed 5. Strasbourg, Council of Europe, 2005.

8 von Herrath D, Schaefer K, Hüfler M, Pauls A, Koch KM: Complications of hemofiltration; in Schaefer, K (ed): Hemofiltration. Contrib Nephrol. Basel, Karger, 1982, vol 32, pp 146–153.
9 Quellhorst E, Hildebrand U, Solf A: Long-term morbidity: hemofiltration versus hemodialysis; in Berland Y, Bonomini V (eds): Dialysis Membranes: Structure and Predictions. Contrib Nephrol. Basel, Karger, 1995, vol 113 pp 110–119.
10 Panichi V, Tetta C, Rindi P, Palla R, Lonnemann G: Plasma C-reactive protein is linked to backfiltration associated interleukin-6 production. ASAIO J 1998;44:M415–M417.
11 Locatelli F, Mastrangelo F, Redaelli B, et al: Effects of different membranes and dialysis technologies on patient treatment tolerance and nutritional parameters. Kidney Int 1996;50:1293–1302.
12 Lornoy W, Becaus I, Billiouw J-M, Sierens L, van Malderen P: Remarkable removal of beta-2-microglobulin by on-line hemodiafiltration. Am J Nephrol 1998;18:105–108.
13 Chaveau P, Nguyen H, Combe C, et al: Dialyzer membrane permeability and survival in hemodialysis patients. Am J Kidney Dis 2005:45:565–571.
14 Ledebo I: On-line hemodiafiltration: technique and therapy. Adv Ren Replace Ther 1999;6:195–208.

Ingrid Ledebo, PhD
Gambro Lundia AB
Box 10101
SE–22010 Lund (Sweden)
Tel. +46 46 16 91 76, Fax +46 46 16 97 77, E-Mail ingrid.ledebo@gambro.com

Ronco C, Canaud B, Aljama P (eds): Hemodiafiltration.
Contrib Nephrol. Basel, Karger, 2007, vol 158, pp 94–102

Hemodiafiltration with Endogenous Reinfusion

Mary Lou Wratten[a], *Paolo M. Ghezzi*[b]

[a]Research Scientist, Sorin Group Italia, Mirandola, and [b]Medical Devices Consultant, Montemassi, Italy

Abstract

Hemodiafiltration (HDF) is well known to increase the solute convective clearance due to increased ultrafiltration but requires substantial amounts of high-quality reinfusion fluid. Initially in the early 90s, individual bags or containers of reinfusion fluid were used and caused many problems related to handling (storage, repeated connections) and costs. Additionally there was an increased risk of circuit contamination. The interest in HDF pushed technological research for online production of sterile and ultrapure reinfusion solutions. Using a 2-chamber filter, it is possible to produce reinfusion fluid from the ultrafiltrate of the patient, which has been 'regenerated' by a sorbent bed, in a closed circuit. This action eliminates any problems of sterility and apyrogenicity, while also providing the possibility of reinfusing physiologically important substances such as bicarbonates and essential and branched-chain amino acids. This HDF method, called hemofiltrate reinfusion (HFR), has been clinically demonstrated to reduce the loss of physiological components and is associated with decreased inflammation and oxidative stress. In addition to its ease of use, the technique is also highly biocompatible. Based on these observations, HFR appears to be a useful technique for patients with complex risk factors such as malnutrition, inflammation and atherosclerosis.

Hemodiafiltration (HDF) was initially proposed as a mixed diffusive-convective technique that offered the advantages of two systems of transmembrane transport: diffusion and convection. This combination allowed better removal of both middle molecules, particularly with respect to hemodialysis (HD), and small uremic toxins when compared to hemofiltration [1, 2].

Although HDF is characterized by processes that can negatively interfere between diffusion and convection, leading to academic and clinical arguments over the choice between pre-, post- or pre-/postdilution, overall the development of HDF offers, without doubt, an important positive evolution in dialytic strategy. Today it is one of the fastest-growing segments for the treatment of chronic uremic patients.

Hemodiafiltration Problems

Hemodiafiltration is associated with 3 problems:

- interference between convection and diffusion;
- quantity and quality of the reinfusion fluid;
- loss of important physiological components in the ultrafiltrate.

Interference between Diffusion and Convection

Convective clearance (and therefore mass transfer) of a diffusible solute in HDF cannot be fully represented by the ultrafiltration flow rate (Q_{UF}) – in that the simultaneous process of both convection and diffusion diminish the solute's concentration. To resolve this problem, Ghezzi et al. [3, 4] proposed a novel form of HDF that used a 2-stage filter, in series, to separate diffusion from convection. The 2 stages permitted simultaneous convection and diffusion, but also offered several benefits over traditional HDF combined in one filter unit. The first stage of the filter used a membrane with high hydraulic permeability for convective solute removal, while the second stage used a membrane with low hydraulic permeability for diffusive solute removal and to control the patient weight. Reinfusion of externally prepared or purchased fluid occurred between the 2 filter stages. This fluid was equal to the Q_{UF}, in order to maintain the effective blood flow rate. The method was called paired filtration dialysis.

Quantity and Quality of the Reinfusion Solutions

The choice of the Q_{UF} depends on several factors. First, from a practical point of view, the Q_{UF} must always be considered within the limits permitted by the Q_{UF}, the hematocrit and total protein fractional filtration. Elevated Q_{UF} improves the depurative efficiency of the treatment, but it also necessitates large quantities of reinfusion solution that must absolutely have a guarantee of safety for the patient. The utilization of ready-to-use reinfusion sacks produced by the pharmaceutical industry is associated with notable problems including handling (repeated connections to the hematic lines, storage) and cost. This has led to interest in online production of reinfusion fluids that can guarantee sterility and allow elevated Q_{UF}, thus leading to economic and practical handling issues to give a good cost/benefit ratio.

Loss of Useful Substances

Every renal replacement treatment has to guarantee optimal depuration, subtraction of excess liquid to achieve the ideal dry weight and correction of electrolyte as well as acid-base abnormalities. Often however, this comes at a price. Many times, very useful beneficial substances are also lost – particularly at high Q_{UF} – and this can lead to severe depletion of substances such as total, essential and branched-chain amino acids, vitamins, hormones and growth factors. Chronic renal failure patients often have high nutritional losses during both convective and diffusive dialytic treatments that may be closely linked to other patient comorbidities or that may aggravate patient health and well-being. HDF is in particular associated with notable losses of amino acids, and it is not surprising that higher losses are found with membranes that have higher hydraulic permeability [5–7].

Development of Hemofiltrate Reinfusion

The easy availability of isolated continuous ultrafiltrate (UF) during paired filtration dialysis led to the hypothesis that the UF could be 'regenerated' and used as an endogenous reinfusion fluid. The first attempt to regenerate the UF was done in the early 90's with 130 ml of noncoated mineral carbon inserted into the ultrafiltration line [8,9]. The method was called hemofiltrate reinfusion (HFR) and is illustrated in figure 1. The technique proved easy to use and offered high treatment tolerance, an optimal balance of bicarbonate (since this is not adsorbed and therefore is reinfused) and was also associated with a diminished inflammatory response often associated with the endogenous reinfusion [10–14].

During the years 1999–2000, HFR was improved by switching to a sorbent cartridge containing 40 ml of a hydrophobic styrenic resin with high affinity for several uremic toxins and middle molecules such as β_2-microglobulin, homocysteine, angiogenin, parathyroid hormone and several chemokines and cytokines [15, 16]. Urea, creatinine, uric acid, Na^+, K^+, phosphate and bicarbonate are not adsorbed and remain unchanged after passage through the cartridge. These can be managed during the second stage of the diffusive sector of the circuit.

Thus, the regenerated UF in the closed circuit is an endogenous reinfusion fluid that is characterized as sterile, ultrapure with a physiological content of bicarbonate and amino acids. In particular with regard to amino acids, HFR has been associated with an amino acid loss similar to that observed with low-flux membranes such as Cuprophan® and surely much lower than that of other high-permeability membranes or HDF which have associated losses as high as 33%. The amino acid loss for HFR and low-flux membranes is approximately 10–11% [17, 18].

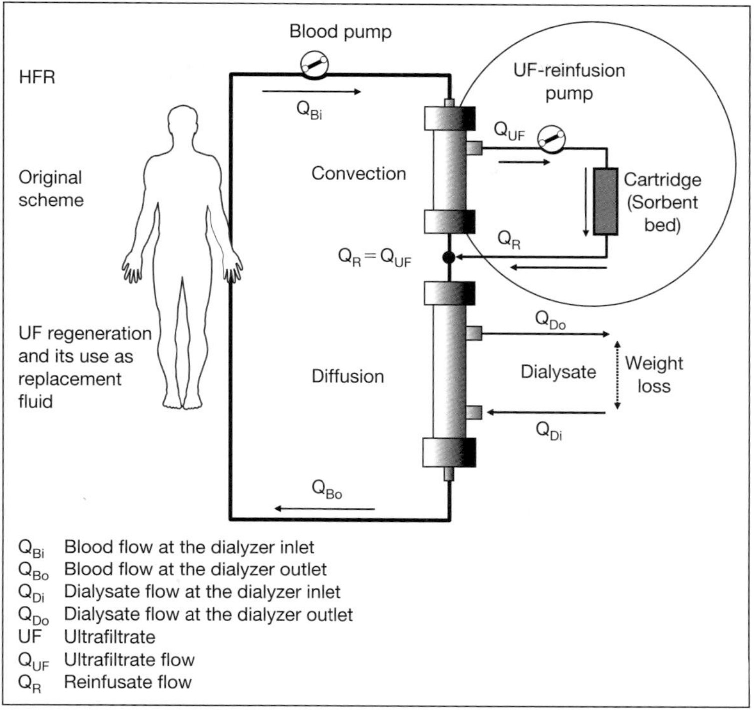

Fig. 1. Original scheme of HFR [9]. Q_{Bi} = Blood flow at the dialyzer inlet; Q_{Bo} = blood flow at the dialyzer outlet; Q_{Di} = dialysate flow at the dialyzer inlet; Q_{Do} = dialysate flow at the dialyzer outlet; Q_R = reinfusate flow.

Ultrafiltrate Characteristics

The UF is a lot more than merely plasma water containing a few uremic toxins. Studies using proteomics and other chromatographic analyses have shown that UF contains over 18,000 proteins and peptides [19–21]. Richter et al. [19] found that the UF, analyzed by matrix-assisted laser desorption ionization/time-of-flight mass spectrometry, consisted of approximately 95% masses that were smaller than 15 kDa. Of these, 55% were found to be fragments from plasma protein fragments (fibrinogen, albumin, β_2-microglobulin, cystatin); 7% were hormones, growth factors and cytokines; 33% consisted of complement, enzymes, enzyme inhibitors and transport proteins. Weissinger et al. [21] also found a significant polypeptide population in a recent study that analyzed UF from uremic patients using either high- or low-flux hemodialyzers. In this study they found a higher number of polypetides in samples obtained from uremic patients with high-flux dialyzers compared to low-flux dialyzers (1,394 polypeptides with high-flux dialyzers vs. 1,046 with low-flux dialyzers) as well as a significant difference if they obtained UF from healthy human donors by filtering plasma through a 5- or 50-kDa filter (590 polypeptides for the high cutoff, 490 polypeptides for the low cutoff). Although the study focused on the characterization of uremic toxins, there are certainly a lot of beneficial substances that are also lost during HDF with high convection. One of the advantages of HFR over classical HDF is that the technique allows the advantages of convection to better remove higher-molecular-weight toxins, but also reinfuses important vitamins, hormones and other physiological compounds.

How Does Hemofiltrate Reinfusion Work?

HFR is a renal replacement therapy that utilizes convection, diffusion and adsorption (fig. 1). It uses a double-stage filter that consists of a high-flux polyethersulfone (Diapes™) filter in the first convective stage and a low-flux polyethersulfone filter (Diapes) in the second diffusive stage. The stages of the filter allow complete separation of convection from diffusion. The convective part of the first stage allows pure UF to pass through a sorbent resin cartridge. The resin is a hydrophobic styrenic resin consisting of many pores and channels adding to its large surface area – approximately 700 m^2/g of resin. The resin has a high affinity for many different uremic toxins. These toxins are adsorbed to the resin beads, and the purified UF is then reinfused to a port between the first and second stages of the filter. The first convective/adsorption stage has no net fluid removal. The blood and reinfused clean UF then undergo traditional dialysis. The second stage works by classical HD. This is also where the patient net fluid loss occurs.

One of the reasons that the UF was chosen to pass through the cartridge instead of direct hemoperfusion, was that the UF has a slower flow rate than the blood and this allows a longer contact time with the resin and a higher toxin adsorption. In addition there are no problems related to hemoincompatibility due to the absence of inflammatory cells and platelets. The cartridge adsorption was maximized by various studies to determine the maximal adsorption at different flow rates for different cartridge diameters and quantities of resin. The treatment is usually performed on the Formula Plus™ dialysis machine (Bellco-Sorin) which has a particular software program that automatically determines the best Q_{UF} based initially on the maximal linear velocity (the flow rate that gives the best adsorption). The machine also determines the patient's hematocrit and transmembrane pressure to adjust the Q_{UF} based on these parameters. Thus, the Q_{UF} is usually higher at the start of the treatment and then adjusts if necessary to reduce the flow rate based on changes in hemoconcentration [22].

Clinical Benefits of Hemofiltrate Reinfusion

There are several studies that show a clinical benefit for patients using HFR. HFR is generally indicated for end-stage renal disease patients with an increased risk of complications related to inflammation, malnutrition and atherosclerosis. This category of patients includes patients with diabetes, high levels of C-reactive protein, elderly patients and patients at higher risk of cardiovascular problems.

Meloni et al. [23, 24] performed a study to determine whether HFR in a postdilution mode would have a benefit in uremic toxin and cytokine removal. They observed high urea and β_2-microglobulin removal, and surprisingly also had efficient cytokine reduction despite the high sieving coefficients associated with interleukin 6 and tumor necrosis factor α. The cartridge is also able to adsorb significant amounts of homocysteine without significant adsorption of vitamin B_{12} or folate as described by Splendiani et al. [25]. They suggest that this mechanism may also be important in reducing cardiovascular risk.

Another study by Bolasco et al. [26] also observed a significant reduction in C-reactive protein in HFR patients compared to when the patients had standard HD. Of interest they also observed improved phosphate removal which they associated with a deceleration in bone turnover and reduced total and bone alkaline phosphatase. Both cytokines and inflammation have been linked to harmful bone metabolism, and alkaline phosphatase has been associated with mortality.

Panichi et al. [27] performed a study to determine whether HFR and online HDF had an effect on inflammatory and nutritional markers. The study was designed as a crossover study with a 1-month washout period of standard HD between a 4-month period of HFR followed by a second period of online HDF (or vice versa). Both techniques significantly improved inflammation indicated by reduced levels of C-reactive protein and interleukin 6 compared to the start from standard HD or during the washout period. In addition they observed increased levels of interleukin 10.

A more recent crossover study comparing HFR to standard HD has recently been completed by Calò et al. [28]. This study not only looked at circulating concentrations of molecules associated with inflammation and oxidative stress, but also determined long-term changes in gene expression in patients undergoing HFR. They observed reduced mRNA production and protein expression of p22phox and plasminogen activator inhibitor 1 (PAI-1) compared with HD. Both p22phox and PAI-1 are implicated in inflammation and oxidative stress

[29–32]. p22phox is an important subunit of the NAD(P)H complex that produces most of the reactive oxygen species in vascular tissue. The p22phox subunit has been implicated in vascular hypertrophy and is often upregulated in atherosclerotic vessels and vessels of diabetic individuals. PAI-1 inhibits fibrinolysis and is also upregulated in insulin resistance. In fact, insulin, glucose and very-low-density lipoprotein triglyceride also stimulate PAI-1 transcription and secretion in endothelial cells. It is thought to be important in progression of coronary syndromes and development of myocardial infarcts, in particular because fibrinolysis can be reduced in venous occlusion. In addition they also observed decreased levels of circulating oxidized low-density lipoprotein compared to no change in standard HD.

Despite good removal of uremic toxins and reduction of inflammatory molecules, HFR is also associated with a sparing of amino acids. Typically high-flux HD or HDF is associated with a 25–30% loss of amino acids which can amount up to a loss of 3–4 g/treatment [5, 33]. Ragazzoni et al. [17] showed a significant sparing in essential, branched and total amino acids during HFR compared to online HDF.

A more recent application has been to optimize sodium balance during the HFR treatment by measuring the conductivity of the isolated UF [34]. Frequently, both HD and HDF are associated with sodium imbalances leading to clinical symptoms such as hypotension, headache and nausea during the dialytic treatment. Ursino et al. [34] developed a mathematical model to predict the solute kinetics, osmolality and fluid volume changes during HFR. The model was validated in a small clinical study that showed good agreement between measured and predicted sodium concentrations. Studies are currently under way to evaluate a biofeedback model.

Conclusions

Although HDF clearly shows increased clinical and survival benefits, chronic renal failure patients continue to have problems associated with inflammation, oxidative stress and cardiovascular morbidity and mortality. Diabetes as a cause of end-stage renal disease is increasing at an alarming rate. The dialysis patient population is also getting older. These factors may be important when considering what type of convective therapy to use. Any type of renal replacement therapy has to be a compromise between optimization of toxin removal and eventual loss of beneficial physiological substances. HFR may be able to offer distinct advantages related to inflammation and nutrition for patients with high levels of comorbidities or syndromes associated with inflammation and cardiovascular complications.

The constant increase in anagraphic patient age and comorbidities for patients requiring renal replacement therapies has translated in a new group of patients with a more fragile clinical profile and, unfortunately, often a poorer quality of life. Renal replacement therapies have made tremendous strides but should aim even further at providing treatment that is not merely aimed at life-sustaining, but rather towards providing an acceptable quality of life. HFR represents a biotechnological response that offers a rationale and adequate treatment that may be useful in limiting (or decreasing) complications related to the new profile of many chronic renal failure patients today.

References

1 Kunitomo T, Lowrie EG, Kumazawa S, et al: Controlled ultrafiltration with hemodialysis: analysis of coupling between convective and diffusive mass tansfer in a new HD-UF system. Trans Am Soc Artif Intern Organs 1977;23:234–243.

2 Leber HW, Wizemann V, Goubeaud G, et al: Simultaneous hemodialysis/hemofiltration: an effective alternative to hemofiltration and conventional hemodialysis in the treatment of uremic patients. Clin Nephrol 1978;9:115–121.

3 Ghezzi PM, Frigato G, Fantini GF, et al: Theoretical model and first clinical results of the paired filtration dialysis (PFD). Life Support Syst 1983;1(suppl 1):271–274.

4 Ghezzi PM, Sanz-Moreno C, Gervasio R, et al: Technical requirements for rapid high-efficiency therapy in uremic patients: paired filtration dialysis (PFD). Trans Am Soc Artif Intern Organs 1987;33:546–550.

5 Ikizler TA, Flakoll PJ, Parker RA, Hakim RM: Amino acid and albumin losses during hemodialysis. Kidney Int 1994;46: 830–837.

6 Navarro JF, Marcen R, Teruel JL, et al: Effect of different membranes on amino-acid losses during hemodialysis. Nephrol Dial Transplant 1998;13:113–117.

7 Navarro JF, Mora C, Leon C, et al: Amino acid losses during hemodialysis with polyacrylonitrile membranes: effect of intradialytic amino acid supplementation on plasma amino acid concentrations and nutritional variables in nondiabetic patients. Am J Clin Nutr 2000;71:765–773.

8 Ghezzi PM, Gervasio R, Tessore V, et al: Hemodiafiltration without replacement fluid: experimental study. Trans Am Soc Artif Intern Organs 1992;38:61–65.

9 Ghezzi PM, et al: Use of the ultrafiltrate obtained in two-chamber hemodiafiltration as replacement fluid. Int J Artif Organs 1991;14:227–234.

10 Arese M, Cristol JP, Bosc JY, et al. Removal of constitutive and inducible nitric oxide synthase-active compounds in a modified hemodiafiltration with on-line production of substitution fluid: the contribution of convection and diffusion. Int J Artif Organs 1996;19:704–711.

11 De Francisco AL, Botella J, Escallada R, et al: Hemodiafiltration with sorbent-regenerated ultrafiltrate as replacement fluid: a multicenter study. Nephrol Dial Transplant 1997;12:528–534.

12 La Greca G, Brendolan A, Ghezzi PM, et al: The concept of sorbents in hemodialysis. Int J Artif Organs 1998;21:303–308.

13 Botella J, Ghezzi PM, Sanz-Moreno C. Adsorption in hemodialysis. Kidney Int 2000;76:S60–S65.

14 De Francisco ALM, Ghezzi PM, Brendolan A, et al: Hemodiafiltration with online regeneration of the ultrafiltrate. Kidney Int 2000;76:S66–S71.

15 De Nitti C, Giordano R, Gervasio R, et al: Choosing new adsorbents for endogenous ultrapure infusion fluid: performances, safety and flow distribution. Int J Artif Organs 2001;24:765–776.

16 Tetta C, Ghezzi PM, De Nitti C, et al: New options for on-line hemodiafiltration; in Ronco C, La Greca G (eds): Hemodialysis Technology. Contrib Nephrol. Karger, Basel, 2002, vol 137, pp 212–220.

17 Ragazzoni E, Carpani P, Agliata S, et al: HFR vs HDF on-line: valutazione della perdita amino-acidica plasmatica. G Ital Nefrol 2004;21(suppl 30):85–90.
18 De Simone W, De Simone M, De Simone A, et al: Aspetti dell'emodiafiltrazione online con rigenerazione e reinfusione dell'ultrafiltrato (HFR). Studio multicentrico. G Ital Nefrol 2004;21(suppl 30):161–167.
19 Richter R, Schulz-Knappe P, Schrader M, et al: Composition of the peptide fraction in human blood plasma: database of circulating human peptides. J Chromatogr B Biomed Sci Appl 1999;726: 25–35.
20 Lefler DM, Pafford RG, Black NA, et al: Identification of proteins in slow continuous ultrafiltrate by reversed-phase chromatography and proteomics. J Proteome Res 2004;3:1254–1260.
21 Weissinger EM, Kaiser T, Meert N, et al: Proteomics: a novel tool to unravel the patho-physiology of uraemia. Nephrol Dial Transplant 2004;19:3068–3077.
22 Wratten ML, Sereni L, Lupotti M, et al: Optimization of a HFR sorbent cartridge for high molecular weight uremic toxins. G Ital Nefrol 2004;21(suppl 30):67–70.
23 Meloni C, Ghezzi PM, Cipriani S, et al: One year of experience in postdilution hemofiltration with online reinfusion of regenerated ultrafiltrate. Blood Purif 2004;22:505–509.
24 Meloni C, Ghezzi PM, Cipriani S, et al: Hemodiafiltration with post-dilution reinfusion of the regenerated ultrafiltrate: a new on-line technique. Clin Nephrol 2005;63:106–112.
25 Splendiani G, De Angelis S, Tullio T, et al: Selective adsorption of homocysteine using an HFR online technique. Artif Organs 2004;28:592–595.
26 Bolasco PG, Ghezzi PM, Ferrara R, et al: Effect of on-line hemodiafiltration with endogenous reinfusion (HFR) on the calcium-phosphorus metabolism: medium-term effects. Int J Artif Organs 2006;29:1042–1052.
27 Panichi V, Manca-Rizza G, Paoletti S, et al: Effects on inflammatory and nutritional markers of haemodiafiltration with online regeneration of ultrafiltrate (HFR) vs online haemodiafiltration: a cross-over randomized multicentre trial. Nephrol Dial Transplant 2006;21:756–762.
28 Calò LA, Naso A, Carraro G, et al: Effect of haemodiafiltration with online regeneration of ultrafiltrate on oxidative stress in dialysis patients. Nephrol Dial Transplant 2007;22:1413–1419.
29 Bonora E: The metabolic syndrome and cardiovascular disease. Ann Med 2006;38:64–80.
30 Yamamoto K, Takeshita K, Kojima T, et al: Aging and plasminogen activator inhibitor-1 (PAI-1) regulation: implication in the pathogenesis of thrombotic disorders in the elderly. Cardiovasc Res 2005;66:276–285.
31 Hoekstra T, Geleijnse JM, Schouten EG, Kluft C: Plasminogen activator inhibitor-type 1: its plasma determinants and relation with cardiovascular risk. Thromb Haemost 2004;91:861–872.
32 Gill PS, Wilcox CS: NADPH oxidases in the kidney. Antioxid Redox Signal 2006;8:1597–1607.
33 Prado de Negreiros Nogueira Maduro I, Elias NM, Nonino Borges CB: Total nitrogen and free amino acid losses and protein calorie malnutrition of hemodialysis patients: do they really matter? Nephron Clin Pract 2007;105:c9-c17.
34 Ursino M, Coli L, Magosso E, et al: A mathematical model for the prediction of solute kinetics, osmolarity and fluid volume changes during hemodiafiltration with on-line regeneration of ultrafiltrate (HFR). Int J Artif Organs 2006;29:1031–1040.

Mary Lou Wratten
Sorin Group Italia
Via Camurana, 1
IT–41037 Mirandola, Modena (Italy)
Tel. +39 0535 29281, Fax +39 0535 29282, E-Mail marylou.wratten@sorin.com

Ronco C, Canaud B, Aljama P (eds): Hemodiafiltration.
Contrib Nephrol. Basel, Karger, 2007, vol 158, pp 103–109

Low- (Classical) and High-Efficiency Haemodiafiltration

Volker Wizemann

Georg-Haas-Dialysezentrum, Giessen, Germany

Abstract

The distinction between high-efficiency haemodiafiltration (HDF), usually applied with online preparation of substitution fluid, and 'classic' low-efficiency HDF (using less than 15 litres of substitution fluid) makes sense since the magnitude of convection (expressed by substitution volume) is important for the claimed benefits of HDF. Many experimental and observational data support the notion that in comparison to conventional low-flux haemodialysis, high-efficiency HDF might have many clinical advantages and might prolong life. Randomized prospective trials, such as a current Dutch trial, are overdue to prove these hypotheses. Low-efficiency HDF is as effective as high-flux haemodialysis in providing convection. Clinical comparisons between high-flux haemodialysis and HDF are sparse. The magnitude of convection is indirectly dependent on the degree of extracorporeal blood flow. With 14-gauge needles, blood flows of >500 ml/min can be safely maintained without haemodynamic or hyperkalaemic consequences. With regard to blood purification kinetics, high-efficiency HDF appears ideal for performing daily short treatments.

Haemodiafiltration (HDF) began to be used in the 1970s [1] under the name 'simultaneous haemofiltration/haemodialysis', which today is still helpful to remember, since HDF aims to combine the advantages of haemofiltration (convection and thereby increased removal of larger substances) with those of haemodialysis (diffusion and thereby increased removal of smaller solutes). Thus the disadvantages of both basic methods are avoided. From the point of view of solute transport and removal, HDF is a win-win method.

In the beginning, the amount of substitution fluid was predetermined by the availability of 1 single brand of 4.5 litres of sterile replacement fluid. HDF was therefore first used with 2 bags(9 litres) of substitution fluid, and later with 4 bags (18 litres). The buffer substance in the bags was lactate, and in the dialysate acetate. When online HDF was introduced experimentally in the 1980s and the restrictive costs of infusion fluid no longer applied, substitution volumes in (postdilution) HDF usually surpassed 20 litres.

Definition of Low-Efficiency and High-Efficiency Haemodiafiltration

The distinction – albeit arbitrary – between the 2 types of postdilution HDF makes sense, since the clearances of the so-called medium- and high-molecular-weight substances primarily depend on the magnitude of convective transport, of which the extent of necessary substitution is an indirect measure. The diffusive part of postdilution HDF is mostly uninfluenced by the magnitude of convection (substitution). Since all potential benefits of HDF over haemodialysis are based on the addition of convection, it is rational to classify HDF according to the magnitude of convection (achieved substitution volume). In an international observational study, high-efficiency HDF (postdilution) was defined when the volume of replacement exceeded 15 l/session [2]. A further argument to accept such a distinction comes from an ongoing prospective randomized trial [3], in which online HDF with substitution volumes of 20–30 litres is compared to low-flux haemodialysis with focus on mortality and morbidity. A third argument for distinguishing high-efficiency HDF from classic low-volume HDF is based on the observation that high-flux haemodialysis (in contrast to low-flux haemodialysis) is a kind of low-volume HDF, since convection and substitution occurs internally within the dialyser, and convection can be as high as 10 l/session [4]. This finding is supported by the findings of Canaud et al. [2] in the European DOPPS population that the relative risk of mortality is identical in low-efficiency (-volume) HDF and high-flux haemodialysis. Thus, subsuming all forms of HDF (with substitution volumes ranging from 3 to 65 litres) as 1 homogeneous treatment form and comparing the outcome with haemodialysis not surprisingly showed no differences [5].

In the following the focus will be on high-efficiency HDF, defined as online HDF requiring 15 litres or more of postdilution volume substitution per session. The postdilution mode was chosen because most observational and prospective trials use this method.

Rationale for High-Efficiency Haemodiafiltration

The reported benefits of HDF on amyloidosis, nutrition, renal anaemia, cardiovascular morbidity, reduction of inflammatory markers and survival are reviewed elsewhere [2, 3, 6–9]. Further recent observational data [10] confirm the DOPPS findings [2]. However, most evidence is class III–V, and despite sophisticated adjustments a bias in patient selection cannot be excluded. Furthermore, HDF patients have often been compared with haemodialysis patients with a questionable quality of treatment, which might rather indicate method-linked side effects such as achieving higher Kt/V scores, sterile dialysate, consequences of more biocompatible membranes and sufficient compensation of acidosis rather than the beneficial effects of convection itself. All these described beneficial effects could also have been achieved by using the full potential of haemodialysis, even low-flux haemodialysis. The European MPO study is a prospective randomized trial comparing high- and low-flux haemodialysis groups of sicker patients (albumin less than 4 g/dl) and the primary objective is survival. Since this study includes only incident patients and the distinction of membrane permeability is clear cut, the outcome might be more conclusive than that of the HEMO study, and if a survival benefit of the high-flux group is found, it might be interesting to learn whether even more convection (with HDF) could surpass the benefits of high-flux dialysis. Today, we are in a similar situation as we have been for 20 years, and we urgently require confirmation of the observational studies by randomized controlled trials such as the ongoing CONTRAST study [3]. The well-known technical versatility of HDF to be applied also in pre- or mixed-dilution mode [for review, see 6] and to advocate HDF in all its modes (according to the rheological situations) as standard therapy appears to be 1 step too many at the present level of hard evidence.

Convection

Less controversial is the statement that the convective part of HDF should be maximized since the clearance of all medium-molecular marker substances directly depends on the magnitude of convection [11, 12]. Figure 1 shows that clearance of β_2-microglobulin can be markedly increased by increased convection (substitution volume is a surrogate), whereas small solutes are influenced only marginally. Figure 2 demonstrates that diffusion is the decisive factor for small-solute clearances.

Magnitude of Blood Flow

Convection and diffusion are both indirectly and directly dependent on the magnitude of blood flow. Absolute diffusive clearances of urea increase with increasing blood flow, whereas β_2-microglobulin as a marker for convective

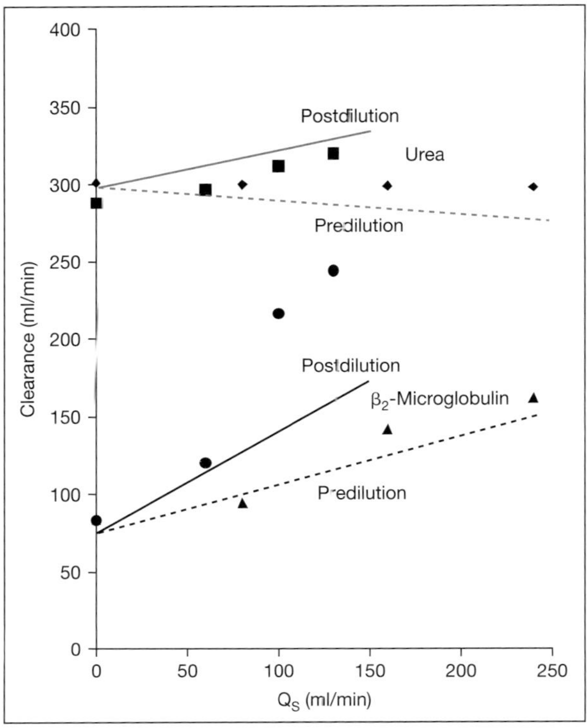

Fig. 1. Clearance as a function of substitution fluid flow Q_S (Fresenius FX60, blood flow 400 ml/min, dialysate flow 800 ml/min). Clearance increase by convection is more pronounced for β_2-microglobulin.

transport is indirectly related to blood flow, because only a fixed proportion (approx. 20%) of the blood entering the dialyser can be filtered safely. The proportion of filtrate is also (to a lesser extent than blood flow) associated with the degree of renal anaemia and the haemorheological situation. Under routine conditions the main determinant for the magnitude of convection is the quantity of blood flow.

For both parts (convection and diffusion) of HDF, high blood flow is a prerequisite for high efficiency. In some European countries, such as Germany, comparatively low blood flows are traditional, and higher extracorporeal blood flows are met with 2 typical arguments, the first being 'results in haemodynamic instability during dialysis'. This topic was already studied in detail 17 years ago by Ronco et al. [13], who demonstrated that increasing blood flow had no influence at all on haemodynamics. We systematically followed 32 haemodialysis patients in whom blood flows of 250 ml/min were compared to 500 ml/min, and no differences were found regarding heart rate, blood pressure or intradialytic

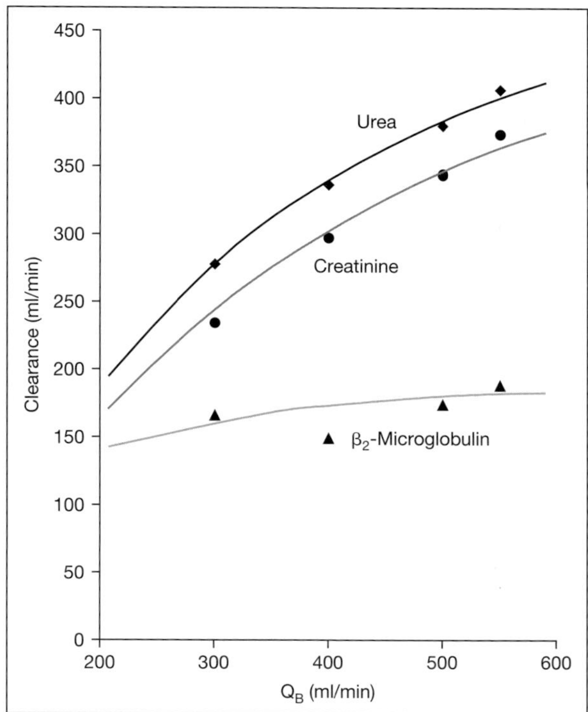

Fig. 2. Clearance as a function of blood flow Q_B (Fresenius FX100, dialysate flow 800 ml/min, substitution fluid flow 60 ml/min, online, postdilution). Clearance of small molecules is strongly increased by higher blood flow rates.

hypotension [Techert et al., in press]. Since increasing blood flow could alter the thermal balance, and since this factor was identified as the cause of the observed haemodynamic stability with convective methods [14], special attention should be paid to achieving a neutral thermal balance during high-efficiency HDF, which not only requires high substitution volumes, but also high blood flows, as thermal factors.

The second argument against higher blood flows – 'leads to haemolysis and hyperkalaemia' – to our knowledge lacks any confirmation in the literature. In our series with 32 patients, blood flow rates of 500 ml/min were associated with identical plasma-free haemoglobin levels at the end of dialysis to treatments with blood flows of 250 ml/min.

It should be noted that the vast majority of arteriovenous fistulas can provide a blood flow of 400–500 ml/min when 14-G needles are used. Under these conditions, negative 'arterial' pressures are even lower than with blood flows of 250 ml/min and use of 17-gauge needles.

Online mixed HDF (substitution pre- and postdilution), controlled by transmembrane pressure ultrafiltration feedback, can further increase the clearances of marker solutes (with the exception of urea) at a given blood flow [15]. The feedback system automatically adjusts the infusion volume and site according to blood flow conditions and internal pressures to maintain a constant and safe filtrate flow. From the aspect of safety it remains open whether a 10% increase in β_2-microglobulin clearance justifies a more than doubling of total infusion volumes.

Variation of High-Efficiency Haemodiafiltration Duration and Frequency

Due to the compartmentalization of the body and the transport properties of larger solutes, an effective blood purification method focusing on such solutes must not necessarily be applied in the same fashion as conventional haemodialysis, which is usually done for 4–5 h 3 times a week. Kinetic studies show that the vascular compartment is already almost depleted of β_2-microglobulin, or substances which behave like 'middle molecules' such as phosphate, when high-efficiency HDF is applied [Beck et al., in press]. In comparison, during conventional haemodialysis the depletion curves are shifted to the right, indicating that longer duration treatment in contrast to HDF makes sense. Thus, the application of high-efficiency HDF of short duration (e.g. for 2–2.5 h) daily would lead to a considerable increase in removal of 'middle-molecular' substances compared to an identical HDF of longer duration but applied only 3 times a week [Beck et al., in press]. Maduell et al. [16] clinically tested a daily schedule of short high-efficiency HDF and found a 21% reduction in pretreatment β_2-microglobulin compared to a conventional high-efficiency schedule of identical weekly duration (3×4 h/week).

Conclusions

High-efficiency (postdilution) HDF is a potent blood purification method, and most published and proposed studies refer to this mode. It remains to be clarified by class I evidence whether HDF is as safe as low-flux and high-flux haemodialysis, and whether there are mortality and morbidity advantages.

References

1 Leber HW, Wizemann V, Goubeaud G, et al: Simultaneous hemofiltration/hemodialysis: an effective alternative to hemofiltration and conventional hemodialysis in the treatment of uremic patients. Clin Nephrol 1978;9:115–120.

2 Canaud B, Bragg-Gresham JL, Marshall MR, et al: Mortality risk for patients receiving hemodiafiltration versus hemodialysis: European results from the DOPPS. Kidney Int DOI: 10.1038/sj.ki.5000447.
3 Penne EL, Blankestijn PJ, Bots ML, et al: Resolving controversies regarding hemodiafiltration versus hemodialysis: the Dutch Convective Transport Study. Semin Dial 2005;18:47–51.
4 Ronco C, Brendolan A, Lupi A, et al: Effects of reduced inner diameter of hollow fibers in hemodialyzers. Kidney Int 2000;58:809–817.
5 Rabindranath KS, Strippoli GFM, Roderick P, et al: Comparison of hemodialysis, hemofiltration, and acetate-free biofiltration for ESRD: systematic review. Am J Kidney Dis DOI: 10.1053/ajkd.2004.11.008.
6 Canaud B, Levesque R, Krieter D, et al: On-line hemodiafiltration as routine treatment of end-stage renal failure: why pre- or mixed dilution mode is necessary in on-line hemodiafiltration today? Blood Purif 2004;22(suppl 2):40–48.
7 Canaud B, Morena M, Leray-Moragues H, et al: Overview of clinical studies in hemodiafiltration: what do we need now? Hemodial Int 2006;10:S5–S12.
8 Maduell F: Hemodiafiltration. Hemodial Int 2005;9:47–55.
9 Kooman JP, van der Sande FM, Beerenhout CM, et al: On-line filtration therapies: emerging horizons. Blood Purif 2006;24:159–162.
10 Jirka T, Cesare S, di Benedetto A, Perera Chang M, et al: Mortality risks for patients receiving hemodiafiltration versus hemodialysis. Kidney Int 2006;70:1524.
11 Wizemann V, Rawer P, Schmidt H, et al: Efficiency of hemodialysis, hemofiltration, hemodiafiltration. Hemodiafiltration – Proceedings 1st Symposium Giessen. Oberursel, Verlag Hygieneplan, 1981.
12 Wizemann V, Külz M, Techert F, et al: Efficacy of haemodiafiltration. Nephrol Dial Transplant 2001;16(suppl 4):27–30.
13 Ronco C, Feriani M, Chiaramonte S, et al: Impact of high blood flows on vascular stability in haemodialysis. Nephrol Dial Transplant 1990;5(suppl):109–114.
14 van der Sande FM, Kooman JP, Konings CJ, et al: Thermal effects and blood pressure response during post-dilution hemodiafiltration and hemodialysis: the effect of amount of replacement fluid and dialysate temperature. Am J Soc Nephrol 2001;12:1916–1920.
15 Pedrini LA, De Christofaro V: On-line mixed hemodiafiltration with a feedback for ultrafiltration control: effect on middle molecule removal. Kidney Int 2003;64:1505–1513.
16 Maduell F, Navarro V, Torregrosa E, et al: Change from thrice weekly on-line hemodiafiltration to short daily on-line hemodiafiltration. Kidney Int 2003;64:305–313.

Prof. Dr. Volker Wizemann
Georg-Haas-Dialysezentrum
Johann-Sebastian-Bach-Strasse 40
DE–35392 Giessen (Germany)
Tel. +49 641 92207 15, Fax +49 641 29187, E-Mail wizemann.volker@phv-dialyse.de

Ronco C, Canaud B, Aljama P (eds): Hemodiafiltration.
Contrib Nephrol. Basel, Karger, 2007, vol 158, pp 110–122

Online Hemodiafiltration

Technical Options and Best Clinical Practices

B. Canaud

Nephrology, Dialysis and Intensive Care Unit, Aider and Renal Research and Training Institute, Lapeyronie University Hospital, Montpellier, France

Abstract

Online production of substitution fluid by 'cold sterilization' (ultrafiltration) of dialysis fluid gives access to virtually unlimited amounts of sterile and nonpyrogenic solution. The incorporation of the online hemodiafiltration (ol-HDF) module into the dialysis proportioning machine hardware simplifies the handling procedure, secures the process by keeping the safety regulation of the monitor and offers virtually unlimited amounts of sterile and nonpyrogenic substitutive solution. The safety of the ol-HDF relies upon use of ultrapure water and strict and permanent highly hygienic rules of use. The use of a specifically designed certified HDF machine is also mandatory. Several forms of ol-HDF have been developed and used to cover specific clinical needs of chronic kidney disease patients. Conventional ol-HDF are classified according to the mode of substitution as post-, pre- and mixed dilution. Alternative-based ol-HDF incorporate push/pull HDF, double high-flux HDF, paired HDF and middilution HDF. A very simple description of these methods is provided in this section. Best clinical practices are summarized in this section to optimize performances of ol-HDF and maximize the safety of the method. It is noteworthy to stress the important role of blood flow, fluid volume exchange, hemodiafilter performances and duration of sessions in the overall treatment efficacy. It is also crucial to insist on the importance of strict hygienic handling, microbiology monitoring and the quality assurance process to ensure the safety of the method. In addition, ol-HDF offers the best technical platform to develop new therapeutic strategies such as daily treatment, total automation of priming and cleansing procedures and biofeedback volume control.

Rationale for Online Hemodiafiltration

Hemodiafiltration (HDF) is an established treatment modality that tends to gain in popularity since it offers now an optimal and affordable form of renal replacement therapy in chronic renal disease patients [1–3]. By enhancing and enlarging the molecular-weight spectrum of uremic toxins removed, HDF improves dialysis efficiency [4–6]. By increasing instantaneous fluxes of various solutes, HDF facilitates the correction of internal milieu disturbances [7]. By improving the global hemocompatibility of the dialysis system (synthetic low-reactive membrane, ultrapure dialysis fluid, protein membrane coating), HDF contributes to reduce side effects and complications of long-term dialysis [8, 9].

The behavior of solute clearances is unique in HDF, since the simultaneous occurrence of diffusive and convective clearances in the same dialyzer tends to cut down the power of each process [10]. Accordingly, the global efficiency of HDF may not be considered as a simple sum of diffusive and convective clearances, it is a more complex relationship. In addition, the site of substitution fluid (post-, pre-, mid- or mixed-dilution mode) affects significantly HDF performances.

Online production of substitution fluid by 'cold sterilization' (ultrafiltration) of dialysis fluid gives access to virtually unlimited amounts of sterile and nonpyrogenic intravenous-grade solution [11–13]. The incorporation of the online HDF (ol-HDF) module into the dialysis proportioning machine hardware is beneficial: first, it simplifies the handling procedure compared to bag use; second, it secures the process by enslaving the infusion module to the safety regulation of the HDF monitor; third, it permits to check regularly the physical integrity of the ultrafilters by means of a built-in air pressure test [14]. This technically advantageous and cost-competitive production of substitution fluid has been employed to develop various forms of high-efficiency HDF modalities (postdilution, predilution, mixed-dilution, middilution). The generic term commonly used to characterize these modalities is ol-HDF [15–17].

Technical Requisite and Hygiene Handling

The safety of the ol-HDF is relying upon strict and permanent conditions of use and handling. Compliance with guidelines is the only way to prevent adverse effects and to warrant success of the ol-HDF program.

The use of ultrapure water (UPW) to feed the HDF machine is a basic requirement for ol-HDF [18]. Several studies have updated our knowledge concerning the water treatment system required [19]. UPW is a high-grade quality water which has been developed mainly to satisfy the needs of the semiconductor industry. For HDF purposes, UPW refers to reverse-osmosis-treated water (one or more stages of reverse osmosis in series) with a resistivity in the range of 0.1–5.0 MΩ/cm with a very low level of bacterial and endotoxin contamination, i.e. >100 CFU/l and endotoxin Limulus amebocyte lysate (LAL) <0.03 endotoxin units (EU)/ml. Production and distribution of UPW to the HDF machine may be achieved with several water treatment options. Distribution pipes must be adequately designed to prevent stagnation, to eliminate dead arms and other recontamination sites. Permanent recirculation of treated water through a closed loop circuit with a microfiltration system is required when a buffer tank is used.

The use of specifically designed HDF and European-Community-certified machines is necessary. Several certified ol-HDF machines are presently available on the European market. Basically, these ol-HDF machines share common features that include an infusion pump with a flow-measuring system, a dialysate ultrafilter module (usually two certified ultrafilters in series) placed onto the hydraulic circuit of the machine and an enslaving system feedback control by the machine alarm detection system. The infusate module is a captive part of the machine which is disinfected simultaneously with each process of the HDF machine. In some machines, a built-in pressure test (bubble point) is performed periodically by the HDF monitor to check the integrity of the ultrafilter membrane. The infusate module consists in an adjustable pump running up to 200 ml/min with a counter calculating the total amount of fluid infused into the patient. The safety of the infusion module is linked to the general alarms of the HDF monitoring system. Ultrapure dialysate flowing into the dialysate compartment of the hemodiafilter is produced through an ultrafilter (UF1) placed just at the exit site of the dialysate [20, 21]. A fraction of the fresh dialysate (100/800 ml/min) produced by the proportioning HDF system is diverted by the infusion pump and infused into the blood of the patient (either postfilter or prefilter infusion). Ultrapurity of the infusate is then secured by a second-stage ultrafiltration (UF2) before being infused into the patient. In this configuration, infusate flow diverted from the inlet dialysate is compensated by an equivalent ultrafiltration flow taken from the patient through the hemodiafilter with the fluid balancing chamber. Ultrafilters are an integral part of the HDF machine that are disinfected after each run and changed periodically.

Online cold sterilization of biological fluids is based on a membrane filtration process (ultrafilter). However, it is important to recall that the retentive capacity of an ultrafilter is restricted to certain conditions of use [22, 23]. The use of UPW, sterile electrolyte concentrates and frequent disinfection of the HDF machine reducing the bacterial contamination level are basic requirements to prevent ultrafilter bacterial overflow.

Hygiene handling is a crucial measure to ensure a permanent safety of the HDF system. Measures needed to maintain the bacterial contamination at a low level have two targets: one is to maintain the ultrapurity of water feeding the HDF machines by means of frequent disinfection of the water treatment system, destruction of biofilm by chemical agents and/or thermochemical disinfection, change of filters and disposable tubings at regular intervals and by permanent recirculation of UPW in the distribution system; the other is to prevent recontamination and bacterial proliferation in the HDF machine by means of frequent disinfection, use of sterile liquid concentrate or powder and periodical changes of ultrafilters.

Quality monitoring of the dialysate and the infusate is mandatory to detect early microbiological contamination of the system. The microbiological inventory of water, dialysate and infusate should be performed according to best practice guidelines and pharmacopeia regulation. Sampling methods, culture media and sensitive microbiological methods have been validated and published elsewhere [24, 25]. Endotoxin content (infusate and dialysate) should be assessed using a sensitive LAL assay with a threshold detection limit of 0.03 EU/ml. Information concerning the microbiological monitoring must be stored to prove the quality of treatment. Such rules must be considered as a part of the good medical practices for ol-HDF.

Hemodiafiltration Treatment Options

Conventional ol-HDF relies on the combination of diffusive and forced convective clearances in the same hemodiafilter module. Basically, the substitution fluid (infusate) is a sterile nonpyrogenic solution produced extemporaneously from fresh dialysate by double ultrafiltration (cold sterilization process) and infused directly into the patient's blood on the venous side. Infusate diverted from the inlet dialysate is extemporaneously compensated by the fluid balancing system of the dialysis machine which is ultrafiltering the same amount of fluid from the patient's blood. A high ultrafiltration rate is achieved by the dialysis machine by increasing adequately the transmembrane pressure (TMP) applied to the hemodiafilter. Weight loss is required to correct patient fluid overload and is achieved in addition by increasing consequently the ultrafiltration rate.

Depending on the infusion site of fluid substitution, several HDF modalities have been described: *postdilution HDF* (infusion after the hemodiafilter); *predilution HDF* (infusion before the hemodiafilter); *mixed HDF* (infusion simultaneously before and after the hemodiafilter) [26]. This is presented in figures 1–3.

HDF requires use of a high-flux dialyzer and achievement of high blood flow (350–450 ml/min) with high dialysate flow (600–800 ml/min). It is recommended to couple the infusion rate to the effective blood flow to reduce the filtration fraction (20–30% maximum). A simple rule of prescribing infusion flow is to use one third of the inlet blood flow in postdilution mode and half of the

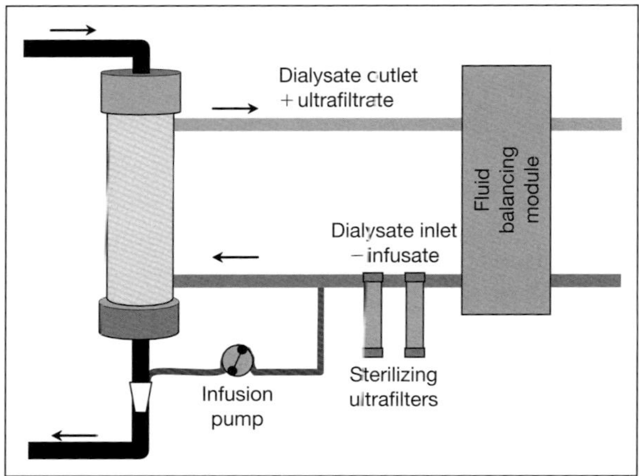

Fig. 1. Postdilution ol-HDF

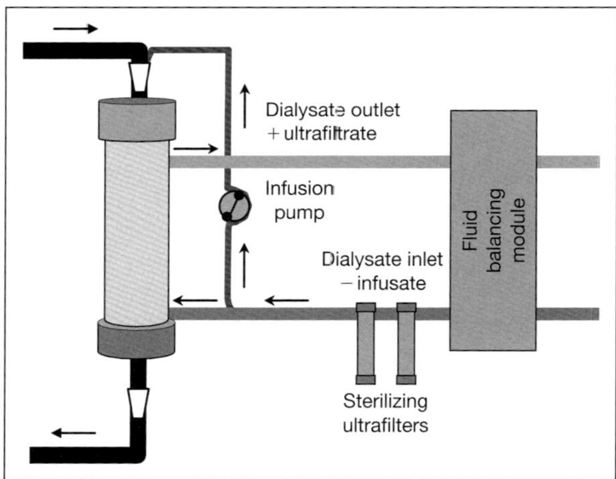

Fig. 2. Predilution ol-HDF.

inlet blood flow in predilution HDF. Typical infusion flow rates are 100 ml/min (24 liters for a 4-hour session) in postdilution HDF and 200 ml/min (48 liters for a 4-hour session) in predilution HDF mode, respectively, to match urea clearance. Mixed pre- and postdilution HDF represents a recently introduced technical option. As it is suggested by recent studies, mixed HDF optimized fluid exchanges by enslaving infusion rate and flow repartition to the TMP trends. Accordingly, one fraction of the substitution fluid is infused in the postdilution site while the other fraction is infused in the predilution site. The ratio of pre-

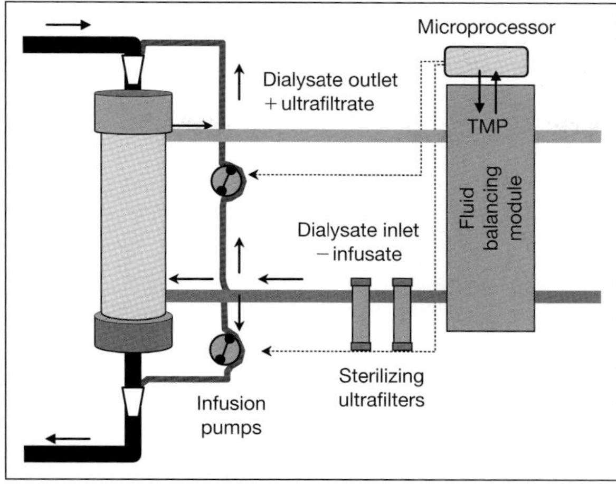

Fig. 3. Mixed-dilution ol-HDF with TMP controlled by microprocessor.

to postinfusion flow is feedback controlled by the HDF monitor (programmed HDF) in order to maintain the TMP in a safe range. Based on this TMP-controlled HDF, it has been shown that significantly higher β_2-microglobulin clearances and lower albumin losses can be achieved [27, 28].

Regarding *alternative-based convective HDF methods,* several variants of HDF have been described over the last decade. All of them claim to be advantageous as compared to the conventional ol-HDF method. They are briefly described in the chronological order of description.

Push/pull HDF is based on a double-cylinder piston pump (push/pull pump) implemented on the effluent dialysate line of the dialysis machine. Based on this alternate pump device, 25 alternate cycles of 20 ml of ultrafiltration (pull) and backfiltration (push) are performed through the hemodialyzer per minute meaning that 120 liters of ultrafiltered plasma water are backfiltered from the fresh inlet dialysate in a 4-hour treatment [29].

Double high-flux hemodialysis consists in two high-flux dialyzers assembled in series while the dialysis fluid irrigates countercurrently the two dialyzers [30]. By means of an adjustable clamp restriction placed on the dialysis fluid pathway between the two dialyzers, ultrafiltration is promoted in the first dialyzer and backfiltration in the second dialyzer [31].

Paired hemofiltration is a double-chamber HDF technique that was initially proposed to separate convective and diffusive solute fluxes in two modules [32] (fig. 4). This method is based on the association of two high-flux dialyzers in series, one with a small surface (e.g. 0.4 m^2) that permits the infusion of substitution fluid (backfiltration) and the second a high-flux hemodialyzer

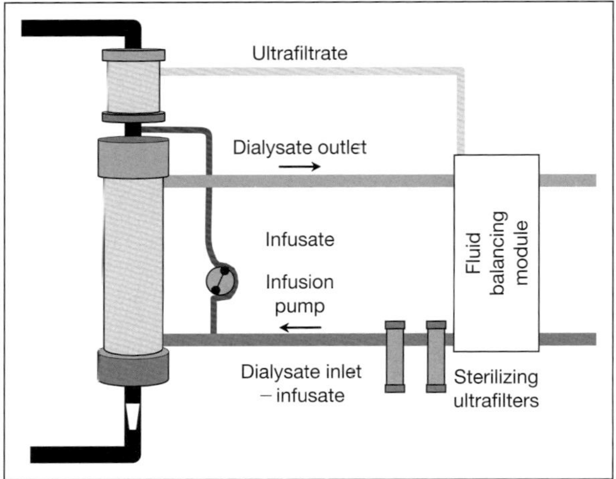

Fig. 4. Paired hemofiltration.

(1.8 m^2) that allows convective and diffusive exchange from dialysate (fig. 4). The substitution fluid produced by cold sterilization from the fresh dialysis fluid is infused either on predilution mode or on postdilution mode according to the position of the dialyzer.

HDF with endogenous reinfusion derives from paired hemofiltration. The main feature of HDF with endogenous reinfusion is the online regeneration of the ultrafiltrate by an adsorbing multilayer device [33]. The regenerated ultrafiltrate is then reinfused as an endogenous substitution fluid (fig. 5).

Middilution HDF is the last option that relies on a newly designed hemodiafilter consisting in two high-flux fiber bundles built in one dialyzer housing. Blood is running countercurrently (ultrafiltration in the first bundle and diffusion in the second bundle) with an infusion performed on the distal head (middle part of the two bundles). In this version the first part of the module ensures the convective transport (ultrafiltration) and the second part of the module the diffusive transport countercurrently with the dialysate after blood has been diluted in the opposite head of the dialyzer (fig. 6).

Online Hemodiafiltration – Best Clinical Practices

Indications for Online Hemodiafiltration

All chronic kidney disease stage 5 (CKD-5) patients requiring a renal replacement therapy support may benefit from ol-HDF. No specific contraindication to ol-HDF therapy has been reported to date.

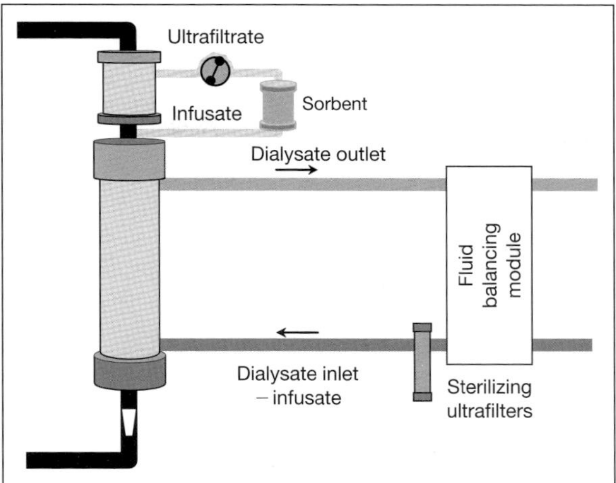

Fig. 5. Hemofiltration with regeneration of infusate.

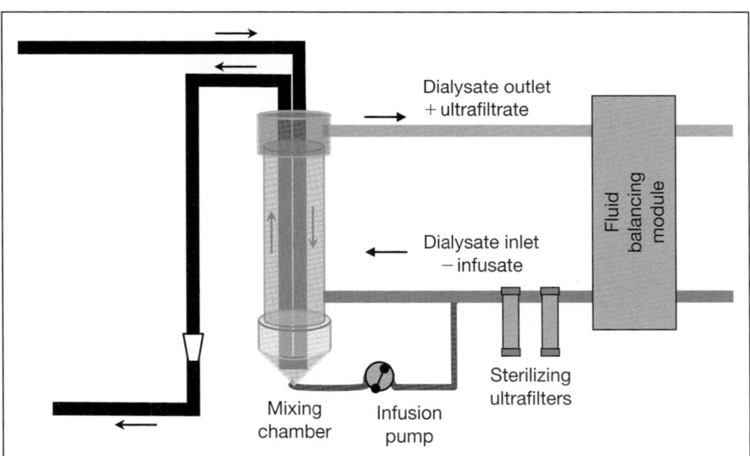

Fig. 6. Middilution ol-HDF.

Two categories of CKD patients are nevertheless particularly suitable for ol-HDF: first, unstable CKD patients presenting with severe cardiovascular risk factors, chronic hypotension, diabetics, elderly and uncompliant patients with large interdialytic fluid gain; second, junior and senior CKD patients requiring a large dialysis dose covering the whole spectrum of uremic toxins or being exposed to prolonged periods of renal replacement therapy. Selection of CKD patients may be justified by the better vascular stability and by the improved biocompatibility provided by the method.

Vascular Access

Patients treated with ol-HDF require an access capable of delivering an extracorporeal blood flow of at least 350 ml/min, and preferably higher, on a reliable basis. High blood rate facilitates the ultrafiltration flow and reduces the TMP problems during the session.

Hemodiafilter

A high-flux, high-efficiency dialyzer is required. The membrane should have a high hydraulic permeability (ultrafiltration coefficient K_{UF} >50 ml/h/mm Hg), high solute permeability (mass transfer-area coefficient K_oA urea >600 and β_2-microglobulin >60 ml/min) and large surface of exchange (1.50–2.10 m^2).

Prescription and Substitution Fluid Volume per Session

The conventional ol-HDF treatment schedule is based on 3 dialysis sessions per week of 4 h (12 h/week). In this relatively short treatment time, it is of paramount importance to ensure high blood flows (400 ml/min) coupled with high dialysate and/or infusate flow rates in order to optimize solute exchange.

By increasing the frequency and/or duration of HDF sessions, it is also possible to achieve a more physiological and more effective treatment.

Follow-Up and Monitoring of Patients Treated with Online Hemodiafiltration

Follow-up and monitoring of ol-HDF-treated patients are strictly equivalent to those of patients treated with regular conventional hemodialysis. Dialysis adequacy targets as recommended by the Kidney Disease Outcome Quality Initiative and the European Best Practice Guidelines should be equivalent in terms of extracellular fluid volume control, blood pressure control, minimum dialysis dose delivered (urea Kt/Vdp >1.2), uremia control, acidosis and hyperkaliemia correction, phosphorus, calcium and parathyroid hormone control, and anemia correction.

On a regular basis, ol-HDF provides a higher solute removal rate as compared to conventional low- and high-flux hemodialysis for low- and middle-size uremic toxins including the β_2-microglobulin. On a long-term basis, this higher efficacy translates in a reduction of the time-averaged concentration of blood β_2-microglobulin concentrations meaning that this middle-size marker should be routinely incorporated in the criteria of dialysis adequacy.

Due to the high volume of fluid exchanged per session (25–50 l/session) it is also recommended to follow on a monthly basis the inflammatory profile of ol-HDF-treated patients (e.g. high-sensitivity C-reactive protein) and the nutritional markers (albumin and transthyretin).

With ol-HDF, achieving a minimum of international adequacy standards is however quite easy due to the better hemodynamic stability and the higher solute removal capacity of the method.

Microbiological Monitoring

The ultrapurity of the bicarbonate-based dialysate and infusate produced by ol-HDF machines relies on three components: first, a well-bioengineered design water production and delivery system; second, a strict control of hygienic rules aiming to maintain regular disinfection procedures of the water treatment system and the proportioning HDF machines; third, a planned microbiological inventory monitoring of the complete chain of treatment.

Disinfection procedures and monitoring frequency of water treatment system and ol-HDF machines may vary from country to country according to specific regulations of the health authorities. The overall aim is to ensure at any time the quality and safety of the ol-HDF method. It is recommended to perform a complete disinfection of the hydraulic circuit of the ol-HDF machine (chemical, heat or mixed) after each run as stated by best clinical practice guidelines. A new sterile tubing set for the infusate line is requested at each new HDF session. Periodical changes of ultrafilters installed on inlet dialysate and infusate lines should be performed according to manufacturer instructions or earlier in case of technical failure. Disinfection of the water treatment system and water distribution circuit should be performed as a minimum on a monthly basis. The type of disinfection (chemical, heat or mixed) and periodicity of disinfection procedures may vary from one center to another but should comply in any cases with the manufacturer recommendations and should be adapted to the microbiological results. More frequent disinfection procedures (daily or weekly) of the water distribution pipe using heat or mixed heat/chemical procedures appear to be the optimal way of preventing bacterial contamination and biofilm formation.

Monitoring the microbiology of the water treatment chain and ol-HDF machines should comply with best practice recommendations and country-specific rules. All recommendations have been reported in detail in the European Best Practice Guidelines. They represent the most comprehensive and update guidelines that should be applied to secure the ol-HDF method [34]. Water feeding the HDF machines should be checked weekly during the validation phase and at least monthly during the surveillance and maintenance period. Dialysate and infusate produced by proportioning ol-HDF machines should be checked at least every 3 months. Microbiological monitoring should include the culture of water and/or dialysate and the determination of endotoxin content. Sampling method, culture media and delay for observation have been published elsewhere. Membrane filtration and culture on a nutrient-poor medium (R2A) are strongly recommended [35, 36]. Cultures are maintained at room temperature (20–22°C) and observed for 7 days. Bacterial colony count and identification should be performed with appropriate methods. Endotoxin content (infusate and dialysate) should be assessed with a sensitive LAL assay with a threshold detection limit of 0.03 EU/ml.

Conclusions

Online HDF modalities offer at the present time the most effective renal replacement modality for CKD-5 patients [37, 38]. High-flux ol-HDF allows delivering a high 'dialysis dose' based on the conventional urea marker. By enhancing the convective fluxes, ol-HDF enlarges the spectrum and increases the uremic toxin mass removed. ol-HDF improves the hemocompatibility profile of extracorporeal renal replacement modalities and reduces inflammation of CKD-5 patients. Online production of substitution fluid reduces the cost of treatment and simplifies the technical aspect of the method. In addition, by giving access to an unlimited amount of high-quality intravenous fluid, the online HDF concept opens new therapeutic options (feedback control of volemia, automation of priming and restitution). These unique properties should give the online HDF a leading position in the CKD-5 therapeutic options to enhance the overall efficacy of renal replacement therapy and to improve the global care of end-stage renal failure patients [39].

References

1 Henderson LW, Besarab A, Michaels A, Bluemle LW: Blood purification by ultrafiltration and fluid replacement (diafiltration). Trans ASAIO 1967;13:216–222.
2 Leber HW, Wizemann V, Goubeaud G, Rawer P, Schutterle G: Hemodiafiltration: a new alternative to hemofiltration and conventional hemodialysis. Artif Organs 1978;2:150–153.
3 Passlick-Deetjen J, Pohlmeier R: On-line hemodiafiltration: gold standard or top therapy? In Ronco C, La Greca G (eds): Hemodialysis Technology. Contrib Nephrol. Basel, Karger, 2002, vol 137, pp 201–211.
4 Sprenger KB: Haemodiafiltration. Life Support Syst 1983;1:127–136.
5 Ofsthun NJ, Leypoldt JK: Ultrafiltration and backfiltration during hemodialysis. Artif Organs 1995;19:1143–1161.
6 Leypoldt JK: Solute fluxes in different treatment modalities. Nephrol Dial Transplant 2000;1:3–9.
7 Ledebo I: On-line hemodiafiltration: technique and therapy. Adv Ren Replace Ther 1999;6:195–208.
8 Canaud B, Bosc JY, Leray H, Stec F, Argiles A, Leblanc M, Mion C: On-line haemodiafiltration: state of the art. Nephrol Dial Transplant 1998;5:3–11.
9 Canaud B, Wizemann V, Pizzarelli F, Greenwood R, Schultze G, Weber C, Falkenhagen D: Cellular interleukin-1 receptor antagonist production in patients receiving on-line haemodiafiltration therapy. Nephrol Dial Transplant 2001;16:2181–2187.
10 Jaffrin MY, Gupta BB, Malbrancq JM: A one-dimensional model of simultaneous hemodialysis and ultrafiltration with highly permeable membranes. J Biomech Eng 1981;103:261–266.

11 Henderson LW, Sanfelippo ML, Beans E: 'On-line' preparation of sterile pyrogen-free electrolyte solution. Trans ASAIO 1978;24:465–467.

12 Shinzato T, Sezaki R, Usuda M, Maeda K, Ohbayashi S, Toyota T: Infusion-free hemodiafiltration: simultaneous hemofiltration and dialysis with no need for infusion fluid. Artif Organs 1982;6:453–456.

13 Canaud B, Flavier JL, Argilés A, Stec F, Nguyen QV, Bouloux C, Garred LJ, Mion C: Hemodiafiltration with on-line production of substitution fluid: long-term safety and quantitative assessment of efficacy. Contrib Nephrol 1994;108:12–22.

14 Canaud B, Nguyen QV, Argilés A, Polito C, Polaschegg HD, Mion C: Hemodiafiltration using dialysate as substitution fluid. Artif Organs 1987;11:188–190.

15 Sternby J: A decade of experience with on-line hemofiltration/hemodiafiltration; in Maeda K, Shinzato T (eds): Effective Hemodiafiltration: New Methods. Contrib Nephrol. Basel, Karger, 1994, vol 108, pp 1–11.

16 Lonnemann G, Behme TC, Lenzner B, Floege J, Schulze M, Colton CK, Koch KM, Shaldon S: Permeability of dialyzer membranes to TNFα-inducing substances derived from water bacteria. Kidney Int 1992;42:61–68.

17 Canaud B, Imbert E, Kaaki M, Assounga A, Nguyen QV, Stec F, Garred LJ, Boström M, Mion C: Clinical and microbiological evaluation of a postdilutional hemofiltration system with in-line production of substitution fluid. Blood Purif 1990;8:160–170.

18 Canaud B, Peyronnet P, Armynot AM, et al: Ultrapure water: a need for future dialysis. Nephrol Dial Transplant 1986;1:110.

19 Canaud BJM, Mion CM: Water treatment for contemporary hemodialysis; in Jacobs C, Kjellstrand CM, Koch KM, Winchester JF (eds): Replacement of Renal Function by Dialysis. Dordrecht, Kluwer Academic Publishers, 1996, pp 231–255.

20 Schindler R, Lonnemann G, Schaffer J, Shaldon S, Koch KM, Krautzig S: The effect of ultrafiltered dialysate on the cellular content of interleukin-1 receptor antagonist in patients on chronic hemodialysis. Nephron 1994;68:229–233.

21 Mion CM, Canaud B: Should hemodialysis fluid be sterile? Semin Dial 1993;6:28–30.

22 Mion CM, Canaud B: 'On-site' preparation of sterile apyrogenic electrolyte solutions for hemofiltration and hemodiafiltration; in Cambi V (ed): Short Dialysis. Boston, Martinus Nijhoff Publishing, 1987, vol 12, pp 261–291.

23 Sundaram S, Barrett TW, Meyer KB, Perrella C, Neto MC, King AJ, Pereira BJ: Transmembrane passage of cytokine-inducing bacterial products across new and reprocessed polysulfone dialyzers. J Am Soc Nephrol 1996;7:2183–2191.

24 Ward RA, Luehmann DA, Klein E: Are current standards for the microbiological purity of hemodialysate adequate? Semin Dial 1989;2:69–72.

25 Pass T, Wright R, Sharp B, Harding GB: Culture of dialysis fluids on nutrient-rich media for short periods at elevated temperatures underestimate microbial contamination. Blood Purif 1996;14: 136–145.

26 Pedrini LA, De Cristofaro V, Pagliari B, et al: Mixed predilution and postdilution online hemodiafiltration compared with the traditional infusion modes. Kidney Int 2000;58:2155.

27 Pedrini LA, De Cristofaro V: On-line mixed hemodiafiltration with a feedback for ultrafiltration control: effect on middle-molecule removal. Kidney Int 2003;64:1505.

28 Kim ST, Yamamoto C, Taoka M, et al: Programmed filtration, a new method for removing large molecules and regulating albumin leakage during hemodiafiltration treatment. Am J Kidney Dis 2001;38(suppl 1):S220.

29 Miwa M, Shinzato T: Push/pull hemodiafiltration: technical aspects and clinical effectiveness. Artif Organs 1999;23:1123.

30 von Albertini B, Miller JH, Gardner PW, Shinaberger JH: Performance characteristics of the Hemoflow F 60 in high-flux hemodiafiltration; in Streicher E, Seyffart G (eds): Highly Permeable Membranes. Contrib Nephrol. basel, Karger, 1985, vol 46, pp 169–173.

31 Pisitkun T, Eiam-Ong S, Tiranathanagul K, Sakunsrijinda C, Manotham K, Hanvivatvong O, Suntaranuson P, Praditpornsilpa K, Chusil S, Tungsanga K: Convective-controlled double high flux hemodiafiltration: a novel blood purification modality. Int J Artif Organs 2004;27:195–204.

32 Ghezzi PM, Botella J, Sartoris AM, et al: Use of the ultrafiltrate obtained in two-chamber (PFD) hemodiafiltration as replacement fluid: experimental ex vivo and in vitro study. Int J Artif Organs 1991;14:327.
33 de Francisco AL, Pinera C, Heras M, Rodrigo E, Fernandez G, Ruiz JC, Tetta C, Arias M: Hemodiafiltration with on-line endogenous reinfusion. Blood Purif 2000;18:231–236.
34 European Best Practice Guidelines for Haemodialysis. Part 1. IV. Dialysis fluid purity. Nephrol Dial Transplant 2002;1(suppl 7):45–62.
35 Ward RA, Luehmann DA, Klein E: Are current standards for the microbiological purity of hemodialysate adequate? Semin Dial 1989;2:69–72.
36 Pass T, Wright R, Sharp B, Harding GB: Culture of dialysis fluids on nutrient-rich media for short periods at elevated temperatures underestimate microbial contamination. Blood Purif 1996;14: 136–145.
37 Golper TA: What technological advances will significantly alter the future care of dialysis patients? Semin Dial 1994;7:323–324.
38 Canaud B, Kerr P, Argilés A, Flavier JL, Stec F, Mion C: Is hemodiafiltration the dialysis modality of choice for the next decade? Kidney Int 1993;43(suppl 41):S296–S299.
39 Henderson LW: Dialysis in the 21st century. Am J Kidney Dis 1996;28:951–957.

Prof. B. Canaud
Nephrology, Dialysis and Intensive Care Unit, Lapeyronie University Hospital
371, avenue du Doyen-Gaston-Giraud
FR–34295 Montpellier (France)
Tel. +33 4 67 33 84 95, Fax +33 4 67 60 37 83, E-Mail b-canaud@chu-montpellier.fr

Ronco C, Canaud B, Aljama P (eds): Hemodiafiltration.
Contrib Nephrol. Basel, Karger, 2007, vol 158, pp 123–130

Mixed-Dilution Hemodiafiltration

Luciano A. Pedrini, Simona Zerbi

Nephrology and Dialysis Department, Bolognini Hospital of Seriate, Seriate, Italy

Abstract

Mixed-dilution hemodiafiltration (mixed HDF) controlled by the transmembrane pressure (TMP) feedback, improves the depurative capacity of the more traditional HDF techniques by fully exploiting the convective mechanism of small- and middle-molecular-weight solute removal. The feedback allows the TMP to be set and profiled from patient and operational parameters recorded online by the machine. It automatically adjusts the infusion ratio between predilution and postdilution at the maximum filtration fraction without reducing the total infusion/ultrafiltration rate and taking into account flow conditions, internal pressures and hydraulic permeability of the dialyzer, and their complex interactions and changes during the session. The application of the TMP profile, while avoiding dangerous hydrostatic pressures within the dialyzer and their negative effects, helps better preserve the permeability of the membrane with the effect of a significantly increased solute removal in a wide molecular range and with minimal protein leakage. In the light of the more recent observations in the literature, the high biocompatibility resulting from the use of synthetic membranes and ultrapure dialysate, combined with the enhanced removal of small- and middle-molecular-weight uremic toxins obtained with high-efficiency HDF, seems to be the best available strategy to prevent or delay the occurrence of long-term dialysis complications and to promote improved survival of dialysis patients. Preliminary results of its application indicate that TMP-modulated mixed-dilution HDF could be one of the most powerful strategies to achieve this goal.

Clinical Benefits and Outcome in Hemodiafiltration

With respect to standard and high-flux hemodialysis (HD), hemodiafiltration (HDF) may induce a sustained increase in removal of both small- and middle-molecular-weight solutes [1–7], several of which are risk factors or markers of severe uremic complications and causes of death in HD patients, such as inflammation, amyloidosis, secondary hyperparathyroidism and accelerated atherosclerosis. Sustained improvement in the uremic toxicity profile may be induced by reducing their level. Lower plasma β_2-microglobulin (β_2-MG) levels were shown to reduce the incidence of bone amyloidosis and carpal tunnel syndrome [8–10] and have recently been associated with reduced mortality in dialysis patients [11]. Controlled studies reported a significant improvement in hemoglobin level and a reduced need for erythropoietin administration in patients on online HDF [2, 12]. Improved control of secondary hyperparathyroidism may be attained in HDF, shown to ensure lower basal levels of phosphate [13, 14] in the long term, which were associated with improved survival in 2 US Renal Data System studies [15].

The HEMO study [16] did not confirm earlier observations of reduced morbidity and mortality in HD patients in association with the use of high-flux membranes [9, 17, 18]. Actually, the difference in β_2-MG clearance between the two groups compared in the HEMO study (low- and high-flux HD, 4 ± 7 vs. 34 ± 11 ml/min) could have been too low to bring to light a significant difference in the overall outcome between groups. Indeed, one of the noteworthy findings of this study was the association between β_2-MG basal levels and death risk in dialysis patients [11]. In HDF definitely higher middle-molecule removal than that in high-flux HD may be attained, provided that HDF is performed with high volume exchange. In randomized studies comparing the two strategies, a significant difference in basal β_2-MG levels only emerged when HDF was performed with a mean filtration volume of 21 l/session [7], but not with a relatively low volume of 8–12 l/session [19]. In the recently published European Dialysis Outcomes and Practice Patterns Study [20], a significantly lower death risk was only observed in patients on HDF when high volume exchange of more than 15 l/session was applied, while no difference was observed in terms of mortality between low-efficiency HDF and conventional or high-flux HD.

Hemodiafiltration Technique and Infusion Modality

HDF is the strategy enabling the high potential of hydraulic and solute permeability of synthetic membranes to be most properly exploited. To optimize its clinical application and achieve the most efficient convective transport, the ultrafiltration flow rate (Q_{UF}) must be forced [3, 20] while maintaining a safe pressure regimen and flow within the dialyzer. The infusion mode highly influences HDF performance [3, 21]. For postdilution, the most efficient infusion mode, there is a limit placed on the Q_{UF} by hemoconcentration, high blood viscosity and resistance to flow, which may result in capillary and dialyzer clotting [22]. Thickness of the secondary protein layer, proportional to the filtration pressure, results in permanent and significant reduction of the membrane permeability, which may compromise the efficiency of the sessions and require the application of increasingly higher and often unpredictable transmembrane pressure (TMP) gradients to maintain the planned ultrafiltration [23]. Control systems implemented on currently available HDF machines are of little help in counteracting the events described above and are unsuited to plan and carry out a session in which ultrafiltration flow or pressure is profiled in order to maintain safe operational conditions [24]. Predilution HDF ensures better rheological and hydraulic conditions than postdilution, and the possibility of higher infusion rates, but at the price of reduced efficiency due to dilution of the solute's concentration available for diffusion and convection.

In search of new and more efficient dialysis strategies, mixed-dilution HDF with a feedback device for Q_{UF} control through TMP has recently been proposed [23, 25, 26] with the aim of improving the efficiency and safety of the HDF technique, while at the same time reducing the shortcomings and risks associated with the traditional HDF infusion modes.

Optimization of Convection

Some observations form the basis of the new technique. At a given blood flow, the maximal efficiency in convective solute removal occurs at the highest achievable filtration fraction (FF) [25]. This is often unpredictable, due to the events described above and to a patient variability, presumably related to the individual refilling capacity as ultrafiltration progresses. At any given blood flow, TMP is exponentially related to FF, and the slope of the curve is a function of the hydraulic permeability of the dialyzer [25]. Above a certain TMP level, the system becomes unstable, and sudden dangerous pressure peaks are likely to result from small changes in blood flow or viscosity, venous pressure or for technical reasons [22]. These events are difficult to prevent or counteract without a feedback system which is able to automatically ensure a constant ultrafiltration and the highest possible FF while maintaining TMP within a safe range.

Principles and Configuration of Mixed-Dilution HDF with TMP Feedback Control

Online mixed HDF was originally performed in our center on a 4008 H online Fresenius system (Fresenius Medical Care, Germany) modified with the application of a Y-shaped infusion line and an additional pump on one Y branch, which diverted part of the total infusion from the postfilter to the prefilter infusion site. A feedback system for TMP control was used in mixed HDF to modulate the predilution/postdilution ratio while maintaining the total

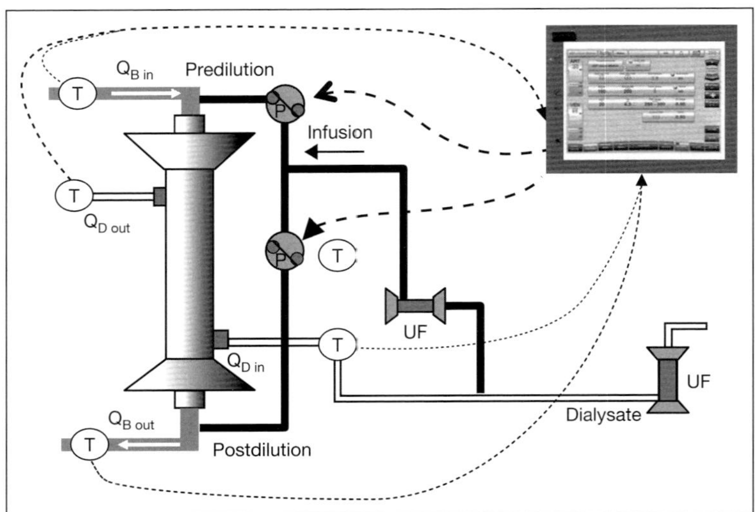

Fig. 1. Online mixed-dilution HDF: schematic representation. Sterile infusion fluid, prepared online with double ultrafiltration (UF), is driven to the infusion ports of the dialyzer by means of 2 peristaltic pumps (P) at relative infusion rates modulated by the TMP feedback through changes of the pumps' speed. TMP, calculated online by means of dedicated software analyzing signals from 4 pressure transducers (T), is forced to follow a definite profile during the session by modulating the ratio between predilution and postdilution in order to optimize the FF.

infusion constant throughout the session (fig. 1). The basic concept is that splitting the infusion between the pre- and postfilter in order to optimize FF guarantees the best possible rheological and hydraulic conditions within the dialyzer at the highest fluid exchange rate and with the most solute removal by convection.

The mean pressure gradient between blood and dialysate compartments along the dialyzer (TMP, mm Hg) is calculated online by means of dedicated software analyzing signals from pressure transducers placed at the inlet and outlet blood and dialysate ports of the dialyzer ($P_{B\ in}$, $P_{B\ out}$, $P_{D\ in}$, $P_{D\ out}$, respectively) using the equation:

$$TMP = 0.5 \cdot [(P_{B\ in} + P_{B\ out}) - (P_{D\ in} + P_{D\ out})] - P_{onc} \quad (1)$$

where P_{onc} (mm Hg) is the mean oncotic pressure exerted by the plasma proteins, set by default to a constant value of 25 mm Hg.

In its last configuration, implemented on the new 5008 Fresenius system, the feedback device operates with internal pressure transducers to monitor and compute TMP. Replacement fluid is driven to the infusion sites of the dialyzer by means of two separate pumps at a speed modulated by the internal software on the basis of the actual TMP value [5].

Setting the Infusion Rate

The system device operates at the start of the mixed HDF session by setting the total infusion rate (Q_S, ml/min) proportionally to the plasma water flow rate of the patient ($Q_{PW\ in}$, ml/min). The total infusion is then split into pre- and postinfusion ($Q_{S\ pre}$, $Q_{S\ post}$, ml/min) at relative infusion rates allowing the desired FF to be obtained.

$Q_{PW\ in}$ is calculated online from the effective blood flow ($Q_{B\ eff} = Q_B$ compensated by means of the arterial pressure), from hematocrit (Hct), monitored online with an integrated device (blood volume monitor, Fresenius Medical Care), and from the water fraction of plasma (Fp), according to the classic equation [27]:

$$Q_{PW\ in} = Q_{B\ eff} \cdot (1 - \text{Hct}/100) \cdot \text{Fp}. \tag{2}$$

FF is defined arbitrarily as the fraction of $Q_{PW\ in}$ ultrafiltered during the passage through the dialyzer, in analogy with a more strict definition [28], as:

$$\text{FF} = (1 - Q_{PW\ out}/Q_{PW\ in}) = Q_{UF}/Q_{PW\ in} \tag{3}$$

where $Q_{PW\ out}$ is the outlet plasma water flow rate.

Initial Q_S is usually set equal to $Q_{PW\ in}$ but , according to the clinical needs and the characteristics of the dialyzer, different values for the $Q_S/Q_{PW\ in}$ ratio may be planned from 0.7 to 1 in steps of 0.05. Different options are also available for the initial FF from 0.3 to 0.5.

On the basis of the planned Q_S and FF, the relative pre- and postinfusion rates are computed by the software device according to the following equations, derived from equation 3:

$$Q_{S\ pre} = (Q_{UF} - \text{FF} \cdot Q_{PW\ in})/\text{FF} \tag{4}$$

$$Q_{S\ post} = Q_S - Q_{S\ pre}. \tag{5}$$

Controlling the Infusion Rate

After the start of the session, the TMP feedback control acts by modulating the ratio between pre- and postdilution in order to gradually achieve and then maintain an optimal and safe TMP value for the entire session (250–300 mm Hg), without affecting the total Q_S nor the planned Q_{UF}. If TMP falls below the lowest value of the range, a small amount of fluid (5–10 ml/min) is diverted from pre- to postinfusion by increasing the postinfusion pump speed, increasing FF (and thus TMP) as a result. Vice versa, the same amount of fluid is diverted from post- to predilution, thus reducing FF, whenever TMP rises beyond its maximum tolerated value. In short, the feedback is aimed at ensuring throughout the sessions the highest FF compatible with the progressive hemoconcentration and loss of hydraulic membrane permeability, which occurs as the session progresses.

Transmembrane Pressure Profiling

High-flux membranes, having generally a cutoff up to 20 kDa, may be responsible for massive protein leakage, mainly when high filtration pressure is applied to the intact membrane in the early phase of the session, and even large molecules such as albumin may be forced into the intact pores and either cross them and get lost in the dialysate or be entrapped inside, with the effect of a permanent and significant reduction of membrane permeability. At a low Q_{UF}, only small peptides and proteins are trapped by the membrane pores and adhere to their inner surface. Compared to the intact membrane, this narrowing of the pore size leads to larger plasma molecules, such as albumin, being rejected, whereas permeability to middle-molecular-weight solutes, such as β_2-MG, is not substantially modified. Based on these observations, in the more recent application of mixed HDF low filtration pressure was applied at the beginning of the session by setting a relatively low FF (0.35–0.40). Then, TMP was allowed to increase gradually up to its optimal value according to an ultrafiltration profile obtained with the help of the TMP feedback with automatic shifts of small amounts of the infusion fluid from the postdilution to the predilution port of the dialyzer without reducing the total Q_{UF}.

Results of Mixed HDF

Due to its experimental characteristic mixed HDF is presently performed in selected centers and the results of its application refer to a limited number of patients. However, the results of the randomized studies published to date show that this infusion mode, when performed at a matched infusion rate, ensures safe hydraulic and flow conditions similar to predilution HDF but may achieve an efficiency in removing small solutes which is definitely higher than that obtained in predilution HDF and similar to that reached in postdilution HDF performed at a maximal ultrafiltration rate [25]. However, the advantage of mixed HDF clearly appears also with respect to middle-molecule removal when higher infusion rates are applied under the control of the TMP feedback, which allows the TMP to be set and modulated according to a defined profile [5, 23]. The feedback automatically adjusts the infusion ratio between pre- and postdilution at the maximum FF without reducing the total infusion and taking into account flow conditions, internal pressures and hydraulic permeability of the dialyzer, and their complex interactions and changes occurring during the sessions. Under these conditions, the highest membrane potential of convective transport is optimized, and online mixed HDF may yield a significantly higher β_2-MG removal than that obtained in postdilution HDF and in middilution HDF [29, 30]. Moreover, the application of the TMP profile, while simultaneously minimizing protein leakage in the first part of the session and dangerous hydrostatic pressures within the dialyzer, helps better preserve the permeability of the membrane in the remaining time of the session, favoring the significantly increased cumulative solute removal typical of this technique.

References

1 Bammens B, Evenepoel P, Verbeke K, Vanrenterghem Y: Removal of the protein-bound solute *p*-cresol by convective transport: a randomized crossover study. Am J Kidney Dis 2004;44:278–285.

2 Lin CL, Huang CC, Chang CT, Wu MS, Hung CC, Chien CC, Yang CW: Clinical improvement by increased frequency of on-line hemodiafiltration. Ren Fail 2001;23:193–206.

3 Lornoy W, Becaus I, Billiouw JM, Sierens L, Van Malderen P, D'Haenens P: On-line haemodiafiltration: remarkable removal of β_2-microglobulin. Long-term clinical observations. Nephrol Dial Transplant 2000;15(suppl 1):49–54.

4 Lornoy W, De Meester J, Becaus I, Billiouw JM, Van Malderen PA, Van Pottelberge M: Impact of convective flow on phosphorus removal in maintenance hemodialysis patients. J Ren Nutr 2006; 16:47–53.

5 Pedrini LA, Cozzi G, Faranna P, Mercieri A, Ruggiero P, Zerbi S, Feliciani A, Riva A: Transmembrane pressure modulation in high-volume mixed hemodiafiltration to optimize efficiency and minimize protein loss. Kidney Int 2006;69:573–579.

6 Schroder M, Riedel E, Beck W, Deppisch RM, Pommer W: Increased reduction of dimethylarginines and lowered interdialytic blood pressure by the use of biocompatible membranes. Kidney Int 2001;59:19–24.

7 Ward RA, Schmidt B, Hullin J, Hillebrand GF, Samtleben W: A comparison of on-line hemodiafiltration and high-flux hemodialysis: a prospective clinical study. J Am Soc Nephrol 2000;11:2344–2350.

8 Gejyo F, Kawaguchi Y, Hara S, Nakazawa R, Azuma N, Ogawa H, Koda Y, Suzuki M, Kaneda H, Kishimoto H, Oda M, Ei K, Miyazaki R, Maruyama H, Arakawa M, Hara M: Arresting dialysis-related amyloidosis: a prospective multicenter controlled trial of direct hemoperfusion with a β_2-microglobulin adsorption column. Artif Organs 2004;28:371–380.

9 Koda Y, Nishi S, Miyazaki S, Haginoshita S, Sakurabayashi T, Suzuki M, Sakai S, Yuasa Y, Hirasawa Y, Nishi T: Switch from conventional to high-flux membrane reduces the risk of carpal tunnel syndrome and mortality of hemodialysis patients. Kidney Int 1997;52:1096–1101.

10 Kuchle C, Fricke H, Held E, Schiffl H: High-flux hemodialysis postpones clinical manifestation of dialysis-related amyloidosis. Am J Nephrol 1996;16:484–488.

11 Cheung AK, Rocco MV, Yan G, Leypoldt JK, Levin NW, Greene T, Agodoa L, Bailey J, Beck GJ, Clark W, Levey AS, Ornt DB, Schulman G, Schwab S, Teehan B, Eknoyan G: Serum β_2-microglobulin levels predict mortality in dialysis patients: results of the HEMO study. J Am Soc Nephrol 2005;17:546–555.

12 Vaslaki L, Major L, Berta K, Karatson A, Misz M, Pethoe F, Ladanyi E, Fodor B, Stein G, Pischetsrieder M, Zima T, Wojke R, Gauly A, Passlick-Deetjen J: On-line haemodiafiltration versus haemodialysis: stable haematocrit with less erythropoietin and improvement of other relevant blood parameters. Blood Purif. 2006;24:163–173.

13 Ding F, Ahrenholz P, Winkler RE, Ramlow W, Tiess M, Michelsen A, Patow W: Online hemodiafiltration versus acetate-free biofiltration: a prospective crossover study. Artif Organs 2002;26:169–180.

14 Minutolo R, Bellizzi V, Cioffi M, Iodice C, Giannattasio P, Andreucci M, Terracciano V, Di Iorio BR, Conte G, De Nicola L: Postdialytic rebound of serum phosphorus: pathogenetic and clinical insights. J Am Soc Nephrol 2002;13:1046–1054.
15 Block GA, Hulbert-Shearon TE, Levin NW, Port FK: Association of serum phosphorus and calcium × phosphate product with mortality risk in chronic hemodialysis patients: a national study. Am J Kidney Dis 1998;31:607–617.
16 Eknoyan G, Beck GJ, Cheung AK, Daugirdas JT, Greene T, Kusek JW, Allon M, Bailey J, Delmez JA, Depner TA, Dwyer JT, Levey AS, Levin NW, Milford E, Ornt DB, Rocco MV, Schulman G, Schwab SJ, Teehan BP, Toto R: Effect of dialysis dose and membrane flux in maintenance hemodialysis. N Engl J Med 2002;347:2010–2019.
17 Leypoldt JK, Cheung AK, Carroll CE, Stannard DC, Pereira BJ, Agodoa LY, Port FK: Effect of dialysis membranes and middle molecule removal on chronic hemodialysis patient survival. Am J Kidney Dis 1999;33:349–355.
18 Port FK, Wolfe RA, Hulbert-Shearon TE, Daugirdas JT, Agodoa LY, Jones C, Orzol SM, Held PJ: Mortality risk by hemodialyzer reuse practice and dialyzer membrane characteristics: results from the USRDS dialysis morbidity and mortality study. Am J Kidney Dis 2001;37:276–286.
19 Locatelli F, Mastrangelo F, Redaelli B, Ronco C, Marcelli D, La Greca G, Orlandini G: Effects of different membranes and dialysis technologies on patient treatment tolerance and nutritional parameters. The Italian Cooperative Dialysis Study Group. Kidney Int 1996;50:1293–1302.
20 Canaud B, Bragg-Gresham JL, Marshall MR, Desmeules S, Gillespie BW, Depner T, Klassen P, Port FK: Mortality risk for patients receiving hemodiafiltration versus hemodialysis: European results from the DOPPS. Kidney Int 2006;69:2087–2093.
21 Pedrini LA, Mercieri A: Pre- and post-dilution hemodiafiltration compared. G Ital Nefrol 2004; 21(suppl 30):S12–S16.
22 Henderson LW: Biophysics of ultrafiltration and hemofiltration; in Maher JF (ed): Replacement of Renal Function by Dialysis, ed 3. Dordrecht, Kluwer Academic, 1989, pp 300–326.
23 Pedrini LA, De Cristofaro V: On-line mixed hemodiafiltration with a feedback for ultrafiltration control: effect on middle-molecule removal. Kidney Int 2003;64:1505–1513.
24 Pedrini LA: On-line hemodiafiltration: technique and efficiency. J Nephrol 2003;16(suppl 7): S57–S63.
25 Pedrini LA, De Cristofaro V, Pagliari B, Sama F: Mixed predilution and postdilution online hemodiafiltration compared with the traditional infusion modes. Kidney Int 2000;58:2155–2165.
26 Pedrini LA, De Cristofaro V, Pagliari B, Filippini M, Ruggiero P: Optimization of convection on hemodiafiltration by transmembrane pressure monitoring and biofeedback; in Ronco C, La Greca G (eds): Hemodialysis Technology. Contrib Nephrol. Basel, Karger, 2002, vol 137, pp 254–259.
27 Sargent JA, Gotch FA: Principles and biophysics of dialysis; in Jacobs C, Kjellstrand CM, Koch KM, Winchester JF (eds): Replacement of Renal Function by Dialysis. Dordrecht, Kluwer Academic, 1996, pp 34–102.
28 Bosch JP, Geronemus R, Glabman S, Lysaght R, Kahn T, von Albertini B: High flux hemofiltration. Artif Organs 1978;2:339–342.
29 Krieter DH, Falkenhain S, Chalabi L, Collins G, Lemke HD, Canaud B: Clinical cross-over comparison of mid-dilution hemodiafiltration using a novel dialyzer concept and post-dilution hemodiafiltration. Kidney Int 2005;67:349–356.
30 Feliciani A, Riva MA, Zerbi S, Ruggiero P, Plati AR, Cozzi G, Pedrini LA: New strategies in haemodiafiltration (HDF): prospective comparative analysis between on-line mixed HDF and mid-dilution HDF. Nephrol Dial Transplant 2007. DOI:10.1093/ndt/gfm023.

Dr. Luciano A. Pedrini
UO Nefrologia e Dialisi, Ospedale Bolognini
Via Paderno 21
IT–24068 Seriate, Bergamo (Italy)
Tel. +39 035 306 3259, Fax +39 035 306 3375, E-Mail nefrologia.seriate@bolognini.bg.it

Ronco C, Canaud B, Aljama P (eds): Hemodiafiltration.
Contrib Nephrol. Basel, Karger, 2007, vol 158, pp 131–137

Paired Hemodiafiltration

F. Pizzarelli

Nephrology and Dialysis Unit, SM Annunziata Hospital, Florence, Italy

Abstract

The feasibility of obtaining low-cost high-quality online reinjection fluids was first explored almost 30 years ago, but regulatory conservatism delayed adoption of the technique for almost 20 years. Online treatments are now commonplace in Europe. The competitive advantages of this treatment modality compared to standard convective treatments include lower costs, better quality assurance, a lower environmental burden and better clinical outcomes. The very high volumes of re-infusion fluids peculiar to online treatment allow a better removal of β_2-microglobulin, and there are claims that survival and anemia are better improved by online treatments than by standard convective treatments. In contrast, the acetate burden and its attendant potential hazards are relevant in patients under online treatment, given the considerable quantity of dialysis fluid injected. Acetate-free paired hemodiafiltration, a new online technique, may further ameliorate performances and clinical outcomes, and may actually cut the gordian knot of the safety of online treatments owing to the implemented safeguards.

Online Treatments

The feasibility of obtaining a sterile and apyrogenic reinfusion fluid using the cold-filtration technique was demonstrated by Henderson and Beans in 1978 [1], and the first report of a clinical application was published a few years later [2].

Many more studies have verified the feasibility and safety of online technology, in both the short [3–7] and the long term [8–12].

These techniques are now rapidly replacing traditional methods in many dialysis centers in Italy and Europe. This spread is mainly due to the facts that sophisticated techniques have ruled out the possibility that the infused fluid could induce cytokine production or inflammation in the patient [11–13], and that the legislative issues involved in online treatments have been resolved [14].

In our center, online treatment has completely replaced standard hemodiafiltration since 1991. In these 15 years, we have performed more than 15,000 treatments, reinfusing almost 500,000 liters of filtered dialysate. Thirty-eight patients have been treated safely for at least 1 year (3 years on average, with a range of 1–10 years).

Although ours is a monocentric clinical experience, and as such liable to errors in case selection, online techniques confirm economic, management and organizational, environmental and clinical advantages as compared to conventional convective techniques using commercially available fluids.

The environmental advantages are not negligible. Online dialysis eliminates the production, transport (almost always by road, in increasingly crowded highways) and disposal of plastic bags. This has particular importance at a time when the problem of environmental pollution is assuming planetary dimensions. With regard only to our center, if we consider that the commercial bags contain 5 liters of solution for reinfusion, we have avoided the production of almost 100,000 plastic containers.

Several comparative studies have indicated that online hemodiafiltration provides an improvement in β_2-microglobulin removal compared with standard hemodialysis, and, consequently, less risk of amyloid-related disease and death [15–18].

In all the studies analyzing survival and comorbidity there is a trend favoring convection, but the data are highly variable, with the effect being more evident in the older studies [19]. A more recent analysis of the European DOPPS database [20] shows a significant reduction in mortality. After adjustment for potential confounders, patients on high-efficiency hemodiafiltration had a 35% lower mortality risk than those receiving low-flux hemodialysis (relative risk = 0.65, p = 0.01). The HEMO study, the only randomized prospective study addressing the question [21], while not demonstrating statistically significant differences in terms of mortality and morbidity between high- and low-flow membranes, did however attribute a marginal advantage to the former. It must be asked whether a possible effect, estimated at 9%, while not statistically significant, would not however be biologically relevant in view of the very hard outcome tested, that is, the survival of the patient. A post-hoc analysis of the HEMO study also provides another interesting piece of data: the link between mortality and levels of β_2-microglobulin; the mortality-related risk grows by 13% for every increase of 10 mg/dl in predialytic levels of β_2-microglobulin, and this correlation is highly significant [22].

With regard to anemia, the results are more heterogeneous, with some papers against [23, 24] and some in favor of a beneficial effect of online hemodiafiltration [25–27].

To summarize, treatments based on convective fluxes, in contrast to standard hemodialysis, offer confirmed advantages in terms of less dialysis-related amyloidosis and some degree of improvement in patient survival and anemia. Although online treatments fall squarely within the definition of 'device' as set forth in the European standards [12, 14], the main concern is still there: in online treatments only a post-hoc assessment of sterility and apyrogenicity of the reinfusion fluid can be made and nephrologists have concerns about the impossibility of testing the purity of the filtered dialysis fluid infused during the course of the treatment.

Paired Hemodiafiltration

Paired hemodiafiltration (PHF; Bellco®) is a new online method offering a response to the above-mentioned concerns [28, 29].

In this technique, which uses a dual stage filter with high-flux membranes in both chambers, diffusion and convection are performed in the larger (1.9 m^2) chamber. Part of the dialysis fluid is diverted by the infusion pump into the infusion line and injected into the patient by backfiltration in the smaller (0.7 m^2) filter chamber (fig. 1).

Interestingly enough, PHF is based on backfiltration, but is derived from paired filtration dialysis (Bellco), a technique conceived by Ghezzi et al. [30] to avoid backfiltration, and its attendant potential microbiological hazards, by physical separation of convection and diffusion. Technological improvements in monitors and quality of the treated water changed the scenario. Backfiltration is no longer a challenge for nephrologists but instead a means to obtain high-quality reinjection fluid.

From this point of view PHF offers some special and unique characteristics.

First, in PHF, the last stage of dialysis fluid ultra-filtration takes place inside the dialyzer, i.e. exactly where the dialysis fluid mixes with blood. Lack of connections or infusion lines beyond the last dialysis fluid ultrafiltration point minimizes any possible source of contamination (fig. 1).

Second, PHF incorporates an online dialyzer membrane integrity check. By reversing the direction of rotation of the infusion pump, instead of injecting fluids into the patient, blood ultrafiltrate is obtained. A standard blood leak detector will detect any red blood cells in that ultrafiltrate, thereby giving an idea of the integrity of the membrane devoted to the last stage of dialysis fluid filtration (fig. 1). We have performed experiments, both in vitro and in vivo, which tested filters in which 1 single fiber was deliberately broken [28]. The system demonstrated high sensitivity to even such minimal damage. The online integrity check is so reliable because it works with leaking blood not diluted with dialysis fluid. The membrane integrity test is performed at the beginning of the treatment and while it is under way, and as often as deemed necessary.

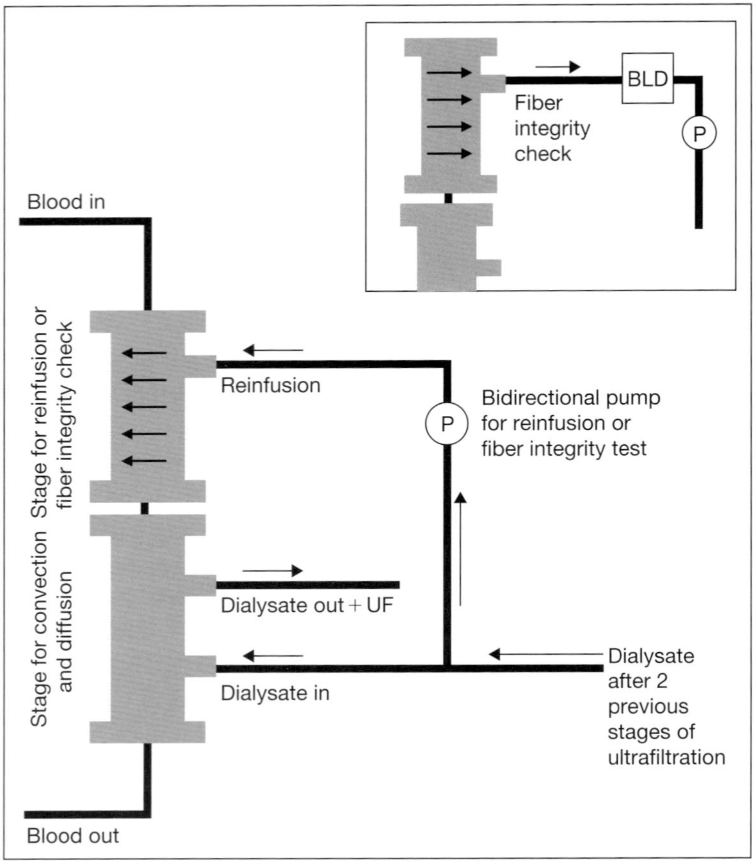

Fig. 1. Graphical representation of PHF circuit. See text for details. BLD = Blood leak detector; UF = ultrafiltrate.

As for clinical outcomes, we have demonstrated for PHF the same peculiarities as other online methods: optimum removal of β_2-microglobulin and no cytokine-inducing capability [28, 29].

We recently tested acetate-free PHF [31]. The background for doing so is that in patients on online convective treatments, given the considerable quantity of dialysis fluid reinfused, the small amount of acetate present in the bicarbonate dialysis fluid as a pH-stabilizing factor may allow a significant transfer of acetate into the patient, which could induce cytokine activation. We found that in comparison with the pretreatment values, plasma acetate levels were unchanged during and after acetate-free PHF, while they were 5–6 times higher in the course of PHF containing acetate in the dialysis fluid; plasma acetate levels returned to basal values 2h after the end of the procedure. The total increase in bases in the patient attributable to acetate was 36%. IL-6 plasma levels were superimposable at the beginning and in the course of the 2 methods compared, but there was a tendency towards a greater increase at an interval of 2h following PHF with acetate.

Conclusions

Online treatments make up an emerging form of dialytic replacement therapy, as is demonstrated by their continually increasing use and the interest shown in the method by the major producers of electromedical devices in the field. We believe that there are clinical, economic and environmental reasons for preferring online treatments to conventional techniques. The analysis of our data and of the literature allows us to conclude that online treatments are just as safe as standard methods in terms of sterility and apyrogenicity of the fluid infused. These methods are in line with applicable standards, provided that the producer clearly defines the limits of safe use of the methods and that the users, the physicians and nurses, ensure that such limits are effectively respected in routine clinical practice.

Among the many different online treatments available today, PHF offers some special and unique characteristics. For the same performance and sterility, PHF is the only online method currently available that makes it possible to verify, in the course of the treatment, the integrity of the ultrafilter membrane in which the final filtration of the dialysis fluid occurs. Acetate-free PHF reduces both acetate burden and cytokine activation. Clinical advantages due to these effects should be evaluated in properly designed prospective studies. Should our data be corroborated in a broader population observed over an appropriate period of time, then acetate-free PHF may become the top standard of convective online treatments.

References

1 Henderson LW, Beans E: Successful production of sterile pyrogen-free electrolyte solution by ultrafiltration. Kidney Int 1978;14:522–525.

2 Ramperez P, Beau MC, Deschodt G, et al: Economic preparation of sterile pyrogen free infusate for haemofiltration. Proc EDTA 1981;18:293–296.

3 Luehmann D, Hirsch D, Collins A, Shapiro F, Keshaviah P: Central on-site preparation of substitution fluid for hemofiltration. Trans ASAIO 1984;30:195–198.

4 Canaud B, Nguyen QV, Lagarde C, Stec F, Polaschegg HD, Mion C: Clinical evaluation of a multipurpose dialysis system adequate for hemodialysis or for postdilution hemofiltration/hemodiafiltration with on-line preparation of substitution fluid from dialysate; in Streicher E, Seyffart G (eds): Highly Permeable Membranes. Contrib Nephrol. Basel, Karger, 1985, vol 46, pp 184–186.

5 Rindi P, Pilone N, Ricci V, Cioni L: Clinical experience with a new hemodiafiltration (HDF) system. Trans ASAIO 1988;34:765–768.
6 David S, Caserta C, Cambi V: Preparazione estemporanea di soluzioni sterili ed apirogene di sostituzione: Liquido di dialisi liquidi di sostituzione. Milano, Wichtig, 1989, pp 59–64.
7 Pizzarelli F, Cerrai T, Dattolo P, Neri V, Maggiore Q: L'emodiafiltrazione con preparazione on-line del reinfusato è fattibile e sicura; in La Greca G, Petrella E, Cioni A (eds): I liquidi nella dialisi. Milano, Ghedini, 1992, pp 131–137.
8 Sternby J: A decade of experience with on-line hemofiltration/hemodiafiltration; in Maeda K, Shinzato T (eds): Effective Hemodiafiltration: New Methods. Contrib Nephrol. Basel, Karger, 1994, vol 108, pp 1–11.
9 Canaud B, Flavier JL, Argils A, Stec F, N'Guyen QV, Bouloux C, Garred LJ, Mion C: Hemodiafiltration with on-line production of substitution fluid: long-term safety and quantitative assessment of efficacy; in Maeda K, Shinzato T (eds): Effective Hemodiafiltration: New Methods. Contrib Nephrol. Basel, Karger, 1994, vol 108, pp 12–22.
10 von Albertini B, Mishkin G, Lew SQ, Velasquez M, Bosch JP: Long-term survival outcome with high efficiency dialysis: effects of time, membrane and reuse. J Am Soc Nephrol 1996;7:1468.
11 Pizzarelli F, Cerrai T, Dattolo P, Tetta C, Maggiore Q: Convective treatments with on-line production of replacement fluid: a clinical experience lasting 6 years. Nephrol Dial Transplant 1998;13: 363–369.
12 Pizzarelli F, Maggiore Q: Clinical perspectives of on-line hemodiafiltration. Nephrol Dial Transplant 1998;13(suppl 5):34–37.
13 Canaud B, Wizemann V, Pizzarelli F, Greenwood R, Schultze G, Weber C, Falkenhagen D: Cellular interleukin-1 receptor antagonist in patients receiving on-line haemodiafiltration therapy. Nephrol Dial Transplant 2001;16:2181–2187.
14 Pirovano D: Regulatory issues for on-line haemodiafiltration. Nephrol Dial Transplant 1998; 13(suppl 5):21–23.
15 van Ypersele de Strihou C, Jadoul M, Malghem J, Maldague B, Jamart J: Effect of dialysis membrane and patient's age on signs of dialysis-related amyloidosis. The Working Party on Dialysis Amyloidosis. Kidney Int 1991;39:1012–1019.
16 Hakim RM, Wingard RL, Husni L, Parker RA, Parker TF: The effect of membrane biocompatibility on plasma β_2-microglobulin levels in chronic hemodialysis patients. J Am Soc Nephrol 1996; 7:472–478.
17 Locatelli F, Marcelli D, Conte F, Limido A, Malberti F, Spotti D: Comparison of mortality in ESRD patients on convective and diffusive extracorporeal treatments. The Registro Lombardo Dialisi e Trapianto. Kidney Int 1999;55:286–293.
18 Lornoy W, Becaus I, Billiouw JM, Sierens L, van Malderen P: Remarkable removal of β_2-microglobulin by on-line hemodiafiltration. Am J Nephrol 1998;18:105–108.
19 Locatelli F, Manzoni C, Di Filippo S: The importance of convective transport. Kidney Int Suppl 2002;80:115–120.
20 Canaud B, Bragg-Gresham JL, Marshall MR, et al: Mortality risk for patients receiving hemodiafiltration versus hemodialysis: European results from the DOPPS. Kidney Int 2006;69:2087–2093.
21 Eknoyan G, Beck GJ, Cheung AK, Hemo Study Group: Effect of dialysis dose and membrane flux in maintenance hemodialysis. N Engl J Med 2002;347:2010–2019.
22 Cheung AK, Levin N, Greene T, et al: Effects of high flux hemodialysis on clinical outcomes: results of the HEMO study. J Am Soc Nephrol 2003;14:3251–3263.
23 Ward RA, et al: A comparison of on-line hemodiafiltration and high-flux hemodialysis: a prospective clinical study. J Am Soc Nephrol 2000;11:2344–2350.
24 Wizemann V, et al: On-line haemodiafiltration versus low-flux haemodialysis: a prospective randomized study. Nephrol Dial Transplant 2000;15(suppl 1):43–48.
25 Maduell F, et al: Change from conventional haemodiafiltration to on-line haemodiafiltration. Nephrol Dial Transplant 1999;14:1202–1207.
26 Bonforte G, et al: Improvement of anemia in hemodialysis patients treated by hemodiafiltration with high-volume on-line prepared substitution fluid. Blood Purif 2002;20:357–363.
27 Vaslaki L, et al: On-line haemodiafiltration versus haemodialysis: stable haematocrit with less erythropoietin and improvement of other relevant blood parameters. Blood Purif 2006;24:163–173.

28 Pizzarelli F, Tetta C, Cerrai T, Maggiore Q: Double chamber online hemodiafiltration: a novel technique with intra-treatment monitoring of dialysate ultrafilter integrity. Blood Purif 2000;18: 237–241.
29 Pizzarelli F, Cerrai T, Tetta C: Paired hemodiafiltration: technical assessment and preliminary clinical results; in Locatelli F, Ronco C, Tetta C (eds): Polyethersulfone: Membranes for Multiple Clinical Applications. Contrib Nephrol. Basel, Karger, 2003, vol 138, pp 99–105.
30 Ghezzi PM, Frigato G, Fantini GF: Theoretical model and first clinical results of the paired filtration dialysis (PFD). Life Support System 1983;1(suppl 1):271–274.
31 Pizzarelli F, Cerrai T, Dattolo P, Ferro G: On-line haemodiafiltration with and without acetate. Nephrol Dial Transplant 2006;21:1648–1651.

Francesco Pizzarelli
Direttore UO Nefrologia e Dialisi, Ospedale SM Annunziata
Via dell'Antella 58
IT–50011 Antella, Firenze (Italy)
Tel./Fax +39 055 2496 223, E-Mail fpizzarelli@yahoo.com

Ronco C, Canaud B, Aljama P (eds): Hemodiafiltration.
Contrib Nephrol. Basel, Karger, 2007, vol 158, pp 138–152

Acetate-Free Biofiltration

Antonio Santoro[a], *Francesco Guarnieri*[b], *Emiliana Ferramosca*[a], *Fabio Grandi*[b]

[a]Department of Nephrology, Dialysis and Hypertension, Malpighi Hospital, and [b]Hospal SpA, Bologna, Italy

Abstract

Acetate-free biofiltration (AFB) is a hemodiafiltration technique that, technically as well as biologically speaking, has all the premises for being a perfectly biocompatible technique capable of satisfying even the demands of critical patients laden with comorbidities. Important clinical benefits to patients have been reported, such as a better correction of acid-base balance, an improved nutritional status and a better hemodynamic stability. In particular, as far as the cardiovascular instability is concerned, several studies have shown that the rationale behind a better hemodynamic stability is the overall absence of acetate usually present in the dialysis bath, which often leads to an impaired vascular tone and a reduced cardiac contractility. One of the powerful features of AFB is its adaptability to new devices and tools which can be easily and safely used. In AFB, potassium modulation in the dialysate is easily achieved. Thus, patients with elevated levels of predialysis potassium and a tendency to develop both intra- and interdialysis arrhythmias benefit most. Lastly, the possibility to associate AFB with devices like Hemocontrol (which allows for a feedback conditioning of blood volume) broadens its practical scope, not only for use with hypotension-prone patients, but also with hypertensive patients with massive increases in their interdialysis body weight. In this category of patients, avoiding the risk of dangerous hypovolemias allows for the achievement of dry body weight, thereby facilitating the control of arterial blood pressure and minimizing the clinical consequences of a chronic fluid overload.

Over the past few years, both the progressive increase in the mean age of patients on chronic dialysis and greater comorbidity, particularly cardiovascular pathologies and diabetes, have significantly increased the critical clinical status of patients undergoing extracorporeal dialysis.

The major repercussions of this clinical complexity can be observed in the symptoms of the hemodialysis (HD) sessions that have seen the return of hemodynamically unstable events and a greater incidence of intradialytic cardiac arrhythmias.

A technological response has followed chiefly by the development of new dialysis techniques and so-called online intradialytic monitoring that seeks to prevent critical situations and to continuously measure various physiological parameters of the patient, both of a hemodynamic and a biochemical kind.

Acetate-free biofiltration (AFB) is a hemodiafiltration technique that, technically as well as biologically speaking, has all the premises for being a perfectly biocompatible technique capable of satisfying the demands even of critical patients laden with comorbidities.

The History of Acetate-Free Biofiltration

The idea of an acetate-free dialysis technique, with no buffer at all, first originated about 25 years ago. The inventors of dialysis with intravenous bicarbonate infusion published their feasibility study in the USA in 1980 [1]. Just 2 years later, in Europe, Zucchelli et al. [2] developed *biofiltration*, a technical and conceptual modification of acetate dialysis, with the aim of decreasing the frequency and severity of some side effects related to acetate, such as intradialytic metabolic acidosis and hemodynamic intolerance to acetate. In 1984, simultaneously in Italy and France, AFB was launched [3].

Currently, almost all dialysis techniques contain some acetate in the dialysis fluid in order to keep it chemically stable. Acetate mainly has a chemical role, allowing for the improvement of the dialysis fluid's electrolytic stability. However, together with bicarbonate, acetate is also a source of buffers that restore the patient's acid-base balance. The proportion of acetate transferred by this mechanism may theoretically reach as much as one third or more of the total buffers transferred by diffusion to the patient [4]. This result has been confirmed by a clinical observation by Agliata et al. [5]. Acetate anions from the dialysis fluid in HD cross the dialysis membrane and the wall of the cell by diffusion. According to the Krebs cycle, acetate may lead to the generation of bicarbonate, increasing this ion's intracellular concentration. Bicarbonate anions from the dialysis bath in HD cross the dialysis membrane and restore the extracellular buffer level, until a concentration gradient is maintained. Meanwhile, bicarbonate from the intracellular space moves to the extracellular space due to the concentration gradient. Despite the small proportion of acetate in bicarbonate dialysis (BD), the level of plasma acetate may rise, as it has been shown by Higuchi et al. [6] in a study comparing AFB and BD. In that study, each patient was his/her own control and the pre and post dialysis plasma acetate levels were

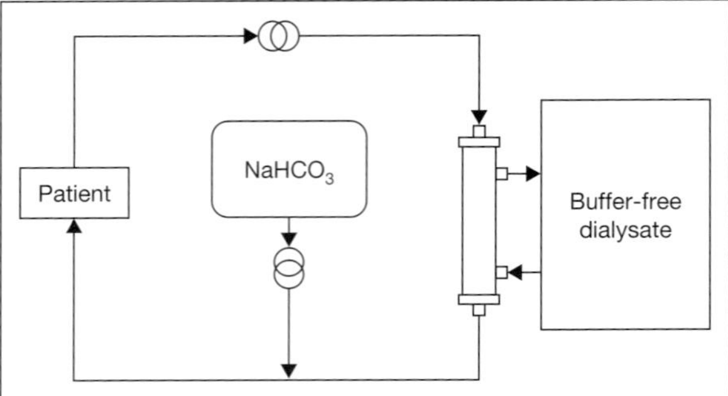

Fig. 1. The AFB technique setting.

0.24 ± 0.08 and 0.28 ± 0.06 mEq/l in AFB, respectively, and 0.3 ± 0.03 mEq/l and 0.42 ± 0.12 mEq/l in BD ($p < 0.05$).

Indeed, acetate is directly and indirectly involved in generating a number of side effects. Among these are hypoxia, vasodilatation and the increased production of inflammatory mediators, such as cytokines. All factors increase the risk of cardiovascular instability.

Technical Aspects of Acetate-Free Biofiltration

AFB is a diffusive-convective dialysis technique characterized by a completely buffer-free dialysis fluid, a highly biocompatible hemodialyzer, i.e. AN69ST, and a sodium bicarbonate substitution fluid infused to the patient in postdilution mode (fig. 1).

Unlike other diffusive-convective dialysis therapies, the absence of a buffer in the dialysis bath makes the correction of the acid-base balance very simple and controllable. The acid-base balance correction in AFB is achieved by the intravenous infusion of sodium bicarbonate. The overall bicarbonate mass balance is straightforward, because the process of bicarbonate removal from the filter and the bicarbonate restoration from the substitution fluid are completely separate so that the steady-state plasma bicarbonate can be computed as the ratio between the infusion flow rate and the bicarbonate clearance multiplied by the bicarbonate concentration of the substitution fluid. In practice, steady-state plasma bicarbonatemia can be preset at the beginning of the dialysis session and controlled during the treatment simply by the infusion and the blood flow rates. The dialysis monitor can be equipped with a surveillance system to supervise the bicarbonatemia recovery process during dialysis, thereby preventing accidental errors, which could potentially lead to patient acidosis or alkalosis states by the treatment end.

In order to better personalize the correction of metabolic acidosis in AFB, the importance of the patient buffer system should be considered during the intravenous administration of bicarbonate. Some authors have studied this system and developed a mathematical model based on the apparent bicarbonate distribution space (ABS), which is the volume of distribution of the bicarbonate. This model explains the relationship between blood pH and acid-base status in chronic dialysis patients. In particular, Fernandez et al. [7] have reckoned that the lower the bicarbonate serum concentration, the larger the ABS (and that the higher the bicarbonate serum level, the smaller the ABS). This model allows for a quantification of the amount of bicarbonate needed to modify the pH and the bicarbonate serum level to a given extent just by knowing the initial bicarbonatemia [8]. This fact then suggests that knowing the predialysis bicarbonate levels is essential when administering bicarbonate to the patient, so as to quantify the ABS and calculate the infusion flow rate of bicarbonate suitable for the patient.

The absence of acetate in the AFB bath is offset by adding an extra amount of chloride to make the bath electrochemically stable. Special attention ought to be paid to the role of chloride anion (Cl^-) concentration on conductivity, since chloride contributes to conductivity as much as the sodium cation. Dialysis fluid conductivity is indeed related to all cations and anions dissolved in the dialysis fluid, and not to sodium alone. A more elevated chloride concentration in the dialysis fluid, as well as for the AFB, affects the conductivity value, thereby triggering its increase. Furthermore, as chloride ions contribute to conductivity more than bicarbonate and acetate anions, the conductivity of the dialysis fluid in AFB is higher than that in BD. In order to achieve the same concentration of sodium in both BD and AFB, a higher value of dialysis fluid conductivity must be set in AFB.

AN69ST Dialysis Membrane for Acetate-Free Biofiltration

AFB, thanks to the highly biocompatible AN69ST dialysis membrane, is different from the other diffusive-convective therapies. The AN69ST membrane is superior in terms of absorption clearances, particularly of high-molecular-weight molecules, which are responsible for severe pathologies. The recent innovative treatment (ST stands for 'surface-treated') applied to the membrane surface by using macromolecules, such as polyethylene imines, allowed for the creation of a more neutral surface, characterized by areas with a high density of electrically positive charges that can absorb heparin molecules in a stable way [9]. This allows for dialysis treatments with a reduced heparin regimen, or with a total absence of heparin as a systemic anticoagulant [10, 11]. AN69ST maintains the same characteristics as the original AN69 membrane in terms of cytokine absorption.

Clinical Results

Since its first clinical application [12, 13], important clinical benefits to patients have been reported, such as a better correction of acid-base balance, an improved nutritional status and a better hemodynamic stability.

Correction of Metabolic Acidosis and Nutritional Status

Metabolic acidosis leads to several important complications, amongst which there is the muscular catabolism stimulus accompanied by a reduction in lean body mass, a progressive loss of calcium and sodium carbonate from the bone and cardiovascular instability, mainly due to an increase in peripheral vascular resistances secondary to a sympathetic reflex. The ease with which uremic acidosis can be corrected is one of the prerogatives of AFB. Santoro and numerous colleagues [4–14] have established statistical models that rapidly allow us to obtain, from the patient's bedside, the desired target values of post-dialysis bicarbonate levels. In a study on 81 patients followed for 67 months, Movilli et al. [15] found that bicarbonatemia seems to be directly correlated with serum albumin ($p = 0.001$) and inversely correlated with the protein catabolic rate ($p = 0.027$). In particular, by clustering the patients into two groups (HCO_3^- <20 mmol and HCO_3^- >23 mmol) the level of serum albumin was around 3.95 and 4.17 g/dl, respectively. The clinical results were very important as far as the so-called fragile patients are concerned, such as the elderly. In this group of patients, AFB offers a better correction of metabolic acidosis, allowing us to achieve a better predialysis blood pH level as compared with standard BD and hemodiafiltration.

Galli et al. [16] have investigated the role of dialysis therapies on cardiovascular stability and nutritional status by comparing AFB and BD in a 1-year longitudinal study on 18 patients. As far as the nutritional status is concerned, they found that the serum albumin level increased from 3.8 to 4.1 g/dl ($p = 0.013$), while postdialysis bicarbonatemia and pH were 30.2 ± 3.6 mmol in AFB and 26.1 ± 3.2 mmol in BD ($p = 0.017$) and 7.44 ± 0.05 in AFB and 7.48 ± 0.04 in BD ($p = 0.038$). Also, Chiappini et al. [17] found that AFB seems to be responsible for a better nutritional status with higher prealbumin values compared to conventional dialysis (118.8 ± 14.3 in AFB vs. 97.8 ± 15.8% of normal value in BD) and lower levels of interleukin 1β (10.3 ± 7.4 in AFB vs. 15.6 ± 7.0 pg/ml in BD).

Acetate-Free Biofiltration and Improvement of Hemodynamic Stability

Both AFB and hemodiafiltration, as compared with standard BD, offer a better dialysis tolerance in elderly patients, as reported by Movilli et al. [18, 19]. Very important are the clinical results related to dialysis patients with cardiovascular and cerebrovascular disease. In such a group, a lower frequency of neurological symptoms in AFB as compared with BD has been reported [20]. The clinical benefits obtained in the diabetic patients were considered by the Italian Society of Nephrology, which set AFB as the gold standard for the treatment of diabetic patients with marked intolerance to conventional dialysis [21].

At the beginning of dialysis, hypotension can be seen as being linked to both nonautonomic and autonomic causes. As said before, one of the causes of cardiovascular instability is intolerance to the acetate present in the dialysis bath. By different mechanisms, the acetate can provoke cardiovascular instability. In particular, increased nitric oxide synthesis provokes a relaxation in the vessel smooth muscles, causing an increase in the internal diameter of the vessel.

The different potential of various dialysis fluids in provoking nitric oxide generation was reported in 1997 by an in vitro study by Amore et al. [22]. Furthermore, the effect of AFB on peripheral vascular disease, in comparison to standard dialysis, was demonstrated by Bufano et al. [23] in 2000. Nitric oxide is also involved in the pathogenesis mechanisms of vascular damage. Amore et al. [24] further assessed the beneficial effects of AFB in reducing the risk of vascular damage.

In that study, the inflammatory status was evaluated by means of the measurement of nitric oxide synthase activity on lymphocytes and monocytes, endothelial cells and smooth muscle cells coming from the blood of healthy donors, after incubation following different simulations of dialysis treatment. All the studied markers showed a higher nitric oxide synthase activity in BD. Furthermore, lymphomonocytes treated with BD activate the smooth muscle cells. Bearing in mind that the different treatments had all been performed using the same dialysis membrane and the same biological quality of the dialysis bath (endotoxin-free), any clinical difference highlighted by this study can only be attributed to the presence or the absence of acetate in the standard dialysis and AFB baths, respectively.

We have analyzed 9 clinical studies on AFB, focusing particularly on cardiovascular stability, specifically on the capacity of AFB to prevent dialysis-related hypotension. Table 1 presents the main qualitative and quantitative information related to these studies [25–30]. The overall population is made up of around 200 patients, and the studies' follow-up is between 4 and 12 months. The pooled analysis started calculating the 'odds ratio' and respective confidence interval at the 95% level in each of the 9 studies. The odds ratio was calculated by computing the proportion of dialyses complicated by hypotension from the data reported in each study. The pooled odds ratio was then calculated by the Peto-Yusuf method (fig. 2). The ratio means the odds ratio of hypotensive symptoms in AFB in relation to BD; hence, values below 1 favor to AFB, while

Table 1. Main characteristics of the studies used in the systematic analysis of hypotension in AFB versus BD

Author	Year	Multi-center	Centers	Study length months	Experi-mental design	Random-ized	PRV	Patients	Male/female	Age years	Time on dialysis months
Ronco et al. [25]	1988	no	1	6	p-g	yes	no	6		55	
Briganti et al. [20]	1991	yes	7	8	c-o	yes	yes	48	29/19	54	62.8
Galli et al. [16]	1992	no	1	6	c-o	no	yes	18	7/11	64.5	22
SCS [26]	1992	yes		12	c-o	no	yes	33	15/18	49	
Kuno et al. [27]	1994	no	1	6	c-o	no	yes	6	3/3	48	158
Movilli et al. [19]	1996	no	1	18	c-o	yes	yes	12	7/5	76	18
Verzetti et al. [28]	1998	yes	13	12	c-o	yes	yes	41	24/17	60	25
Schrander-van der Meer et al. [29]	1999	no	1	12	p-g	yes	no	24	11/9	65	68
Cavalcanti et al. [30]	2004	no	1	4	c-o	yes	no	12	4/8	73.8	4
Overall								*200*			

PRV = Primary response variable; patients = number of enrolled patients; p-g = parallel group; c-o = cross-over; SCS = Spanish Cooperative Study.

values above 1 favor to BD. The probability of intradialysis hypotension in AFB is about 40% of the probability of dialysis hypotension in BD.

The Evolution of Acetate-Free Biofiltration

Potassium-Profiled and Blood-Volume-Tracking in Acetate-Free Biofiltration

Potassium-profiled AFB (AFBK) is a recently introduced modified AFB whose purpose is to prevent sudden variations in plasma potassium that can be potentially risky for the onset of arrhythmias during dialysis.

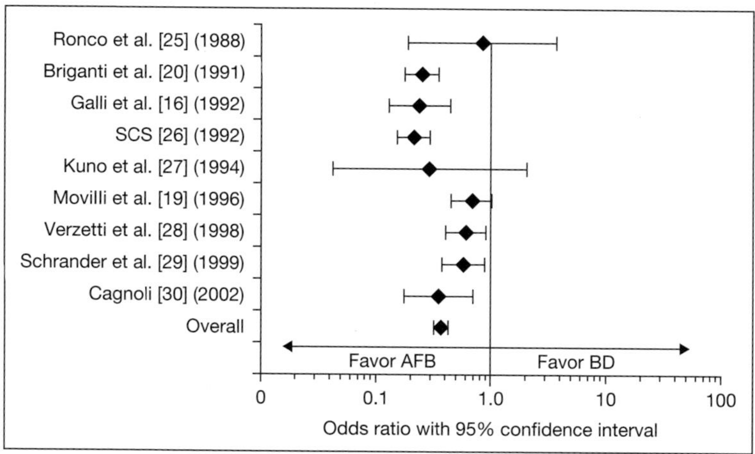

Fig. 2. Systematic analysis of the peer-reviewed data from the literature on hypotension in AFB versus BD. The value of the overall odds ratio calculated by Mantel-Haenszel statistics is 0.4.

AFBK is based on conventional AFB, but the dialysate potassium decreases over time from an initial to a final value in a exponential-like pattern (fig. 3). This potassium profile can be established by the use of 2 independent concentrate fluid pumps connected with the dialysis monitor and a double-compartment concentrate bag, containing potassium-rich AFB concentrate in the small compartment and potassium-free concentrate in the large one. During AFBK the potassium level is reduced while the other electrolytes (sodium, calcium, magnesium) remain constant in the course of the treatment. This facilitates the achievement of the desired potassium mass balance in the patient by a smoother potassium removal rate since the concentration gradient between the blood and the dialysis fluid is kept more constant over the treatment time. Thus, equivalent overall potassium removal has been shown to be obtained by adjusting the initial and final dialysate potassium levels [31]. A more constant potassium concentration gradient also limits the negative effects of extracellular potassium removal on the electrophysiology of cardiac cells.

The clinical indications for end-stage renal disease patients on dialysis to undergo AFBK is hyperkalemia, and patients who are highly prone to intradialysis and interdialysis arrhythmias, such as those with diabetes mellitus, hypertension and cardiomyopathy, may also benefit significantly from this therapy.

The major prevalence of diabetes, anemia, hyperparathyroidism and hypertension among chronic dialysis patients engenders structural heart disease. Moreover, fluid overload and metabolic abnormalities such as metabolic aci-

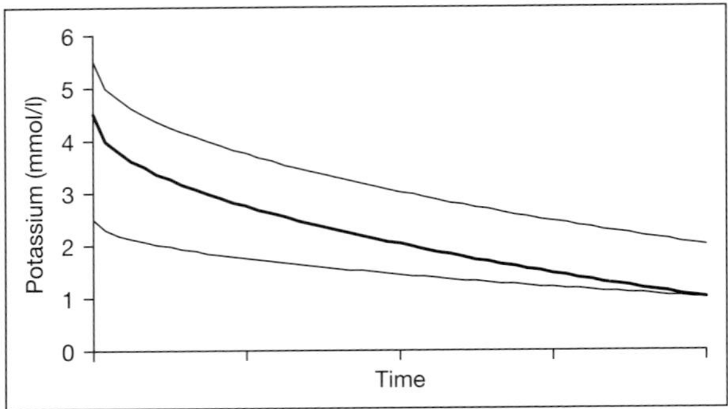

Fig. 3. Dialysate potassium profiles in AFBK. The upper and lower limits assure that the patient cannot be exposed to harmful concentrations of dialysate potassium. By adjusting the values at the beginning and at the end of the dialysis, the overall potassium removal can be set prior to the beginning of the dialysis.

dosis, dyskalemia or dysmagnesemia lead to an increased risk of clinically significant ventricular arrhythmias and sudden cardiac death. During the dialysis procedure, the dialysis patients present a nonhomogeneous repolarization, and this is confirmed by the increase in Q–T duration and Q–T dispersion [32]. The dialysis-related sudden variations in extracellular potassium, calcium and pH may be corroborating factors in the genesis of an electrical disequilibrium in myocardial cells. One of the potential therapeutic options is indeed the adjustment of the dialysis fluid composition. A multicenter crossover clinical study aimed at investigating the electrical behavior of two different K^+ removal rates upon myocardial cells (risk of arrhythmia and ECG alterations) has recently been performed [31]. Conventional AFB and AFBK were used in a patient sample to understand the effect on premature ventricular contraction (PVC) and on repolarization indices. The study was divided into two phases: phase 1 was a pilot study to evaluate K^+ kinetics and to test the effect on the electrophysiological response of the two procedures. The second phase was set up as an extended crossover multicenter trial in a patient subset prone to arrhythmias during dialysis.

The main result of the phase 1 of the study was that serum potassium showed a marked decrease in conventional AFB during the first half of dialysis, greater than in AFBK. The greatest difference in serum potassium was achieved at 60 min after the start of dialysis (4.1 ± 0.4 mEq/l in AFBK vs. 3.8 ± 0.4 mEq/l in AFB) while the final values were equivalent in both treatments. Despite this difference in serum potassium, the final potassium removed by AFB and AFBK was comparable (88 ± 15 mEq in AFBK vs. 92 ± 19 mEq in AFB).

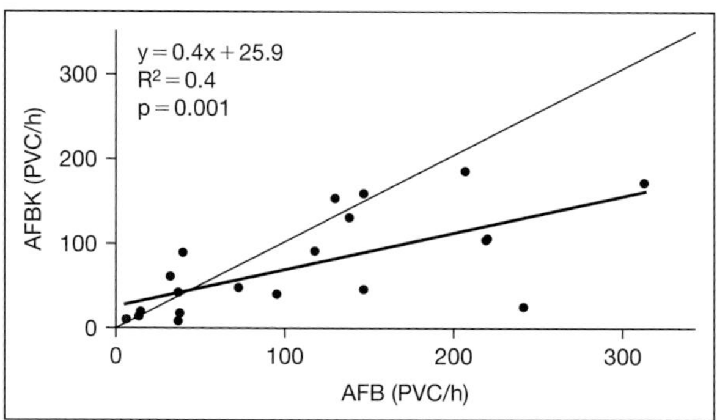

Fig. 4. Scatter plot of PVC per hour in AFBK against standard AFB. The thin line is the identity line, the thick one is the regression line [32].

The ANOVA for repeated measures applied to the PVC per hour did not show any statistical differences ($p = 0.428$), but in a patient subgroup (at least within grade II of Lown grading, i.e. number of PVC per hour >30) these were consistently lower in AFBK than in AFB ($p = 0.02$, Wilcoxon test).

During phase 2 the PVC again increased in both AFB and AFBK, although less so in the latter halfway through dialysis (fig. 4). By plotting the PVC per hour in AFBK against the those in AFB, most of the values lie below the bisector indicating a marked reduction in arrhythmias in AFBK. By means of this study, it was possible to show that it is not the K^+ removal rate alone that may be destabilizing from an electrophysiological standpoint, but rather its removal dynamics. This is all the more evident in patients with arrhythmias who benefit from the K^+ profiling during their dialysis treatment.

A possible explanation for this finding has recently been published by Buemi et al. [33], who investigated the clinical effects of AFBK as compared with conventional AFB on the repolarization indexes (Q–T interval corrected, $Q–T_c$, and $Q–T_c$ dispersion) in 28 patients (fig. 5). The indexes were assessed in the midweek dialysis at the times 0, 15, 45, 90, 120 and 240 min during dialysis. It is worth noting that the time patterns of the parameters were different between the two therapies with a rapid increase in AFB and a stable behavior in AFBK. Again, as previously reported by Santoro et al. [31], the discriminant was the different plasma potassium time pattern. In fact, plasma potassium decreased more slowly in AFBK than in BD. The highest difference was found at 15, 45 and 90 min after the start of dialysis ($p < 0.01$), which could partly explain the related effect on the ventricular repolarization.

The blood volume tracking (BVT) system is a tool designed to prevent a severe fall in blood volume during HD that potentially exposes patients to

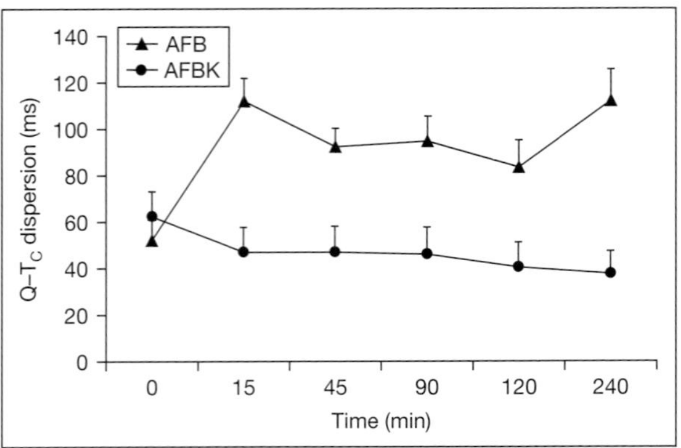

Fig. 5. Repolarization index Q–T_c dispersion in AFBK compared to AFB [34]. Significant differences were found at 45, 90 and 120 min ($p < 0.05$). However, AFB showed a fast increase in the first part of dialysis not observed in AFBK, the values of which remained stable throughout the session.

volume-dependent hypotension. The main goal of BVT is to drive the actual patient's blood volume along an ideal blood volume trajectory by a continuous adjustment of two dialysis parameters: the ultrafiltration rate and the dialysis fluid conductivity. The ideal trajectory is chosen in a way that the blood volume will decrease less during dialysis with BVT than during a number of test dialyses in which dialysis hypotension developed. BVT has two further goals: the achievement of total weight loss and the prevention of sodium overload in the patient. It is clear that the three different goals are mutually contradictory, so the BVT system continuously searches for the best solution or compromise among these three goals. To do so efficiently, the system is given some tolerances, with adjustable width, as regards each of the three goals.

A number of publications highlight that BVT dialysis leads to a decrease in both the frequency and the severity of dialysis hypotension, particularly in the hypotension-prone patient. In the meantime, there have also been some reports on the benefits of BVT in patients experiencing dialysis hypotension only incidentally.

The above-mentioned studies were all aimed at understanding the relative role played by BVT alone in preventing dialysis-related hypotension. Nevertheless, BVT only acts on one factor involved in intradialytic symptoms, such as volume-dependent hypotension. Then, to further improve dialysis tolerance, the idea of combining BVT and AFB seems to be promising, as AFB acts on other factors, namely vascular resistance and cardiac output.

The first attempt to show an improvement in the treatment tolerance was made by Ronco et al. [34] who compared AFB and BVT-AFB in 12 patients with frequent dialysis hypotensions. That study showed that in the presence of similar weight loss rates (3,646 ± 684 ml without BVT vs. 3,710 ± 710 with BVT, p = n.s.), cardiovascular tolerance significantly improved in the biofeedback-driven sessions (hypotension episodes 59/72 without BVT vs. 24/72 with BVT, $p < 0.001$). That study also showed a possible positive effect of the improved cardiovascular stability on urea kinetics and treatment efficiency (equilibrated Kt/V 1.03 ± 0.01 without BVT vs. 1.12 ± 0.05 with BVT, $p < 0.001$), accounted for as the result of an improved tissue perfusion highlighted by a reduced urea rebound (14.2 ± 2.7% without BVT vs. 6.4 ± 2.3% with BVT, $p < 0.001$).

Further evidence emerged from a study by Santoro et al. [31], aimed at investigating the cardiovascular compensatory response to hypovolemia in a population of 12 HD patients, by means of a model-based computer analysis of BVT-AFB against conventional dialysis. A novel result was that the critical blood volume threshold (i.e. the relative blood volume change at which acute hypotension appeared) was significantly lower in BD than in BVT-AFB, that is to say less negative (−7.9 ± 2%) in BD than BVT-AFB (−10.9 ± 2.6%, $p < 0.05$). As direct consequence, hypotensive events occurred earlier in BD than in BVT-AFB (collapse time 123 ± 41 min in BD vs. 183 ± 25 min in BVT-AFB, $p < 0.01$).

Differences in the effectiveness of compensation to hypovolemia were evident in the control of microvascular resistance and the efficacy of inotropic control on cardiac contractility. The result of the computer-based analysis is that the estimated total peripheral resistance increased twice as much in BVT-AFB than in BD (change in total peripheral resistance 9.1 ± 9.4% in BD vs. 18.9 ± 6.6% in BVT-AFB, $p < 0.05$), whereas the decrease in the estimated stroke volume was twice as high in BD (change in stroke volume −19.1 ± 8.2% in BD vs. −10.7 ± 7.8% in BVT-AFB, $p < 0.01$).

A deeper insight into the same experiment was gained by the analysis of heart rate variability [35]. This revealed that the low-frequency component in BD, after an initial increase, slowly became depressed (from 0.56 ± 0.19 nU at the beginning of dialysis to 0.56 ± 0.22 at the end in BD, yet from 0.59 ± 0.14 nU at the beginning to 0.67 ± 0.12 nU at the end of dialysis in BVT-AFB, $p < 0.05$).

The low-frequency component of heart rate variability reflects the autonomic activation of the mechanisms controlling the cardiovascular functions. The lowering of the low-frequency component in BD is therefore consistent with a worsened effectiveness of vasoconstriction and cardiac contractility even in the presence of significant adrenergic activation (heart rate increase from 72 ± 9 at the beginning to 75 ± 10 beats/min at the end in BVT-AFB, vs. 73 ± 10 at the beginning to 85 ± 10 beats/min at the end in BD, $p < 0.05$).

Conclusions

AFB is definitely one of most user-friendly hemodiafiltration techniques. Indeed, the chance to modify the composition of the dialysis bath and the bicarbonate solution to be infused either alternatively or simultaneously gives it a versatility that is not at all typical of the online techniques. As a matter of fact, in the online techniques the composition of the dialysis liquid cannot be separated from that of the infusion liquid. This is a major drawback that often undermines their adaptability to the patient's needs. In AFB, the potassium modulation in the dialysate is easily achieved and is starting to bear its fruits in clinical terms. Patients with elevated levels of predialysis potassium and a tendency to develop both intra- and interdialysis arrhythmias benefit most. Lastly, the chance to associate AFB with devices such as Hemocontrol (which allows for a feedback conditioning of the blood volume) broadens its practical scope, not only for hypotension-prone patients, but also hypertensive patients with massive increases in their interdialysis body weight. In this category of patients, avoiding the risk of dangerous hypovolemias allows for the achievement of dry body weight, thereby facilitating the control of arterial blood pressure and minimizing the clinical consequences of a chronic fluid overload.

References

1 Van Stone JC, Mitchell A: Hemodialysis with base-free dialysate. Proc Dialysis Transplant Forum 1980;10:268–271.

2 Zucchelli P, Santoro A, Raggiotto G, Degli Esposti E, Sturani A, Capecchi V: Biofiltration in uremia: preliminary observations. Blood Purif 1984;2:187–195.

3 Buoncristiani U, Ragaiolo M, Petrucci V, Bruni F, Pala E, Damiani C, Brugnano R: Biofiltration with buffer-free dialysate. Int J Artif Organs 1986;9(suppl 3):9–14.

4 Santoro A, Spongano M, Ferrari G, Bolzani R, Augella F, Borghi M, Briganti M, Cagnoli L, Docci D, Feletti C, et al: Analysis of the factors influencing bicarbonate balance during acetate-free biofiltration. Kidney Int 1993;41(suppl):S184–S187.

5 Agliata S, Atti M, Fortina F, Airoldi G, Baroni A, Ragazzoni E, Schweiger C, Cavagnino A: Acetate in the dialysate in bicarbonato dialysis (abstract); in Ward RA, Golper TA (eds): Abstracts of the Tenth Annual Meeting of the International Society of Blood Purification, Louisville, October 1992. Blood Purif 1992;10(special issue).

6 Higuchi T, Kuno T, Takahashi S, Kanmatsuse K: Chronic effect of long-term acetate-free biofiltration in the production of interleukin 1β and interleukin-1 receptor antagonist by peripheral blood mononuclear cells. Am J Nephrol 1997;17:428–434.

7 Fernandez PC, Cohen RM, Feldman GM: The concept of bicarbonate distribution space: the crucial role of body buffers. Kidney Int 1989;36:747–752.

8 Pacitti A, Casino FG, Pedrini l, Santoro A, Atti M: Prescription and surveillance of the acetate-free biofiltration sessions: the bicarbonate cycle. Int J Artif Organs 1995;18:722–725.

9 Renaux JL, Atti M: The AN69ST dialysis membrane; in Ronco C, La Greca G (eds): Hemodialysis Technology. Contrib Nephrol. Basel, Karger, 2002, vol 137, pp 111–119.

10 Chanard J: Assessment of heparin-binding to the AN69 ST hemodialysis membrane. I. Preclinical study. ASAIO J 2005;51:342–347.

11 Lavaud S: Assessment of the heparin binding AN69 ST hemodialysis membrane. II. Clinical studies without heparin administration. ASAIO J 2005;51:348–351.
12 Bandiani G, Camaiora E, Nicolini MA, Perotta U: Tolerance and adequacy of acetate-free biofiltration (AFB): two years clinical experience (abstract). Proc EDTA Congr, Madrid, 1988, p 148.
13 Bandiani G, Camaiora E, Nicolini MA, Perotta U: The acid-base balance during acetate-free biofiltration (AFB) (abstract). Proc EDTA Congr, Madrid, 1988, p 148.
14 Santoro A, Ferrari G, Spongano M, Badiali F, Zucchelli P: Acetate-free biofiltration: a viable alternative to bicarbonate dialysis. Artif Organs 1989;13:476–479.
15 Movilli E, Bossini N, Viola BF, Camerini C, Cancarini G, Feller P, Strada A, Maiorca R: Evidence for an independent role of metabolic acidosis on nutritional status in hemodialysis patients. Nephrol Dial Transplant 1998;13:125–131.
16 Galli G, Bianco F, Panzetta G: Acetate free biofiltration: an effective treatment for high-risk dialysis patients; in Man NK, Rotella J, Zucchelli P (eds): Blood Purification in Perspective: New Insight and Future Trend. Cleveland, ICAOT Press, 1992, No 320, vol 2.
17 Chiappini MG, Moscatelli M, Batoli R: Effects of different hemodialysis methods on the nutritional status of HD patients. Ren Fail 1990;12:277–278.
18 Movilli E, Gaggiotti M, Maiorca R: Hemodiafiltration in hypotension-prone elderly uremic patients. Geriatr Nephrol Urol 1995;4:183–187.
19 Movilli E, Camerini C, Zein H, D'Avolio G, Sandrini M, Strada A, Maiorca R: A prospective comparison of bicarbonate dialysis, hemodiafiltration and acetate-free biofiltration in the elderly. Am J Kidney Dis 1996;27:541–547.
20 Briganti M, Borghi M, Cagnoli L, Feletti C, Fusaroli M, Sanna G, Santoro A, Stallone C, Zucchelli P: Valutazione clinica e neurologica della biofiltrazione senza acetato: studio multicentrico. G Ital Nefrol 1991;8:291–297.
21 Fuiano G, Zoccali C: Linee guida per la diagnosi e la terapia della nefropatia diabetica. G Ital Nefrol 2003;20(suppl):S96–S108.
22 Amore S, Cirina P, Mitola S, Peruzzi L, Bonaudo R, Gianoglio B, Coppo R: acetate intolerance is mediated by enhanced synthesis of nitric oxide by endothelial cells. J Am Soc Nephrol 1997;8: 1431–1436.
23 Bufano G, Grandi F, Ariano R, Atti M: Plasma levels of nitric oxide (NO) and peripheral vascular resistances (PVR) during hemodialysis (abstract 1358). J Am Soc Nephrol 2000, Abstr 33rd Annu Meet ASN, Toronto, p 258A.
24 Amore A, Cirina P, Bonaudo R, Conti G, Chiesa M, Coppo R: Bicarbonate dialysis, unlike acetate-free biofiltration, triggers mediators of inflammation and apoptosis in endothelial and smooth muscle cells. J Nephrol 2006;19:57–64.
25 Ronco C, Fabris A, Chiaromonte S, De Dominicis E, Feriani M, Brendolan A, Brigantini L, Milan M, Dell'Aquila R, La Greca G: Comparison of four different short dialysis techniques. Int J Artif Organs 1988;11:169–174.
26 Junco E, Aljama P, Arias M, Bocal J, Rotella J, Caralps A, Castello D, Luno J, Martin de Francisco AL, Martin Malo A, Montenegro J, Perez R, Sanz C, Saracco J, Teixido J, Valderrabano F, Madero R: Acetate free biofiltration: Spanish Cooperative Study; in Man NK, Rotella J, Zucchelli P (eds): Blood Purification in Perspective: New Insight and Future Trend. Cleveland, ICAOT Press, 1992, No 320, vol 2.
27 Kuno T, Kikuchi F, Yanai M, Nagura Y, Takahashi S: Clinical advantages of acetate-free biofiltration; in Maeda K, Shinzato T (eds): Effective Hemodiafiltration: New Methods. Contrib Nephrol. Basel, Karger, 1994, vol 108, pp 123–130.
28 Verzetti G, Navino C, Bolzani R, Galli G, Panzetta G: Acetate-free biofiltration versus bicarbonate hemodialysis in the treatment of patients with diabetic nephropathy: a cross-over multicentric study. Nephrol Dial Transplant 1998;13:955–961.
29 Schrander-van der Meer AM, Ter Wee PM, Kan G, Donker AJ, Van Dorp WT: Improved cardiovascular variables during acetate-free biofiltration. Clin Nephrol 1999;51:304–309.
30 Cavalcanti S, Ciandrini A, Severi S, Badiali F, Bini S, Gattiani A, Cagnoli L, Santoro A: Model based study of the effects of the hemodialysis technique on the compensatory response to hypovolemia. Kidney Int 2004;65:1499–1510.

31 Santoro A, Mancini E, Gaggi R, Cavalcanti S, Severi S, Cagnoli L, Badiali F, Perrone B, London G, Fessy H, Mercadal L, Grandi F: Electrophysiological response to dialysis: the role of dialysate potassium content and profiling; in Ronco C, Brendolan A, Levin NW (eds): Cardiovascular Disorders in Hemodialysis. Contrib Nephrol. Basel, Karger, 2005, vol 149, pp 295–305.

32 Cupisti A, Galetta F, Caprioli R, Morelli E, Tintori GC, Franzoni F, lippi A, Meola M, Rindi P, Barsotti G: Potassium removal increases the QTc interval dispersion during hemodialysis. Nephron 1999;82:122–126.

33 Buemi M, Aloisi E, Coppolino G, et al: The effect of two different protocols of potassium haemodiafiltration on QT dispersion. Nephrol Dial Transplant 2005;20:1148–1154.

34 Ronco C, Brendolan A, Milan M, Rodeghiero MP, Zanella M, La Greca G: Impact of biofeedback-induced cardiovascular stability on hemodialysis tolerance and efficiency. Kidney int 2000;58: 800–808.

35 Severi S, Ciandrini A, Grandi E, Cavalcanti S, Bini S, Badiali F, Gattini A, Cagnoli L: Cardiac response to hemodialysis with different cardiovascular tolerance: heart rate variability and QT interval analysis. Hemodial Int 2006;10:287–293.

Antonio Santoro, MD
Department of Nephrology, Dialysis and Hypertension, Malpighi Hospital
Via P. Pelagi, 9
IT–40138 Bologna (Italy)
E-Mail santoro@aosp.bo.it

Ronco C, Canaud B, Aljama P (eds): Hemodiafiltration.
Contrib Nephrol. Basel, Karger, 2007, vol 158, pp 153–160

Mid-Dilution: An Innovative High-Quality and Safe Haemodiafiltration Approach

Jacky Potier

Centre Hospitalier Louis-Pasteur, Cherbourg, France

Abstract

Mid-dilution (MidD) is a new concept allowing post- and predilution in the same dialyser (Olpur® MD 190). The aim of the study was to compare, in 6 patients, MidD with post- and predilution wird regard to purification tests, such as reduction ratios and instantaneous whole-blood clearances, of urea, creatinine and phosphorus as examples of low-weight molecules and of β_2-microglobulin as an example of a middle molecule (MM). The aim was also to indicate directions for the use of this new dialyser, taking into account our own experience and the few observations already published. It was concluded that MidD, under excellent safety conditions, in spite of increased intradialyser pressures, offers a very high purification performance, particularly for MM, because of high convective volumes exceeding the recommended objectives for a better survival in dialysis.

Traditionally, there are 2 methods of haemodiafiltration (HDF): postdilution (PostD) and predilution (PreD), each with counter-indications determined by their potential risks. PostD, because of haemoconcentration on the outlet side of the dialyser, increases the risks of coagulation and increase in the transmembrane pressure (TMP), the more so when the blood flow (Q_B) is low or the haematocrit (Hct) is high. PreD decreases the purification of the small molecules because of haemodilution in the dialyser, unless a high substitution flow (Q_S) is used. The idea of a joint use of the 2 methods is the origin of mixed dilution [1]. The variation of the 2 substitution fluid flow rates, PostD and PreD, throughout the session is subjected to an objective of TMP and leads to use first the purifying capacity of PostD, then at the end of dialysis the protective advantage of PreD. The joint association of the 2 methods is also at the origin of mid-dilution (MidD), a new concept based on the Olpur MD 190 dialyser (Nephros Inc., New York, N.Y., USA), already available and usable on all monitors equipped with an online production of dialysate for HDF.

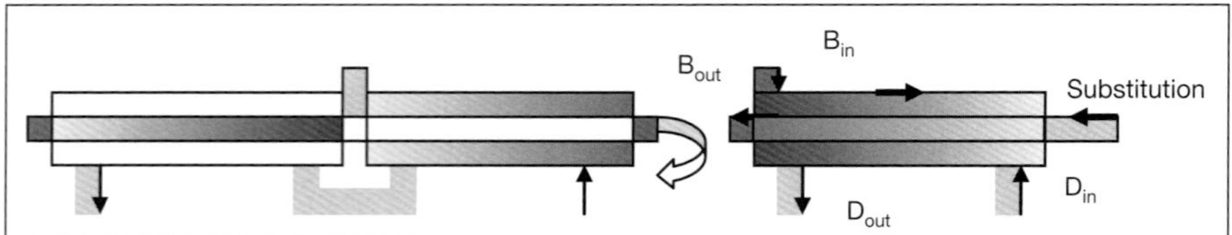

Fig. 1. Origin of Olpur MD 190 from 2 dialysers in series, the first (PostD) without its peripheral fibres and the second (PreD) without its central fibres. The 180-degree rotation of the second on the first results in a single dialyser with 2 blood stages, in which the dialysate flows with the blood in the second PreD stage and against the blood in the PostD stage. B_{in} = Inlet blood; B_{out} = outlet blood; D_{in} = inlet dialysate; D_{out} = outlet dialysate.

Concept

The initial principle (fig. 1) is to use in series 2 dialysers, with a first stage in PostD and a second in PreD. For practical reasons, a single dialyser was used thanks to a 180-degree rotation of the PreD component.

The Olpur 190 MD is thus the manufactured product resulting from this new concept. It is composed of polyethersulphone fibres (wall thickness = 35 µm, inner diameter = 210 µm) with a total surface of 1.90 m^2. In its initial configuration, 1.10 m^2 were devoted to PostD (peripheral fibres) and 0.80 m^2 to PreD (central fibres).

In fact, the first clinical trials in this configuration highlighted an instability of the pressures in the dialyser, manifested by a high TMP and a necessary reduction of the total convection volume, manifestly lower than the target expected by the system's designer.

The first modification [2] consisted in inverting the blood connections – an operation called simple reverse (SR) – the PreD stage becoming PostD and vice versa. The internal haemodynamic dialyser conditions were thus manifestly improved, allowing a Qs >200 ml/min. It is also possible to perform a reverse dialysis in a double reverse (DR) modality, with identical purification results, in particular for a better adaptation to the Fresenius 5008 monitor (unpubl. data).

Principles of Use

In this 2-stage system, the PostD stage is the more effective, but also the limiting factor in terms of Q_S, since it is responsible for the haemoconcentration phenomenon.

If it is assumed that the PostD/PreD ratio of the convection is close to the ratio of their surfaces, then the PostD convection is 0.8/1.9, i.e. 42% of the total convection. In addition, it is generally recommended in PostD not to exceed a filtration fraction (FF) of 50% [3] of the plasmatic water flow (Q_{PW}). If $Q_B = 350$ ml/min with Hct = 33% and total protides (Pt) = 70 g/l, then Q_{PW} is estimated as $Q_{PW} = Q_B \times (Q_B - Ht \times 0.01) \times (Q_B - Pt \times 0.00017)$, i.e. 200 ml/min. Q_S authorized in PostD thus equals $200 \times 0.5 = 100$ ml/min, and total Q_S including PostD and PreD could then be $100 \times (100/42) = 238$ ml/min.

We published a table [4] allowing Q_S to be determined for each Q_B and according to Hct, and were able to check in vivo the relevance of these recommendations. More simply, with $Q_B > 320$ ml/min and Hct $< 36\%$, Q_S can be fixed at 225 ml/min without exceeding a monitor TMP of 250 mm Hg.

The complexity of diffusion and convection in such a dialyser makes their modelling delicate [5], and for the moment leads to more assumptions than certainties, thus placing paramount importance on clinical experimentation.

Methods

Six stable patients on renal replacement therapy were submitted to 1 session of MidD in its DR configuration, 1 of PreD and 1 of PostD. All sessions were carried out under similar operating conditions with a Fresenius 5008 dialysis system (Fresenius Medical Care, Bad Homburg, Germany). The hollow-fibre dialysers employed were an Olpur MD 190 in MidD and an FX80 (Fresenius Medical Care) in PostD and PreD. Effective Q_B as calculated by the machine was set at 320 ml/min (equivalent to a Q_B pump of 360 ml/min), dialysate flow (Q_D) at 500 ml/min and Q_S at 225 ml/min for MidD, 100 ml/min for PostD and 200 ml/min for PreD. The same usual patient low-molecular-weight heparin anticoagulation therapy was applied.

Treatment efficacy was determined by measuring reduction ratios (RR), equilibrated Kt/V (EqKt/V) and instantaneous whole-blood clearances (K) after 60 min.

$$RR = (1 - C_{Post}/C_{Pre}) \times 100$$

with C_{Pre} and C_{Post} being the plasma concentrations before the start and at the end of each treatment session. RR was determined for the small solutes urea, creatinine and phosphorus, and for the middle molecule (MM) β_2-microglobulin (β_2-MG).

$$K = Q_B \times (C_{Art} - C_{Ven}/C_{Art}) + Q_{UF} \times (C_{Ven}/C_{Art})$$

with C_{Art} and C_{Ven} being the plasma concentrations of the blood samples obtained from the arterial and venous blood lines, respectively, of the extracorporeal circuit. Q_{UF} is the ultrafiltration rate, which was set at 600 ml/min during sampling. K was determined for urea, creatinine and β_2-MG. It was impossible to evaluate phosphorus clearance because of the too low value of the venous sample, under the lowest limit of the laboratory method used.

Comparative statistical analyses were assessed with the t test for paired data (StatView).

Table 1. Comparison of RR (%) and instantaneous whole-blood clearance (ml/min) between MidD, PostD and PreD

	MidD	PostD	PreD
Total convection, litres	54.5±2.3	25.2±1.2	47.7±1.4
RR urea	78.3±5.6[a]	80.3±4.9[a, b]	76.8±7.4[b]
RR creatinine	69.0±5.7[a]	70.3±4.6[b]	66.3±6.1[a, b]
RR phosphorus	63.8±7.8	61.1±6.3	57.3±13.3
RR β_2-MG	82.3±3.8[a]	80.9±4.1[b]	74.6±4.1[a, b]
K urea	273.6±12.7[a]	288.8±10.0[b]	264.5±5.3[a, b]
K creatinine	215.5±20.9[a]	232.5±17.8[b]	199.8±9.3[a, b]
K β_2-MG	172±11.5[a]	165.6±10.3[b]	125.5±9.2[a, b]
EqKt/V	1.55±0.25[a]	1.66±0.26[a, b]	1.52±0.27[b]

Values with same superscripts within rows indicate significant differences, with $p < 0.05$.

Results

Results are presented in table 1.

Low-Weight Molecules

Generally, for high-flux (HF) membranes, the performances of diffusive purification of low-weight molecules (LM) depend above all on Q_B and the gradient of concentration between blood and dialysate. The simultaneous convection improves further the performances in PostD but tends to diminish them proportionally in PreD because of haemodilution [6].

In addition, with MidD, dialysate is at co-current in PreD and even if it is with countercurrent in PostD, it is also partially 'polluted' by PreD. Thus, it is difficult to predict the resultant between these diffusive conditions, a priori unfavourable, and the important favourable convective participation up to 50 liters.

For urea, K is intermediate in MidD (271.6 ml/min), between PostD (288.8 ml/min) and PreD (254.5 ml/min). It is correlated with RR: MidD = 78.3%, PostD = 80.3% and PreD = 76.8%, and with EqKt/V: MidD = 1.55%, PostD = 1.66% and PreD = 1.52%.

For creatinine, we found similar K values, with MidD (215.5 ml/min) between PostD (232.5 ml/min) and PreD (199.8 ml/min), but also RR with MidD = 69.0%, PostD = 70.3% and PreD = 66.3%.

For phosphorus, RR, under the same conditions, was more favourable in MidD (63.8%) than in PostD (61.1%) and PreD (57.3%).

Middle Molecules

The purification of the MM depends above all on the convective flow and, to a lesser degree, on the surface of the membrane, with PostD providing an advantage. With the Olpur MD 190 and the FX80 having comparably sized surface areas (1.9 and 1.8 m^2, respectively), and taking into account the increase in the total convective flow in MidD, compensating for the pejorative effect of the predominant PreD participation, it is logical to find comparable values for the RR of β_2-MG between MidD (82.3) and PostD (80.9), rather higher than PreD (74.6).

Safety of Use

As regards safety, it should be recognized that the evaluation known as '2 points' by the monitors of the TMP, using the ingoing blood pressure ($P_{B\ in}$) and the outgoing dialysate pressure ($P_{D\ out}$) cannot be used with this type of dialyser.

In the initial configuration, the TMP was found to be, depending on various conditions of use [2, 7], between 611 and 713 mm Hg in the PostD stage and between 293 and 307 mm Hg in the PreD stage, with $P_{B\ in}$ between 731 and 902 and $P_{B\ out}$ between 116 and 189 mm Hg.

In SR [2], these results drop to 422 ± 90 in the PostD stage and 188 ± 54 in the PreD stage. However, there are neither clinical nor technical consequences with these high modes of pressure. We had, in our experience, neither membrane rupture nor abnormal frequency of coagulation.

On the other hand, the use of the Fresenius 5008 monitor, with convective flows >200 ml/min, and the joint use of blood temperature monitor (BTM) and online clearance monitor (OCM) modules, makes it necessary to use the DR mode to avoid unforeseen alarms or monitoring module failures.

The impact of a high-pressure system on albumin losses is nil, with an average of 1.6 g/session with SR or DR configurations (unpubl. data with partial collected dialysate) with Q_S between 150 and 225 ml/min.

Discussion

MidD has the advantage of offering within the same dialyser, without any specific machine, the complementary methods of PostD and PreD, allowing adequately large Q_S favourable to the MM and compensating for the diffusive conditions which are largely rather unfavourable for purification of the LM.

Besides, it is difficult to compare results from different papers, given the different protocols used, notably in terms of Q_B (derived from the pump speed or estimated by the monitor), Q_Dd (with flow entirely or partially passing through the dialyser, depending on the substitution flow monitor management), sampling time, ultrafiltration (standardized or not during sampling) etc.

In any case, the results obtained are well beyond the requirements in terms of purification of the PM, and even promising for phosphorus.

For MM, the penalizing effect of PreD, more important in the SR and DR configurations than in the initial configuration, has undoubtedly no clinical consequences [8, 9].

In fact, the amount of convective volumes needed for their purification are well beyond the 15 litres recommended [10] and, anyway, the β_2-MG plasma water clearance exceeds its intercompartmental clearance estimated at 82 ml/min, suggesting that only a different strategic approach in duration and frequency will allow a better purification [11].

Some data give an indication of a better per dialysis purification of cystatin C (CyC), retinol-binding protein (RBP) or leptin compared to PostD [9, 10] or angiogenin and RBP compared to high-flux haemodialysis [12].

More interesting will be measurements of purification of these potential uraemic toxins, not only in terms of clearance, but also in residual blood concentration in the long term.

A multicentric study [13] has already confirmed that MidD had a more beneficial effect on CyC and RBP than PostD.

A particular observation is that PostD and PreD association in the same dialyser could allow patients with limited vascular access [14] to benefit from adequate convective fluid.

The particular configuration of the Olpur MD 190 also leads to an increase in pressure, in particular in the blood compartment and thus of the TMP, irrespective of the values of the various monitors. However, the 2 years' experience in various dialysis centres does not reveal any noxious effect. With a larger surface of 2.2 m^2, the Olpur MD 220, soon to be available, will have 1 m^2 (45% of the total surface) allotted to the first PostD stage, which is supposed to minimize the TMP by allowing the same Q_S in a more significant number of fibres, but also to increase purification, notably of MM.

Anyway, in order to achieve a high-quality convective transfer with complete peace of mind, we strongly recommend choosing the SR or DR configuration of the Olpur MD 190, depending on the monitor used, knowing that the studies, still unpublished, have not shown any difference in purification between these two modes.

Conclusion

The Olpur MD 190 is a dialyser of innovating design, allowing the joint and successive use, within the same dialyser, of both PostD and PreD HDF, determining the MidD modality. It offers very high purification performance with, for MM, an apparent advantage compared to PostD, but which remains to be confirmed in the long term for other potentially noxious substances still insufficiently studied.

Therefore, one can only recommend this HDF modality which guarantees, under excellent safety conditions, a quality of dialysis which largely exceeds the objectives of purification recommended for a better survival in dialysis.

References

1 Pedrini LA, Cozzi G, Faranna P, et al: Transmembrane pressure modulation in high-volume mixed hemodiafiltration to optimize efficiency and minimize protein loss. Kidney Int 2006;69:573–579.

2 Santoro A, Ferramosca E, Mancini E, Monari C, Varasani M, Sereni L, Wratten M: Reverse mid-dilution: new way to remove small and middle molecules as well as phosphate with high intrafilter convective clearance. Nephrol Dial Transplant 2007 April 3, E-pub ahead of print. DOI: 10.1093/ndt/gfm101.

3 Henderson LW: Biophysics of ultrafiltration and hemofiltration; in Maher JF (ed): Replacement of Renal Function by Dialysis. Dordrecht, Kluwer Academic, 1989, pp 300–326.

4 Potier J, Renaux JL: OLPUR 190MD: practical user recommendations for optimal performances. Am Soc Nephrol Congr, 863A–864A, 2006.

5 Garred LJ: Mathematical modeling of the fluid mechanics in a mid-dilution hemodiafiltration device. Am Soc Nephrol Congr, 861A, 2006.

6 Wizemann V, Külz M, Techert F, Nederlof B: Efficacy of hemodiafiltration. Nephrol Dial Transplant 2001;16(suppl 4):27–30.

7 Feliciani A, Riva MA, Zerbi S, Ruggiero P, Lati AR, Cozzi G, Pedrini LA: New strategies in haemodiafiltration (HDF): prospective comparative analysis between on-line mixed HDF and mid-dilution HDF. Nephrol Dial Transplant, 2007 March 8, E-pub ahead of print. DOI: 10.1093/ndt/gfm023.

8 Krieter DH, Falkenhain S, Chalabi L, Collins G, Lemke HD, Canaud B: Clinical cross-over comparison of mid-dilution hemodiafiltration using a novel dialyzer concept and post-dilution hemodiafiltration. Kidney Int 2005;67:349–356.

9 Krieter DH, Collins G, Summerton J, Spence E, Leray Moragues H, Canaud B: Mid-dilution on-line haemodiafiltration in a standard dialyser configuration. Nephrol Dial Transplant 2005;20:155–160.

10 Canaud B, Bragg-Gresham JL, Marshall MR, Desmeules S, Gillespie BW, Depner T, Klassen P, Port FK: Mortality risk for patients receiving hemodiafiltration versus hemodialysis: European results from the DOPPS. Kidney Int 2006;69:2087–2093.

11 Ward RA, Greene T, Hartmann B, Samtleben W: Resistance to intercompartmental mass transfer limits β_2-microglobulin removal by post-dilution hemodiafiltration. Kidney Int 2006;69:1431–1437.

12 Santoro A, Conz PA, De Cristofaro V, Acquistapace I, Gaggi R, Ferramosca E, Renaux JL, Rizziolo E, Wratten ML: Mid-dilution: the perfect balance between convection and diffusion; in Ronco C,

Brendolan A, Levin N (eds): Cardiovascular Disorders in Hemodialysis. Contrib Nephrol. Basel, Karger, 2005, vol 149, pp 107–114.
13 Krieter DH, Nicoud P, Christensson A, Fadel B, Wambergue F, Valentin R, Potier J, Collins G, Canaud B: Long-term multicenter trial comparing post- to mid-dilution online HDF: effects on low-molecular weight (LMW) proteins. Am Soc Nephrol Congr, 410A, 2006.
14 Renaux JL, Graziani G, Borlandelli S, Badalamenti S, Della Cà C, Alli A, Imbasciati E, Varasani M, Mandolfo S: Evaluation of dialytic efficiency of mid dilution hemodiafiltration for patients with limited vascular access. Am Soc Nephrol Congr, 722A, 2006.

Dr. Jacky Potier
Service d'Hémodialyse et de Néphrologie
Rue du Val de Saire
FR–50102 Cherbourg (France)
Tel. +33 6 80 92 12 68, E-Mail j.potier@ch-cherbourg.fr

Ronco C, Canaud B, Aljama P (eds): Hemodiafiltration.
Contrib Nephrol. Basel, Karger, 2007, vol 158, pp 161–168

Double High-Flux Hemodiafiltration

Beat von Albertini

Clinique Cecil et Division de Néphrologie, Centre Hospitalier Universitaire Vaudois, Lausanne, Suisse

Abstract

Hemodiafiltration (HDF) can augment the efficiency of removal of small and large solutes for renal replacement therapy. Double high-flux HDF was developed in 1984 with the objective to shorten treatment time compared to conventional therapy. It consists of a serial pair of dialyzers in the extracorporeal circuit for optimal diffusion and filtration, with substitution by backfiltration of bicarbonate dialysate under volumetric control. Used in conjunction with high blood and dialysate flow rates and high-flux membranes, unmatched high rates of simultaneous diffusive and convective solute transport can be obtained clinically with double HDF. A favorable long-term clinical outcome in comparison with conventional hemodialysis was observed with this therapy, despite shorter treatment times.

Hemodiafiltration (HDF) describes an intermittent renal replacement therapy of combined simultaneous diffusive and convective solute transport, in which the total volume of ultrafiltration largely exceeds the desired weight loss for the patient and is in part replaced with a physiological solution. Substitution occurs either by administration of extraneous parenteral solutions, as introduced by Leber et al. [1], or by online filtered dialysate [2]. The treatment presented here, termed high-flux HDF in the original report of 1984, is based on a serial pair of filters for optimized diffusion and filtration, with substitution by controlled backfiltration of bicarbonate dialysate in the extracorporeal circuit [3, 4]. It was designed to introduce an unprecedented efficiency of total solute transport and thereby to provide simultaneously a better renal replacement therapy with shorter treatment times. It can be performed with standard modern dialysis equipment with volumetric ultrafiltration control and is better known in routine clinical use among patients and staff by the colloquial term 'double high-flux'.

Prior Work

Since the successful demonstration of its feasibility, improvement of renal replacement therapy, in terms of efficiency of small- and large-solute transport, has been a central preoccupation of investigators and has fostered progress in clinical understanding and technical development in this field. Given the limitations of diffusive hemodialysis with cellulosic membranes for large-solute transport, hemofiltration, a purely convective renal replacement therapy approximating the range of solutes filtered in the human glomerulus, was introduced in 1967 [5]. An important innovation with this therapy was online filtration for the production of sterile and pyrogen-free solutions for substitution [6]. More efficient simultaneous small- and large-solute removal in dialysis was demonstrated in 1972 with polyacrylonitrile, a membrane with enhanced diffusive and hydraulic permeability. To prevent excessive ultrafiltration with the clinical use of this membrane, an apparatus for closed-circuit volume control of dialysate was developed, which forms an integral part of modern dialysis machines with programmable weight loss for the patient [7]. The clinically obtainable efficiency of solute transport in dialysis at that time was nevertheless primarily limited by the rate at which the acetate buffer, gained from the then used dialysate, could be metabolized by the patients, resulting in clinical intolerance and vascular instability at blood flow rates higher than 250–300 ml/min [8]. The development of bicarbonate dialysis in 1976 [9] effectively removed this barrier, but the potential for increasing treatment efficiency clinically remained unrecognized for some time [10, 11]. A serendipitous discovery, made with hemofiltration, was that high blood flow rates (up to 500 ml/min), introduced in an effort to obtain small-solute removal similar to control hemodialysis without prolonging treatment time, were observed not only to be available from vascular access, but also to be well tolerated by the patients [12]. The critical importance of appropriate small-solute removal was highlighted in 1983 by the outcome of the National Cooperative Dialysis Study, incidentally demonstrating the validity of the concept of reciprocity of efficiency versus time for prescription of small-solute removal with dialysis [13]. Shorter treatments with HDF were introduced in 1983 but later abandoned [14].

Method

A configuration of 2 high-flux dialyzers is used in the extracorporeal circuit, as depicted schematically in figure 1 (on the left). Its key functional features for HDF are a flow restrictor between the serial dialyzers in the countercurrent dialysate circuit (in the middle) and the

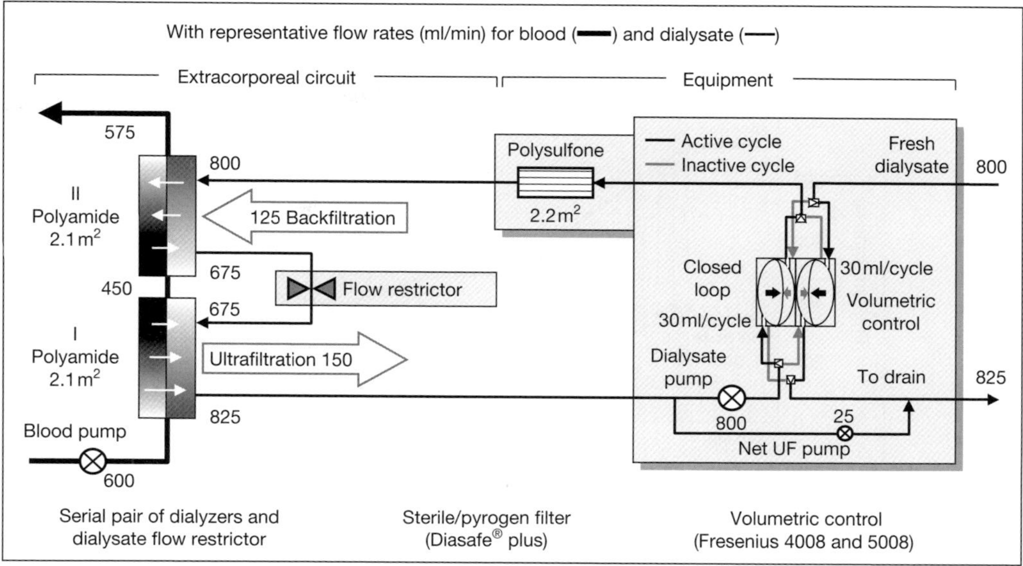

Fig. 1. Configuration for double HDF with representative flow rates occurring during clinical operation.

volumetric control of the standard equipment (on the right), which also contains a filter for online sterile and pyrogen filtration of fresh bicarbonate dialysate.

The volumetric control of dialysate, a standard feature of modern dialysis machines, consists of a closed hydraulic circuit, in which the volume of degassed dialysate entering the extracorporeal circuit is precisely matched to that leaving the circuit by volume displacement. This is technically achieved by 2 identical loops within the machine, which are alternately opened and closed by a set of control valves and pumps. Each loop contains a fixed-volume chamber which is separated into 2 compartments by a flexible membrane. In one circuit, one of these 2 compartments is filled with inflowing freshly prepared dialysate, while the other compartment, filled in a previous cycle with spent dialysate, is thereby emptied into the drain. Simultaneously, in the other loop, one compartment is filled with spent dialysate and thereby empties the other compartment, filled with fresh dialysate, into the dialyzer circuit. To achieve the desired weight loss during the treatment, a predetermined volume is continuously removed from the effluent dialysate by a programmable pump and bypasses the volume control mechanism. The resulting volume deficit lowers the hydrostatic pressure in the closed circuit and thereby augments the pressure gradient across the dialyzer membrane (transmembrane pressure, TMP). Ultrafiltration of plasma water occurs in response to the self-adjusting TMP, at a rate matching the volume of dialysate removed from the closed circuit.

The principle of self-adjusting TMP under volumetric control is exploited for HDF in this configuration of 2 serial dialyzers with high hydraulic permeability. Figure 2 depicts the pressure profile for blood and dialysate in the countercurrent extracorporeal circuit, as typically encountered during clinical treatments. Pressure in the blood circuit (from left to right)

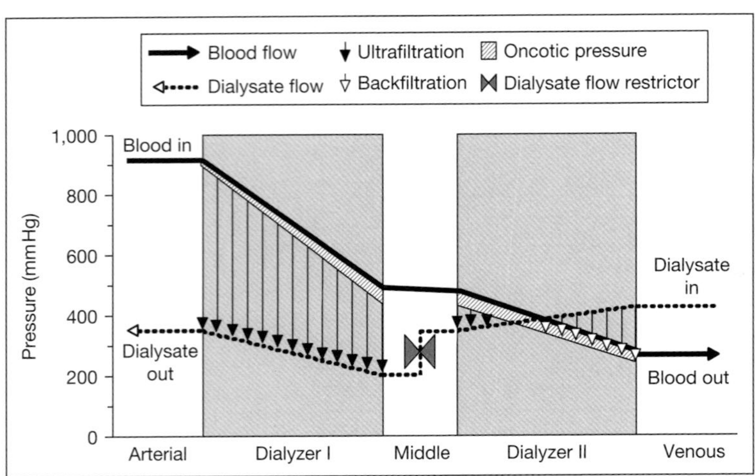

Fig. 2. Pressure profile and transmembrane fluxes in the extracorporeal circuit of double HDF, typically encountered during clinical operation.

diminishes gradually from a high initial pressure, generated by the high rate of the blood pump and the flow resistance of the serial dialyzers, to the pressure in the venous blood line returning to the patient. Pressures in the countercurrent dialysate circuit (from right to left) are modified by the flow restrictor between the serial dialyzers, resulting in higher pressures upstream than downstream of the restriction. The flow restrictor is a very simple device, consisting of a clamp and a calibrated bore in the dialysate line. Once the clamp is manually closed, all dialysate is forced through the restrictive bore until the clamp is opened at the end of treatment.

During treatment, an important hydrostatic pressure gradient exists between blood and dialysate compartments of the first and in part of the second dialyzer, resulting in high ultrafiltration of plasma water to dialysate and thereby increasing the blood oncotic pressure. The higher dialysate and lower blood compartment hydrostatic pressures result in a reverse TMP towards the end of the second dialyzer and transfer of fluid from dialysate to blood. This backfiltration is facilitated by oncotic pressure, which diminishes as the concentrated blood is rediluted. The pressures in the configuration are continuously self-adjusting by the volumetric control of the equipment, maintaining optimal transmembrane fluxes during treatment. The magnitude of these fluxes is evident from the representative clinical flow rates given in figure 1. Blood flow diminishes during passage of the first filter (in this example from 600 to 450 ml/min), due to ultrafiltration (150) and is rediluted in the second filter (to 575) by backfiltation (125), the difference being the net weight loss rate (25), programmed for the treatment in the conventional fashion. Conversely, countercurrent dialysate flow diminishes in the second filter (from 800 to 675 ml/min), due to backfiltation (125) and increases again in the first filter (to 825), due to addition of ultrafiltered plasma water (150). The entire system is self-contained and functions automatically: all that is required for operation is that the blood flow and weight loss rate be set and the flow restrictor clamp be closed at the onset of treatment and the patient and equipment be monitored in the conventional manner.

Results

Used in conjunction with high blood and dialysate flow rates and dialyzer membranes with high diffusive and hydraulic permeability, substantial rates of simultaneous diffusive and convective solute transport can be obtained with this configuration. A variety of membranes have been used for this purpose [15], made of cellulose acetate, polymethylmethacrylate, polysulfone, acrylonitrile and polyamide, which is now routinely used in our center. A recent clearance study, made with two Gambro Polyflux® 21R dialyzers (2.1 m^2) in series, revealed at an effective blood flow rate of 533 ml/min and a dialysate flow rate of 808 ml/min (with ultrafiltration in the first filter of 167 ml/min, backfiltration in the second of 150 ml/min and net weight loss rate of 25 ml/min) an average of whole-blood and dialysate determined clearances of 449 ml/min for urea, 420 ml/min for creatinine and 370 ml/min for phosphate, respectively, and an average of plasma and dialysate clearances for β_2-microglobulin of 168 ml/min in the extracorporeal circuit [unpubl. data].

From its inception, good clinical tolerance was observed with double HDF, despite higher weight loss rates during treatment. Shortened treatment times did not negatively affect blood pressure control in the patients [16]. The long-term clinical outcome with double HDF has recently been analyzed in comparison with other high-efficiency hemodialysis treatments in a total of 183 patients over 6 years [17]. Patient survival was overall favorable with all high-efficiency therapy in comparison to the national registry (US Renal Data System), matched for patients' age, race and etiology of end-stage renal disease. The best outcome was observed in the group treated with double HDF, which incidentally was the one with the shortest treatment times. Analysis by standardized mortality rate revealed a 59% better outcome in comparison to the registry for this group, which was the only one reaching a statistically significant difference by this analysis [18].

Discussion

The development of this treatment must be placed in the historical context in which it occurred, which was towards the conclusion of a period which can now be considered to have probably been the 'golden years' for the development of renal replacement therapy. Based on earlier fundamental contributions establishing feasibility, therapy was particularly moved forward during this time by a large number of seminal contributions, which enhanced clinical understanding and led to most of the technical developments incorporated into modern dialysis. In this stimulating period, interaction within the relatively small international community of clinicians and investigators was intense and open-minded, and clinical research in this field was encouraged by funding agencies, namely the NIH.

The primary goal of intermittent renal replacement therapy is to improve the human condition of patients with end-stage renal disease by maintaining relative well-being and enabling the pursuit of a functional life. Well-being is largely proportional to the quantity of and quality of dialytic therapy, relating to the absence of intra- and interdialytic side effects. Quantity of dialysis is determined by the total clearance volumes of metabolic solutes approximating those excreted by the natural kidneys; technically it is effected by the product of treatment efficiency and treatment time. Time spent on treatment, on the other hand, impacts negatively on the one available for more enjoyable activities, which also define quality of life for a patient. It was in this perspective that the attempt was made in 1984 to combine all known elements of the state-of-art of the time, relevant for efficiency and clinical tolerance for optimization of treatment, with the set objective to substantially shorten the treatment time over conventional therapy without a reduction of removal of small and large solutes.

Double HDF effectively more than doubled the rates of solute transport over conventional therapy. A configuration of paired dialyzers had previously been used for hemodialysis [19] and, in a serial configuration, for HDF with self-generation of substitution fluid [20, 21]. The progress made with double HDF stems from the conjunction of this configuration with the unprecedented high blood flow rates and bicarbonate dialysate during clinical treatments. The former were found to be readily available from most patients' vascular access, and the latter contributed to the observed good clinical tolerance of high treatment efficiency.

It is estimated that close to 100,000 treatments with double HDF have been performed up to now in the USA, Europe and Asia without notable complications. The treatment is well liked by patients and staff for the good clinical tolerance it provides, even at high net ultrafiltration rates (up to 30 ml/min), for its shorter treatment times and ease of operation. For the clinician, it is a valued tool to provide patients with high body weight with a treatment meeting guidelines for treatment adequacy. Further application is limited by the need for double filters, which is economically unfavorable without reuse.

Acknowledgements

The author wishes to acknowledge the stimulation and encouragement he was privileged to receive from the contributions of and the personal contact with many investigators, who cannot all be listed here. He wishes in particular to express his gratitude to his mentors and collaborators, namely the late James H. Shinaberger and Joseph H. Miller of Los Angeles, without whom the development of this treatment could not have been realized, and Juan P. Bosch and Viroj Barlee in Washington, D.C. and Jacky Berger in Lausanne, without whom it could not have been implemented clinically.

References

1 Leber HW, Wizemann V, Goubeaud G, Rawer P, Schuetterle G: Hemodiafiltation: a new alternative to hemofiltration and conventional hemodialysis. Artif Organs 1978;2:150–153.

2 Canaud B, Nguyen A, Argiles C, Polito C, Polaschegg HD, Mion C: Hemodiafiltration using dialysate as substitution fluid. Artif Organs 1987;11:188–190.

3 von Albertini B, Miller JH, Gardner PW, Shinaberger JH: High-flux hemodiafiltration: under six hours/week treatment. Trans Am Soc Artif Intern Organs 1984;30:227–231.

4 Miller JH, von Albertini B, Gardner PW, Shinaberger JH: Technical aspects of high-flux hemodiafiltration for adequate short (under two hours) treatment. Trans Am Soc Artif Intern Organs 1984; 30:377–381.

5 Henderson LW, Besarab A, Michaels AS, Bluemle LW: Blood purification by ultrafiltration and fluid replacement (diafiltration). Trans Am Soc Artif Intern Organs 1967;16:216–222.

6 Henderson LW, Beans E: Successful production of sterile pyrogen-free electrolyte solution by ultrafiltration. Kidney Int 1978;14:522–525.

7 Funck-Brentano JL, Sausse A, Man NK, Grangier A, Roudon-Nucete M, Zingraft J, Jungers P: A new method for hemodialysis combining a high permeability membrane for the medium molecules and a dialysis bath in a closed circuit. Proc Eur Dial Transplant Assoc 1972;9:55–66.

8 Kveim M, Nesbakken R: Utilization of exogenous acetate during hemodialysis. Trans Am Soc Artif Intern Organs 1975;21:138–143.

9 Graefe U, Multinovitch J, Follete WC, Vizzo JE, Babb AL, Scribner BH: Less dialysis-induced morbidity and vascular instability with bicarbonate in the dialysate. Ann Intern Med 1978;88:332–336.

10 von Albertini B, Petersen J: Comparison of high blood flows in bicarbonate vs acetate hemodialysis (abstract). National Kidney Foundation Scientific Meeting Program and Abstracts. Am J Kidney Dis 1983;p32.

11 Keshaviah P, Collins A: Rapid high-efficiency bicarbonate hemodialysis. Trans Am Soc Artif Intern Organs 1986;32:17–23.

12 Geronemus R, von Albertini B, Glabman S, Kahn T, Moutoussis G, Bosch JP: High-flux hemodiafiltration: further reduction in treatment time. Proc Clin Dial Transplant Forum 1979;9:125–127.

13 Parker TF, Laird NM, Lowrie EG: Comparison of the study groups in the National Cooperative Dialysis Study and a description of morbidity, mortality and patient withdrawal. Kidney Int Suppl 1983;13:S42–S49.

14 Wizemann V, Kramer W, Knopp G, Rawer P, Mueller K, Schuetterle G: Ultrashort hemodiafiltration: efficiency and hemodynamic tolerance. Clin Nephrol 1983;19:24–30.

15 von Albertini, B, Miller JH, Gardner PW, Shinaberger JH: Performance characteristics of high-flux hemodiafiltration. Proc Eur Dial Transplant Assoc 1984;21:447–453.

16 Velasquez M, von Albertini B, Lew SQ, Mishkin G, Bosch JP: Equal levels of blood pressure control in ESRD patients receiving high-efficiency hemodialysis and conventional hemodialysis. Am J Kidney Dis 1998;31:618–623.

17 Bosch JP, Lew SQ, Barlee V, Mishkin GJ, von Albertini B: Clinical use of high-efficiency hemodialysis treatments: long-term assessment. Hemodial Int 2006;10:73–81.

18 Wolfe RA, Gaylin DS, Port FK, Held PJ, Wood CL: Using USRDS generated mortality tables to compare local ESRD mortality rates to national rates. Kidney Int 1992;42:991–996.

19 Kuruvila KC, Cadnapaphornchai P, Leasor G, Popovitzer M, Alfrey A, Schrier RW: A model for evening home hemodialysis. Am J Med 1974;57:706–713.

20 Shinzato T, Sezaki R, Matsatune U, Maeda K, Ohbayashi S, Toyota T: Infusion-free hemodiafiltration: simultaneous hemofiltration and dialysis with no need for infusion fluid. Artif Organs 1982; 6:453–456.
21 Cheung AC, Kato Y, Leypolt JK, Henderson LW: Hemodiafiltration using a hybrid membrane system for self-generation of diluting fluid. Trans Am Soc Artif Organs 1982;28:61–65.

Dr. Beat von Albertini
Centre de dialyse Cecil
Avenue de Savoie 10
CH–1003 Lausanne (Switzerland)
Tel. +41 21 343 01 82, Fax +41 21 343 01 81, E-Mail Beat.vonalbertini@hirslanden.ch

Ronco C, Canaud B, Aljama P (eds): Hemodiafiltration.
Contrib Nephrol. Basel, Karger, 2007, vol 158, pp 169–176

Push/Pull Hemodiafiltration

Toru Shinzato, Kenji Maeda

Daiko Medical Engineering Research Institute, Nagoya, Japan

Abstract

Push/pull hemodiafiltration is characterized by alternate filtration and backfiltration, while sterile pyrogen-free dialysate is flowing through a hemodiafilter. During the filtration phase, uremic substances are eliminated not only by diffusive, but also by convective transport. During the backfiltration phase, dialysate is quickly pushed to the blood side (i.e. backfiltration) so as to make up for the excessive reduction in body fluid that has developed during the immediately preceding filtration phase. In the most recently improved version of push/pull hemodiafiltration, the body fluid replacement volume is over 120 liters during a 4-hour treatment. This replacement of a large amount of body fluid may be due to the increased filtration rate in the hemodiafilter resulting from failure of the complete formation of a protein gel layer on the blood side surface. The filtration time in push/pull hemodiafiltration is so short that the also short backfiltration to follow may take over before the protein gel layer is completely formed on the membrane surface. Since the filtration and backfiltration times are much shorter in push/pull hemodiafiltration than the time for blood to pass through the hemodiafilter, it is concentrated and diluted many times (approx. 25 times) before it leaves the hemodiafilter. Therefore, push/pull hemodiafiltration is functionally similar to a predilution hemodiafiltration. The reduction rate of β_2-microglobulin was greater by push/pull hemodiafiltration than by hemodialysis, when a high-flux polysulfone hemodiafilter was employed. However, the difference in the reduction rate was rather small between them, because of the improved hemodiafilters, which remove so much β_2-microglobulin only by dialysis. Nevertheless, restless legs syndrome, irritability, insomnia and pruritus were alleviated after switching the treatment modality from hemodialysis to push/pull hemodiafiltration. This may indicate that these symptoms are caused by the accumulation of uremic substances larger than β_2-microglobulin.

In online hemodiafiltration, a hemodiafiltration method gaining widespread acceptance, a part of the dialysate is infused into blood tubing as a substitution fluid through a line from the dialysate pathway connected to the blood tubing [1]. On the other hand, in push/pull hemodiafiltration, which has been in use in Japan for more than 20 years, filtration and backfiltration are repeated alternately in the hemodiafilter; uremic substances are eliminated by diffusion and convection during the filtration phase, while during the backfiltration phase the dialysate is quickly pushed to the blood side as a substitution fluid in the hemodiafilter [2].

This chapter reviews the mechanical and functional characteristics of push/pull hemodiafiltration and discusses the clinical effectiveness of this treatment modality.

Principles

By definition, push/pull hemodiafiltration is an alternate filtration and backfiltration that takes place while a sterile pyrogen-free dialysate is flowing through a hemodiafilter. During the filtration phase, a certain volume of fluid is filtered from the blood side to the dialysate side, so as to eliminate uremic substances by not only diffusive, but also convective transport. During the backfiltration phase, almost the same volume of dialysate is quickly pushed to the blood side to compensate for the excessive reduction in body fluid that has developed during the filtration phase just before.

Push/Pull Machines

The alternate repetition of filtration and backfiltration by pushing and pulling dialysate in and out of the dialysate flow pathway is done by straightforward push/pull machine action. The push/pull machine itself was developed in 1982 [2] and improved largely in 1994 [3]. In the original version of this push/pull machine, the push/pull volume of the dialysate was 200 ml as compared with the mere 16.7 ml with the more recently improved machine.

With each alternate filtration and backfiltration, the blood efflux from the hemodiafilter decreases or increases, respectively, when either the original or a more recently improved machine is used. To assure a constant flow of blood back to the patient's body, with the original machine, a blood volume equivalent to the volume of alternately occurring filtration and backfiltration is pulled out from the blood tubing into the plastic bag reservoir and then pushed back from the reservoir into the blood tubing downstream of the hemodiafilter, in synchrony with the backfiltration and filtration. With the more recently improved machine, on the other hand, air is also pulled out from the venous chamber and then pushed back into the chamber alternately, in synchrony with the backfiltration and filtration, to assure a constant flow of blood back to the patient's body.

Mechanism of the Push/Pull Machine

Since the original one is rarely used today, we focus here on the mechanism of the recently improved push/pull machine.

Constant Flow of Blood Back to the Body

The key component of the push/pull machine is a double-cylinder piston pump with a discharge volume of 16.7 ml in either direction. This 2-way pump pulls dialysate out from the dialysate removal pathway so as to develop filtration in the hemodiafilter and simultaneously pushes air into the venous chamber so as to lower the air-fluid level therein. Next, the piston pump pushes the dialysate back into the dialysate removal pathway so as to develop backfiltration and simultaneously pulls air from the venous chamber so as to elevate the air-fluid level in the chamber, when a volumetric ultrafiltration controller is employed. With push/pull hemodiafiltration performed using this approach, the variation in the blood flow returned to the patient's body, which is due to alternate filtration and backfiltration, is made constant by lowering and elevating the air-fluid level in the venous chamber.

Control of Transmembrane Pressure

The membrane water permeability changes depending on the kind of membrane material and decreases progressively during hemodiafiltration treatment. In the push/pull hemodiafiltration machine, the pump operation of the double-cylinder piston pump is automatically controlled so that the transmembrane pressure (TMP) is consistently maintained at a preset level (i.e. usually the highest level in the safety range) throughout treatment according to the following mechanism.

The pressure difference between the blood side and dialysate side cylinders of the double-cylinder piston pump is almost equivalent to the TMP in the hemodiafilter, as shown in figure 1, because the pressure (P_D) on the dialysate side cylinder is equal to the pressure in the dialysate tubing, and the pressure (P_B) in the blood side cylinder is equal to the pressure in the venous chamber.

$$TMP = P_B - P_D. \quad (1)$$

We may express the force (F) opposing the piston movement as the product of the cross-sectional area (S) and the pressure difference between the blood side and the dialysate side cylinders which is almost equal to the TMP:

$$F = (P_B - P_D) \times S. \quad (2)$$

Since the reciprocation of the double-cylinder piston pump is translated from the cam rotation, by appropriately controlling the force which rotates the cam (i.e.

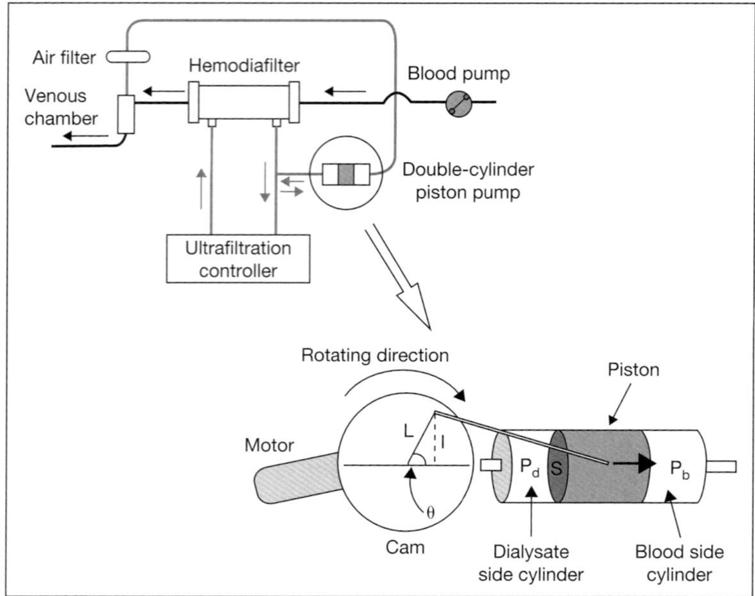

Fig. 1. Schematic diagram of the push/pull hemodiafiltration system. P_D and P_B indicate the pressures in the dialysate and blood compartments of the cylinder, respectively, S the cross-sectional area of the piston, and L the distance from the center of the cam and I the distance from the straight line passing through the center of the cam to the connecting point of the cam and piston.

the torque of the cam), one can apply a constant force on the piston. Figure 1 also shows the cam and double-cylinder piston pump. The torque of the cam can be expressed by the following equation:

$$T = I \times F \tag{3}$$

where T is the cam torque and I is the distance from the straight line passing through the center of the cam (which is parallel to the reciprocation direction of the piston pump) to the connecting point of the cam and piston.

In the following equation, I is obtained:

$$I = L \sin \theta \tag{4}$$

where L indicates the distance from the center of the cam to the connecting point of the cam and piston, and θ denotes the angle of the straight line passing through the center of the cam (which is parallel to the reciprocation direction of the piston), and the straight line passing through the center of the cam and the connecting point of the cam and piston.

The combination of equations 1–4 yields the following equation, by which the cam torque is obtained:

$$T = TMP \times S \times L \sin \theta. \qquad (5)$$

The cam torque is proportional to the voltage applied to the DC motor connected to the cam. Therefore, in a push/pull machine, the DC motor has been improved so that the cam torque can be controlled at $TMP \times S \times L \sin \theta$ at any moment by changing the voltage applied to the motor in relation to the continuously monitored θ value. The TMP is thus maintained at a preset constant value during both the filtration and backfiltration phases, usually 400 mm Hg during the filtration phase and −400 mm Hg during the backfiltration phase.

A rigid, braid-reinforced silicone tubing must be used instead of the conventional dialysate tubings to prevent the dialysate tubings from absorbing a significant portion of the push/pull volume of dialysate with this machine.

Functional Characteristics of Push/Pull Hemodiafiltration

Replacement Volume

The times for filtration and backfiltration are approximately 0.8 and 0.7 s, respectively, and the filtration rate from the blood is around 2.8 ml/mm Hg/min when the TMP is set at the maximum permissible level within the safety range throughout treatment, whether during the filtration or backfiltration phase. Due to this high filtration rate, which is almost equivalent to the filtration rate of tap water (3.3 ml/mm Hg/min), the body fluid replacement volume will exceed 120 liters during a 4-hour push/pull hemodiafiltration.

The resulting increased filtration rate may be due not only to the maximum permissible TMP during the filtration and backfiltration phases, but also to the failure of the protein gel layer [4–6] to form completely on the blood side surface of the hemodiafilter membrane during the filtration phase. As mentioned earlier, in push/pull hemodiafiltration, the filtration time is so short that the short backfiltration to follow may take over before the protein gel layer is completely formed on the membrane surface.

Replacement Mode

Since the filtration and backfiltration times in push/pull hemodiafiltration are much shorter at 0.8 and 0.7 s, respectively, than the time (40 s) for extracorporeally circulating blood to pass through the hemodiafilter, it is concentrated and diluted many times (approx. 25 times) before it leaves the hemodiafilter. Therefore, the push/pull hemodiafiltration is functionally similar to a predilution hemodiafiltration.

Preparation of Dialysate

Since dialysate is infused as a substitution solution in push/pull hemodiafiltration, just as with online hemodiafiltration, the finally infused dialysate must be of intravenous quality. Therefore, dialysate is prepared so as to be sterile and nonpyrogenic in the push/pull hemodiafiltration system.

The dialysate preparation process in the push/pull hemodiafiltration system is virtually the same as for the online hemodiafiltration system [7].

Solute Removal

According to our recent unpublished data, the reduction rate of β_2-microglobulin was greater by push/pull hemodiafiltration than by hemodialysis, when a high-flux polysulfone hemodiafilter (i.e. PS-1.9UW®, Kawasumi Co. Ltd., Tokyo, Japan) was employed with a volumetric ultrafiltration controller (DCS-26®, Nikkiso Co. Ltd., Tokyo, Japan). However, the difference in the reduction rate was rather small ($71.5 \pm 6.5\%$ with push/pull hemodiafiltration against $62.5 \pm 5.8\%$ with hemodialysis; $p < 0.05$). This is due to the vastly improved hemodiafilter, which even in conventional hemodialysis can remove a huge amount of β_2-microglobulin.

We wish to remove great amounts of low-molecular-weight protein, typified by β_2-microglobulin, with a minimized loss of albumin. However, although albumin (60,000 Da) and β_2-microglobulin (12,000 Da) have a great difference in molecular weight, there is only a small difference in their molecular radius. At the time when the original or present push/pull machine was developed, no membrane was available which could screen albumin and β_2-microglobulin very effectively. At that time, when the membrane albumin sieving coefficient (SC) was kept at 0.01, the SC for β_2-microglobulin could only be increased to 0.3. However, nowadays membranes have been developed with which the albumin SC can be kept to 0.006, while the SC for β_2-microglobulin can be increased to over 0.8. Of course, this type of membrane also shows a marked increase in its ability to eliminate β_2-microglobulin by diffusion. Moreover, when such membranes are incorporated in a recent hemodiafilter, the removal of β_2-microglobulin is more remarkable due to enhanced internal filtration [8].

Therefore, as long as the recent hemodiafilter incorporating such membranes is used, there may not be much difference in β_2-microglobulin removal between hemodialysis and push/pull hemodiafiltration, or between hemodialysis and online hemodiafiltration.

Although the reduction rate of β_2-microglobulin is greater by push/pull hemodiafiltration to some extent than by hemodialysis, the urea reduction rate is comparable between them.

Clinical Effectiveness

Although the reduction rate of β_2-microglobulin was greater by push/pull hemodiafiltration than by hemodialysis, the difference was rather small between them, because of the new and vastly improved hemodiafilters, which remove so much β_2-microglobulin only by dialysis. Nevertheless, restless legs syndrome, irritability, insomnia and pruritus were clearly alleviated after switching the treatment modality from conventional hemodialysis to push/pull hemodiafiltration according to our observations. This may indicate that these symptoms could be due to accumulation of uremic substances larger than β_2-microglobulin.

Treatment Cost

The final pyrogen filter on the substitution fluid line branching out from the dialysate pathway and connected to the blood tubing is essential to online hemodiafiltration. In push/pull hemodiafiltration, on the other hand, the hemodiafilter also serves as the final pyrogen filter. Therefore, when the final pyrogen filter must be disposable in online hemodiafiltration, push/pull hemodiafiltration is more cost-effective.

References

1 Canaud B, N'Guyen QV, Lagarde C, Stec F, Polaschegg HD, Mion C: Clinical evaluation of a multipurpose system adequate for hemodialysis, for postdilution hemofiltration/hemodiafiltration with on-line preparation of substitution fluid from dialysate; in Streicher E, Seyffart G (eds): Highly Permeable Membranes. Contrib Nephrol. Basel, Karger, 1985, vol 46, pp 184–186.

2 Usuda M, Shinzato T, Sezaki R, Kawanishi A, Maeda K, Kawaguchi S, Shibata M, Toyoda T, Asakura Y, Ohbayashi S: New simultaneous HF and HD with no infusion fluid. Trans Am Soc Artif Organs 1982;28:24–27.

3 Shinzato T, Fujisawa K, Nakai S, Miwa H, Kobayakawa H, Takai I, Morita H, Maeda K: Newly developed economical and efficient push/pull hemodiafiltration; in Maeda K, Shinzato T (eds): Effective Hemodiafiltration: New Methods. Contrib Nephrol. Basel, Karger, 1994, vol 108, pp 79–86.

4 Dorson WJ, Pizziconi VB, Allen JM: Transfer of chemical species through a protein gel. Trans Am Soc Artif Organs 1971;17:287–292.

5 Porter MC: Concentration polarization with membrane ultrafiltration. Ind Eng Chem Prod Res Dev 1972;11:234–248.

6 Colton CK, Henderson LW, Ford CA, Lysaght MJ: 1. In vitro transport characteristics of a hollow-fiber blood ultrafilter. J Lab Clin Med 1975;85:355–371.
7 Canaud B, Flavier JL, Argil SA, Stec F, N'Guyen QV, Bouloux CH, Garred LJ, Mion C: Hemodiafiltration with on-line production of substitution fluid: long-term safety and quantitative assessment of efficacy; in Maeda K, Shinzato T (eds): Effective Hemodiafiltration: New Methods. Contrib Nephrol. Basel, Karger, 1994, vol 108, pp 12–22.
8 Dellanna F, Wuepper A, Baldamus CA: Internal filtration-advantage in haemodialysis? Nephrol Dial Transplant 1996;11(suppl 2):83–86.

Toru Shinzato
Daiko Medical Engineering Research Institute
4–16–23, Daiko, Higashi-ku
Nagoya-shi, Aichi-ken 461-0043 (Japan)
Tel. +81 52 711 8889, Fax +81 52 711 8808, E-Mail shinzato@xj8.so-net.ne.jp

Ronco C, Canaud B, Aljama P (eds): Hemodiafiltration.
Contrib Nephrol. Basel, Karger, 2007, vol 158, pp 177–184

Principles and Practice of Internal Hemodiafiltration

Gianfranco Beniamino Fiore[a], *Claudio Ronco*[b]

[a]Dipartimento di Bioingegneria, Politecnico di Milano, Milan, and
[b]Department of Nephrology, St. Bortolo Hospital, Vicenza, Italy

Abstract

It has recently been suggested that the potentials of modern high-flux membranes could be exploited with the so-called internal hemodiafiltration (iHDF) technique. In principle, iHDF works just as high-flux hemodialysis but requires the convective dose to be clinically relevant, quantifiable and possibly adjustable by the operator. In this chapter, we briefly survey the theoretical, technological and practical aspects of iHDF, focusing on the mechanism ensuring its convective potential, i.e. the internal filtration/backfiltration (IF/BF) phenomenon. Based on theory, it is highlighted that the enhancement of the convective dose during iHDF relies upon a wise design of the hemodialyzer, both in terms of membrane performance and of hydrodynamics, whereas the adjustment of convection is feasible by proper regulation of the treatment parameters. IF/BF measurements appear to be feasible by indirect means; however, investments are needed to bring technology from the mere research field to the clinical practice. An alternative approach to IF/BF quantification is using mathematical models provided that the developed calculation tools are handy enough for the clinician, or even be implemented in the dialysis machine itself. IF/BF 'calculators' also represent a means to make the clinical staff conscious of the filtration phenomena that take place inside a high-flux hemodialyzer. It is concluded that iHDF is a possible complementary, simplified technique which could increase the clinical diffusion of high-flux convective treatments in the near future.

It is a widely accepted concept that an appropriate combination of convective solute transport to diffusive solute transport enhances the potentials of hemodialysis. The growing success of the clinical use of hemodiafiltration (HDF) [1–3] is evidence of this: HDF is the convective treatment par excellence, because it allows the convective dose to reach very high levels (up to 4.5–5.0 l/h in postdilution) and to be under the operator's direct control. On the other hand, HDF suffers from some practical disadvantages (basically, its cost and the complication of the hardware and procedures involved) which potentially limit its clinical spread.

Convective transport is the leading benefit of high-flux dialysis, too. But high-flux dialysis is based on letting convective transport happen spontaneously within the dialyzer, thanks to the internal filtration/backfiltration (IF/BF) mechanism [4, 5]. As detailed below, in the usual countercurrent setting, direct cross-filtration (DF) happens in the proximal part of the device, which provides for convective solute removal since DF is discharged with the exhausted dialysate. Distal BF of fresh dialysate acts as a 'spontaneous reinfusion' phenomenon, intrinsically ensuring fluid balance. Exploiting BF implies a need for good water quality, just as for the online version of HDF, but it introduces an additional screen for the reinfused fluid (i.e. the dialyzer's membrane itself); moreover, it avoids the need for substitution fluids or additional technology. High-flux dialysis thus has enough practical advantages to be appealing to the clinician as a 'hidden HDF'. We proposed that high-flux dialysis could be reconsidered as a simplified, 'internal' HDF technique (iHDF) [6], provided that the following conditions are met: (1) the attainable convective dose should be clinically relevant; (2) the convective dose should be under the operator's control or, at least, be quantifiable in the clinical theater.

Increasing the Amount of Convection in Internal Hemodiafiltration

IF/BF is governed by hydraulic and oncotic pressures, as sketched in figure 1. Locally, the amount of membrane filtration depends on local transmembrane pressure (TMP) and on the membrane's water permeability, according to the relation:

$$J_{UF}(x) = L_P\,(p_b(x) - p_d(x) - \Pi(x)) = L_P\,(TMP(x)) \qquad (1)$$

where J_{UF} is the local ultrafiltration flux, L_P is the membrane's hydraulic permeability, p is hydrostatic pressure, Π is the blood's oncotic pressure and x is the axial coordinate along the device; subscripts b and d refer to the blood and dialysate compartments, respectively. In the countercurrent arrangement, pressures in the two compartments decay with opposite slopes. Hence BF may occur at distal portions of the device if TMP becomes negative [or the total pressure on the blood side ($p_b[x] - \Pi[x]$) falls below the pressure on the dialysate side]. Thus, in the presence of BF, the device's net ultrafiltration rate Q_{UF} is due to the difference between the DF rate Q_{DF} and the BF rate Q_{BF}:

$$Q_{UF} = Q_{DF} - Q_{BF} \text{ or } Q_{DF} = Q_{UF} + Q_{BF}. \qquad (2)$$

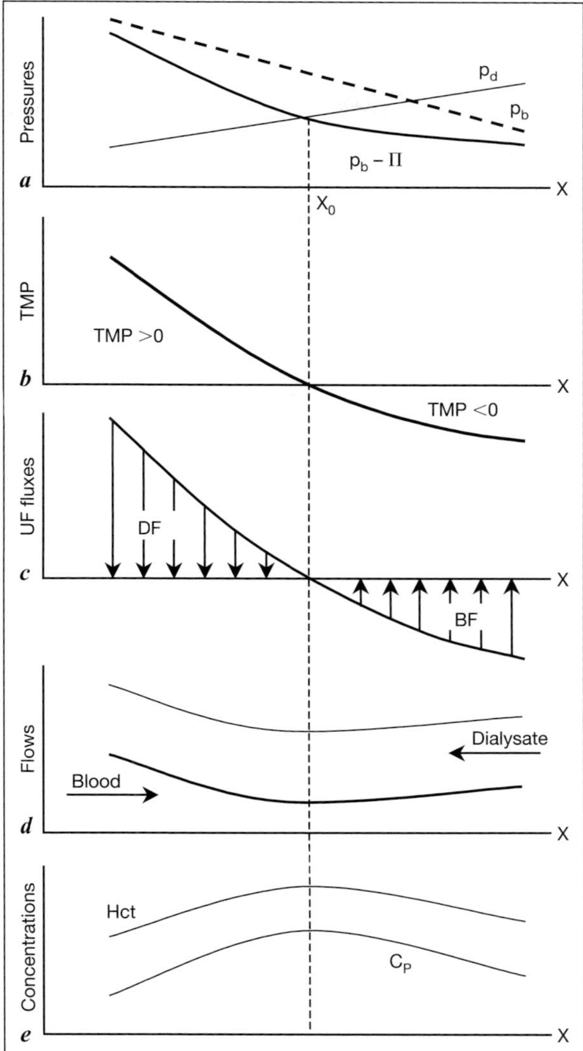

Fig. 1. Schematic diagrams of relevant quantities, plotted against the axial coordinate of the hemodialyzer, x, in the presence of IF/BF. ***a*** The pressure behavior; p_b = Hydraulic pressure in the blood compartment; p_d = hydraulic pressure in the dialysate compartment; Π: oncotic pressure. ***b*** The behavior of transmembrane pressure (TMP). ***c*** The behavior of ultrafiltration (UF) fluxes. ***d*** The behavior of fluid flow (blood flows left to right; dialysate fluid flows right to left). ***e*** The behavior of blood concentrations; Hct = hematocrit; C_P = plasma protein concentration.

The term IF is associated with BF to signify that the real filtration behavior occurring inside the device is not visible: the total convection amount *(Q_{DF})* may not be evaluated measuring the net Q_{UF} only.

For a zero-balance condition ($Q_{UF} = 0$), it is $Q_{DF} = Q_{BF}$. But, for a permeability high enough (as for high-flux membranes), IF persists even when drawing a net Q_{UF} (such as in fig. 1). The overall Q_{BF} is given by:

$$Q_{BF} = \int_{x_0}^{L} L_P \; TMP(x)\, p_f \; dx \tag{3}$$

where p_f is the total fiber perimeter along a cross-section, L is the device's active length and x_0 is the axial position where TMP = 0 (fig. 1). The integral on the right-hand side of equation 3 is represented by the BF area of figure 1c: the overall amount of IF/BF therefore increases with the TMP at the extremities of the dialyzer (which in turn is influenced by the pressure drops along the filter both in the blood and dialysate compartments), and on the membrane's water permeability: the amount of convection obtainable by the IF/BF mechanism is limited by oncotic effects but may be enhanced by a wise exploitation of the hydrodynamic pattern.

The matter of increasing the convective dose has therefore to be tackled by properly orienting the dialyzer design in terms of membrane permeability and hydraulic pressure drops. As for the former, the technical challenge is finding a compromise between enhancing L_P and maintaining an appropriate sieving effect. High-flux polysulfone membranes are normally reported to have a pure-water permeability in the range of 100–400 ml/(h · mm Hg · m^2), with peaks of 700 ml/(h · mm Hg · m^2) for enhanced high-flux membranes [6].

As for the pressure behavior, in the past researchers have already proposed to enhance pressure drops by acting on the dialyzer's design. For the dialysate side, the inclusion of spacer yarns or path constrictors or the increase in fiber density were proposed [7–9]. For the blood side, fiber diameter shrinking [7, 8] or fiber length increase were proposed. At a careful analysis, the latter shows to be a safer choice for the limitation of the hemolytic potential [6].

Measurement of Internal Filtration

Quantification of the convective dose during clinical iHDF is not trivial. IF takes place *within* the dialyzer: at the current state of the technology, there is no way to measure DF or BF directly (even if their difference, i.e. the net Q_{UF}, is measured). Methods for indirect measurement have been proposed, but their application was confined to in vitro studies. One chance is measuring the local concentration of a marker molecule in the blood path [10, 11] or in the dialysate compartment [12]. Indeed, one 'side effect' of the IF/BF phenomenon is a relevant concentration/dilution behavior taking place along the dialyzer (fig. 1, bottom panel). Hence, when the inlet value and the peak value for a marker molecule concentration are measured, a simple formula [10] allows one to deduct the actual DF and/or BF rates taking place inside the device. Amounts of convection of 1,800–3,000 ml/h were measured in vitro by such methods in polysulfone dialyzers [10, 11]. However, the direct transfer of such methods to the clinical use is unfeasible, either due to safety reasons (e.g. when using radioactive or potentially harmful molecules) or to practical reasons (e.g. cumbersome equipment, complex procedures).

One second chance is using Doppler measurements of blood velocity within the dialyzer fibers [13]. The DF of blood in the proximal part of the dialyzer causes erythrocytes to travel more slowly around the x_0 section than at the entrance (fig. 1d), and particularly the peak decrease in blood flow rate (estimated measuring the peak percent decrease in Doppler velocity) equals DF. With this method, amounts of convection up to 2,300 ml/h were indirectly measured in vitro in a polysulfone high-flux dialyzer [13]. The use of such a method during real treatments appears more feasible; however, it is not credible that a common hemodialysis unit would invest so much in the iHDF concept as to be supplied with Doppler equipment and with personnel skilled for its daily use.

Other measuring principles might be explored for indirect quantification of IF/BF with the state-of-the-art sensors. But apart from technical considerations, it seems clear that IF/BF measurement may become a clinical practice in the near future only if this challenge is accepted by the manufacturing companies as an option to provide their dialysis equipment with a technologically oriented added value.

Mathematical Estimation of Internal Filtration

An alternative approach is resorting to the mathematical quantification of convection based on a mathematical model, designed to accept clinically measured quantities as input values and to yield the dialyzer's filtration behavior as its output. An extensive literature exists on the mathematical modeling of fluid and/or solute transport in hollow-fiber dialyzers: a comprehensive review was reported by Eloot et al. [14]. A sound engineering approach consists in tackling the complete continuum problem by means of computational fluid dynamics techniques, which allow for very comprehensive, 3-dimensional, non-Newtonian descriptions of local flow/filtration dynamics and rheology. However, this approach cannot be widely applied for the systematic quantification of real clinical cases, due to the technical competences, the computational times and the costs requested by computational fluid dynamics analyses. At the opposite end, in the past, estimation of BF was proposed by means of elementary calculations, based on neglecting the changes in blood viscosity and protein concentration that take place with blood concentration and dilution [15]. Such early attempts, justified by the need to avoid BF in a period when bad water quality was a threat, were reasonable for low-flux dialyzers. With modern high-flux devices, having a simple analytical formula available for IF/BF estimation is mere fancy, because neglecting oncotic limitation causes greater and greater estimation errors at increasing hydraulic permeability.

The ideal solution in today's scenario would be to supply the clinician with an advanced simulation tool, as easy as a pocket calculator in its use but strong enough in its theoretical basis to yield trustworthy estimations. In an attempt towards this direction, we have recently pursued a 1-dimensional theoretical approach, coupled with the possibility of precharacterizing the devices in vitro [16]. Modeling choices were driven by the aim of building a lightweight calculation tool, usable by a clinician as a support in the quantitative interpretation of practical cases and as a tool to help dialysis prescription. A semiempirical mathematical model describing dialyzer hydrodynamics and membrane filtration was hence developed, and the necessary hydraulic characteristics of commercial hemodialyzers were derived experimentally with 3 hollow-fiber polysulfone devices of different sizes. Both the model and the in vitro characterization were implemented into an easy-to-use PC-based software tool aimed at estimating cross-filtration and IF/BF as a function of the machine settings as well as blood hematocrit and plasma protein concentration. In practice, the clinical user would run simulations related to a patient when the hematochemical data for that patient are available, so as to estimate the possible convective dose achievable for that subject with different devices and/or settings for the dialysis machine. Prospectively, a similar tool could be implemented in future dialysis machines with appropriate software adaptations.

Model results obtained for an IF/BF-prone device (the Toray BS-1.8UL), at normal operating conditions and blood parameters, showed an overall convection around 2,850 ml/h which may be obtained by virtue of IF/BF at zero net ultrafiltration; values up to 3,600 ml/h are reached when the net Q_{UF} is increased to 1,200 ml/h. Results also showed that options exist for the operator to enhance convection by adjusting either blood or dialysate flow rates, with blood flow rate achieving the greater effect. Moreover, model results showed an excellent agreement with experimental results obtained in purposely performed in vitro scintigraphic tests, with only a 3% prediction error.

Internal Hemodiafiltration: A Competitor of Hemodiafiltration?

Most of the considerations summarized above lead to the conclusion that technology is ripe enough to introduce iHDF as a well-grounded technique.

The convective effect achieved cannot be compared with the high convection rates achieved in online HDF, since the amount of convection is limited by the mechanics of the fluids involved in the treatment and the intrinsic nature of the hemodialyzer. But convection figures are high enough to possibly yield visible clinical effects, as recently reported [17].

Quantification of the convective dose appears to be feasible. Even if its clinical measurement is not available for now, the use of appropriate IF/BF calculators could represent a temporary bridge to a future setting in which investments from the industry will have made the necessary technology a reality. Moreover, mathematical modeling has a role in clarifying the mechanisms of filtration and BF, making the capacity of convective transport by a specific device and membrane fully understood and possibly exploited at best, with machine settings used as regulation tools.

In conclusion, rather than considering iHDF a competitor for HDF, it should be included as a possible alternative to extend the conscious clinical application of the convective principle, with lesser potentials than HDF but with lower costs and easier requirements.

References

1 Canaud B, Bragg-Gresham JL, Marshall MR, Desmeules S, Gillespie BW, Depner T, Klassen P, Port FK: Mortality risk for patients receiving hemodiafiltration versus hemodialysis: European results from the DOPPS. Kidney Int 2006;69:2087–2093.

2 Canaud B, Morena M, Leray-Moragues H, Chalabi L, Cristol JP: Overview of clinical studies in hemodiafiltration: what do we need now? Hemodial Int 2006;10(suppl 1):S5–S12.

3 Penne EL, Blankestijn PJ, Bots ML, van den Dorpel MA, Grooteman MP, Nube MJ, van der Tweel I, ter Wee PM, the CONTRAST study group: Effect of increased convective clearance by online hemodiafiltration on all cause and cardiovascular mortality in chronic hemodialysis patients – The Dutch Convective Transport Study (CONTRAST): rationale and design of a randomised controlled trial (ISRCTN38365125). Curr Control Trials Cardiovasc Med 2005;6:8.

4 Leypoldt JK, Schmidt B, Gurland HJ: Net ultrafiltration may not eliminate backfiltration during hemodialysis with highly permeable membranes. Artif Organs 1991;15:164–170.

5 Baurmeister U, Travers M, Vienken J, Harding G, Million C, Klein E, Pass T, Wright R: Dialysate contamination and back filtration may limit the use of high-flux dialysis membranes. ASAIO Trans 1989;35:519–522.

6 Fiore GB, Ronco C: Internal hemodiafiltration (iHDF): a possible option to expand hemodiafiltration therapy. Int J Artif Organs 2004;27:420–423.

7 Ronco C, Brendolan A, Lupi A, Metry G, Levin NW: Effects of a reduced inner diameter of hollow fibers in hemodialyzers. Kidney Int 2000;58:809–817.

8 Mineshima M, Ishimori I, Ishida K, Hoshino T, Kaneko I, Sato Y, Agishi T, Tamamura N, Sakurai H, Masuda T, Hattori H: Effects of internal filtration on the solute removal efficiency of a dialyzer. ASAIO J 2000;46:456–460.

9 Ronco C, Orlandini G, Brendolan A, Lupi A, La Greca G: Enhancement of convective transport by internal filtration in a modified experimental hemodialyzer: technical note. Kidney Int 1998;54: 979–985.
10 Ronco C, Brendolan A, Feriani M, Milan M, Conz P, Lupi A, Berto P, Bettini M, La Greca G: A new scintigraphic method to characterize ultrafiltration in hollow fiber dialyzers. Kidney Int 1992; 41:1383–1393.
11 Sakai Y, Wada S, Matsumoto H, Suyama T, Ohno O, Anno I: Nondestructive evaluation of blood flow in a dialyzer using X-ray computed tomography. J Artif Organs 2003;6:197–204.
12 Leypoldt JK, Schmidt B, Gurland HJ: Measurement of backfiltration rates during hemodialysis with highly permeable membranes. Blood Purif 1991;9:74–84.
13 Sato Y, Mineshima M, Ishimori I, Kaneko I, Akiba T, Teraoka S: Effect of hollow fiber length on solute removal and quantification of internal filtration rate by Doppler ultrasound. Int J Artif Organs 2003;26:129–134.
14 Eloot S, De Wachter D, Van Tricht I, Verdonck P: Computational flow modeling in hollow-fiber dialyzers. Artif Organs 2002;26:590–599.
15 Soltys PJ, Ofsthun NJ, Leypoldt JK: Critical analysis of formulas for estimating backfiltration in hemodialysis. Blood Purif 1992;10:326–332.
16 Fiore GB, Guadagni G, Lupi A, Ricci Z, Ronco C: A new semiempirical mathematical model for prediction of internal filtration in hollow fiber hemodialyzers. Blood Purif 2006;24:555–568.
17 Lucchi L, Fiore GB, Guadagni G, Perrone S, Malaguti V, Caruso F, Fumero R, Albertazzi A: Clinical evaluation of internal hemodiafiltration (iHDF): a diffusive-convective technique performed with internal filtration enhanced high-flux dialyzers. Int J Artif Organs 2004;27:414–419.

Gianfranco B. Fiore, PhD
Dipartimento di Bioingegneria, Politecnico di Milano
Piazza Leonardo da Vinci, 32
IT–20133 Milano (Italy)
Tel. +39 02 2399 3337, Fax +39 02 2399 3360, E-Mail gianfranco.fiore@polimi.it

Ronco C, Canaud B, Aljama P (eds): Hemodiafiltration.
Contrib Nephrol. Basel, Karger, 2007, vol 158, pp 185–193

Clinical Aspects of Haemodiafiltration

Francesco Locatelli, Salvatore Di Filippo, Celestina Manzoni

Department of Nephrology and Dialysis, A. Manzoni Hospital, Lecco, Italy

Abstract

Standard haemodialysis is not a very efficacious treatment of chronic uraemia and patient mortality rate is still very high. The 2002 results of the HEMO study showed that alternative treatments such as 'high-efficiency haemodialysis' and 'high-flux haemodialysis' are associated with a non-significant reduction in the relative risk of mortality (4 and 8%, respectively). In an attempt to define the clinical impact of haemodiafiltration, we review some of the efficacy data from clinical studies in light of a number of factors that may be related to the high mortality among haemodialysis patients.

Uraemia is a pathological condition caused by the retention of solutes that are normally excreted by the kidneys. The aim of haemodialysis (HD) is to remove these solutes, but standard HD is not very efficacious, and patient morbidity and mortality rates are still very high (15–25% per year).

Nearly 20 years ago, the hypothesis that the extremely high morbidity and mortality rates were associated with inadequate removal of 'middle molecules' led to proposals for two alternative methods: high-efficiency HD [1] and high-flux HD [2]. At the same blood and dialysate flows, and using membranes that have the same low permeability as those used for standard HD but a larger surface area, high-efficiency HD increases vitamin B_{12} clearance by about 50% in vitro; high-flux HD uses high-permeability membranes that increase the clearance of solutes with a molecular weight of about 1,500 Da and also remove solutes with a molecular weight of about 11,000 Da, such as β_2-microglobulin.

Observational studies have consistently shown that high-flux treatments have positive effects on the morbidity and survival of HD patients. However, the 2002 results of the HEMO study [3], a prospective, randomized study aimed at

Table 1. Cardiovascular risk factors in chronic kidney disease

Traditional risk factors	Non-traditional risk factors
Older age	Albuminuria/proteinuria
Male gender	Homocysteine
Hypertension	Anaemia
Higher low-density lipoprotein cholesterol levels	Abnormal calcium-phosphate metabolism
Low high-density lipoprotein cholesterol levels	Extracellular fluid overload
Diabetes	Oxidative stress
Smoking	Inflammation
Physical inactivity	Malnutrition
Menopause	
Family history of cerebrovascular disease	
Left ventricular hypertrophy	

verifying the advantages of high-efficiency and high-flux HD over standard HD, were very surprising and in some way disappointing insofar as they showed that greater urea removal non-significantly reduces the relative risk of mortality by only 4% and that high-flux HD was associated with a non-significant reduction of 8%. The major criticisms of the HEMO study design were that it included prevalent instead of only incident patients, reused dialysers and used high-flux dialysers with low convective clearances.

The preliminary results of the Membrane Permeability Outcome (MPO) study [4] seem to be very promising in terms of the first 2 aspects (on the basis of a presentation by the principal investigator at the investigators' meeting); as far as the third is concerned, it is possible to increase convection by means of haemodiafiltration (HDF) as Schneider and Streicher [5] have already shown that, even when using the same membrane, it significantly increases middle-molecules clearance in comparison with HD.

In an attempt to define the clinical impact of HDF, we will review some of the efficacy data from clinical studies in the light of a number of factors that may be related to the high mortality among HD patients. It is well known that cardiovascular disease is the major cause of death, and we will analyse the impact of HDF on some of the main cardiovascular risk factors listed in table 1.

Hyperphosphataemia

Hyperphosphataemia has been associated with an increased risk of all-cause mortality, including cardiovascular mortality [6].

Zehnder et al. [7] compared the transmembrane solute mass removal and clearance of phosphate in 16 patients who underwent high-flux HD for 1 week followed by 1 week's postdilutional online HDF. The results strongly suggested that HDF increases phosphate clearance, and the authors concluded that it should be considered an additional treatment option for dialysis patients with uncontrolled hyperphosphataemia. However, because it was so short, this study does not give any information concerning the possible difference in long-term predialysis phosphataemia levels of the two treatments.

Anaemia

Together with hypertension, anaemia is the main cause of ventricular hypertrophy in dialysis patients.

Maduell et al. [8] evaluated the difference between conventional HDF (mean fluid replacement 4 l/session), in which the extent of convection is roughly comparable with that of high-flux HD, and online HDF (mean fluid replacement 22.5 l/session) in 37 patients over a period of 1 year. The most interesting result was that online HDF led to the better correction of anaemia with lower erythropoietin doses, possibly because the greater elimination of medium-sized molecules reduced the erythropoietin response, although the role of the better quality of dialysate due to online treatment cannot be ruled out. This possibility is further suggested by the results of a study by Schiffl et al. [9] which clearly support the hypothesis that the use of ultrapure (filtered, pyrogen-free and sterile) dialysate reduces the recombinant human erythropoietin doses required to maintain haemoglobin levels as a result of a reduction in systemic inflammatory processes.

Cardiovascular Stability

Cardiovascular instability is the most frequent clinical problem that occurs during both acute and long-term HD. Preventing intradialytic hypotension is of great importance not only to deliver an adequate dialysis dose, but also to achieve the target patient dry body weight, as hypertension in dialysis patients is largely due to fluid overload.

A retrospective study by Pizzarelli et al. [10] compared the results obtained during online HDF with those obtained during standard bicarbonate HD. Online

HDF led to a better cardiovascular tolerance to fluid removal, with a significantly lower incidence of episodes of symptomatic hypotension requiring the administration of saline and/or hypertonic solutions.

A prospective, randomized trial by Lin et al. [11] also found that online HDF led to better haemodynamic stability. They treated 111 patients, who were randomly divided into 4 groups receiving different frequencies of online HDF and/or high-flux HD: HDF 3 times a week; HDF twice and high-flux HD once a week; HDF once and high-flux HD twice a week; high-flux HD 3 times a week. There were fewer episodes of symptomatic hypotension and lower mean saline infusion volumes at greater frequencies of online HDF, which also significantly reduced the amount of erythropoietin required, and improved intra- and interdialysis symptoms. It is interesting that higher predialysis natraemia levels (2.3 mEq/l) were observed in the patients receiving more frequent online HDF, thus suggesting that a reduced sodium removal during HDF was at least partially responsible for the better cardiovascular stability. The same is true for the results of Maduell et al. [8].

Altieri et al. [12] compared the effects of online haemofiltration and online HDF on cardiovascular stability and blood pressure in a randomized trial involving 39 patients and concluded that both treatments allow the good control of intrasession symptoms and blood pressure in stable patients.

According to the original observation by Maggiore [13] that a better haemodynamic protection is provided by a dialysate temperature of about 35°C in comparison with the standard dialysate temperature of 37–38°C, an alternative hypothesis to explain the decrease in hypotensive episodes during online HDF has been suggested by Donauer et al. [14], who identified blood cooling as the main factor. They found that enhanced energy loss occurred within the extracorporeal system despite identical dialysate and substitution fluid temperature settings, which meant that the blood returning to the patient was cooler during online HDF than during HD. The use of cooler, temperature-controlled HD led to an incidence of symptomatic hypotension that was similar to that observed during online HDF.

β_2-Microglobulin

In order to verify the impact of online HDF, Wizemann et al. [15] conducted a 24-month controlled prospective study in which 44 chronic dialysis patients were randomized to low-flux HD or online HDF. There were no differences in morbidity, blood pressure, dialysis-associated hypotensive episodes, haematocrit or erythropoietin dose between the groups, nor any differences in body weight and nutrition parameters. As expected, plasma β_2-microglobulin concentrations did not change in the HD group throughout the 2 years but decreased from similar values to 18 mg/l before dialysis ($p < 0.01$) during the first 6 months of HDF treatment, and then remained constant until the end of the study. However, it is possible that the clinical reversal of the situation by convective methods takes a long time, including the effects of a reduction in β_2-microglobulin levels.

Ward et al. [16] carried out a prospective clinical trial involving 44 patients randomized to online postdilution HDF or high-flux HD for 12 months, and found a similar decrease in pretreatment plasma β_2-microglobulin levels despite the apparent difference in the removal of β_2-microglobulin indicated by the significantly greater pre- to posttreatment reduction in the HDF group. It should be remembered that a change in the concentration of a solute is a good indicator of removal only in the case of solutes distributed in a single pool including plasma, whereas the fact that a substantial rebound in posttreatment plasma β_2-microglobulin levels has been reported suggests that a single-pool model is inadequate to describe β_2-microglobulin kinetics. Intrabody mass transfer rates limit β_2-microglobulin removal, and so the pre- to posttreatment change in concentration overestimates the actual removal.

Emerging Cardiovascular Risk Factors

It has been shown that hyperhomocysteinaemia is independently associated with an increase in cardiovascular risk in dialysis patients.

Arnadottir et al. [17] studied the effects of standard HD on the plasma concentrations of total homocysteine (tHcy) and creatinine in 56 patients, and found that the dialysis-induced reduction in tHcy was less than the reduction in creatinine, despite their similar molecular weight and distribution volumes (0.45 l/kg [18] and 0.48 l/kg [19]). An alternative explanation is that tHcy is partially protein bound and the bound fraction cannot be removed by either low- or high-flux HD; furthermore, as the problem lies in the permeability of the membrane, it cannot be expected that different methods will lead to different results. Support for this hypothesis comes from a 3-month randomized trial by House et al. [20], who examined the effect of maintenance HD with high-flux polysulphone versus low-flux polysulphone on predialysis tHcy levels in 48 patients. More permeable superflux dialysers designed to maximize convective transport are the only ones capable of significantly removing tHcy [21].

Chronic inflammation and oxidative stress are highly prevalent in patients with chronic kidney disease and end-stage renal disease, and may contribute to the high mortality rates associated with cardiovascular disease [22].

In addition, advanced glycation end products (AGEs) may represent a novel class of uraemic toxins with significant implications for long-term dialysis-related pathological states. A study by Lin et al. [23] analysed long-term changes in serum AGE levels using various dialysis modalities. Eighty-one patients with chronic uraemia were divided into 3 groups receiving conventional HD, high-flux HD or online HDF. During the 6-month study period, predialysis serum AGE levels were significantly lower in the patients treated with online HDF than in those treated with conventional or high-flux HD. In line with this, Gerdemann et al. [24] found that predialysis AGE levels in patients treated with HDF and haemofiltration are significantly lower than those of patients treated with high-flux HD using standard dialysis fluid, but the difference was not significant when ultrapure dialysis fluid was used. This suggests that factors other than removal (including ultrapure dialysis fluid and water quality) are responsible for the lower pretreatment AGE levels found in patients treated with HDF compared to HD.

Survival

It is a matter of fact that survival, together with the quality of life, is the most important outcome.

The characteristics and outcomes of patients from 5 European countries receiving HDF or HD in the Dialysis Outcomes and Practice Patterns Study [25] were published in 2006. From 1998 to 2001, the study analysed 2,165 patients stratified into 4 groups: low- and high-flux HD (63.1 and 25.2% of all patients), and low- and high-efficiency HDF (7.2 and 4.5% of all patients). The patients undergoing high-efficiency HDF had a 35% lower relative mortality risk ($= 0.65$; $p = 0.01$) than those receiving low-flux HD, whereas those on low-efficiency HDF showed a non-significant 7% reduction (relative risk $= 0.93$; $p = 0.68$). These results are very impressive but only demonstrate an association: as the authors themselves acknowledged, the benefits of HDF must be tested in controlled clinical trials before any recommendations can be made for clinical practice.

This is particularly true when considering discrepancies between the results of observational and randomized studies. One prospective randomized trial [26] involving 380 patients compared low-flux HD, high-flux HD and HDF in order to evaluate possible advantages in terms of treatment tolerance, nutritional parameters and pretreatment β_2-microglobulin levels. However, it was not found that convection and/or membrane biocompatibility improved cardiovascular stability during dialysis, mainly because the incidence of intradialytic hypotension was very low in the study population as a whole, i.e. the study was underpowered to find possible differences. Moreover, the same trial did not find any difference in survival related to membrane biocompatibility or flux, but it was not primarily designed and powered for that.

An observational study by Hornberger et al. [27] showed that patients treated by high-flux HD had a 65% lower relative risk of mortality than those treated with standard HD, and other observational studies indicate that HD with high-flux dialysers is associated with less morbidity and mortality than HD with low-flux dialysers. In a large observational study comparing convective and diffusive treatments, a non-significant 10% better survival rate was observed in favour of convective treatments [28]. The very large, prospective randomized HEMO study of flux and survival found a non-significant 8% better survival rate in the patients treated with high-flux membranes, although a statistical reduction in cardiovascular morbidity in favour of high-flux dialysis was found in a post hoc analysis.

A systematic review of randomized controlled trials comparing HD, haemofiltration, HDF and acetate-free biofiltration to assess their clinical effectiveness has been published [29], but, because the assessed trials were not powered adequately and their methodological quality was suboptimal, no definite conclusions can be drawn as to which is the best replacement therapy [30].

As the number of randomized prospective trials comparing HDF and standard HD is still limited, no conclusive data are available concerning the effect of HDF on survival and morbidity in patients with end-stage renal disease. However, 2 further studies are currently exploring the potential beneficial effect of convection. An Italian prospective multicentre study [31] is comparing online convective treatments (haemofiltration and HDF) with standard low-flux HD, taking cardiovascular stability and blood pressure control as the primary end points, and impact on symptoms, morbidity and mortality as the secondary end points. The Dutch Convective Transport Study, which was started in the second quarter of 2004 [32], is being conducted in more than 20 centres in the Netherlands and will randomize approximately 800 incident and prevalent HD patients to low-flux HD or online HDF for 3 years in order to investigate the effect of increased convective transport by online HDF on all-cause and cardiovascular mortality in chronic HD patients.

At present, some results of the HEMO study (decreased cardiac mortality) [33] and the preliminary data of the MPO study (principal investigator presentation at MPO investigator meeting [4]) with a significant reduction in mortality in patients with serum albumin levels of less than 4 g/dl (primary end point) as well as in diabetic patients (secondary analysis) make a strong case in favour of high-flux treatments. A large, randomized controlled study is now needed to evaluate the clinical advantages of online HDF.

References

1 Keshaviah P, Collins A: Rapid high-efficiency bicarbonate hemodialysis. Trans Am Soc Artif Intern Organs 1986;32:17.

2 Von Albertini B, Miller JH, Gardner PW, Shinaberger JH: High-flux hemodiafiltration: under six hours/week treatment. Trans Am Soc Artif Intern Organs 1984;30:227–231.

3 Eknoyan G, Beck GJ, Cheung AK, Daugirdas JT, Greene T, et al, for the Hemodialysis (HEMO) Study Group: Effect of dialysis dose and membrane flux in maintenance hemodialysis. N Engl J Med 2002;347:2010–2019.

4 Locatelli F, Hannedouche T, Jacobson SH, La Greca G, Loureiro A, Martin-Malo A, Papadimitriou M, Vanholder R: The effect of membrane permeability on ESRD: design of a prospective randomised multicentre trial. J Nephrol 1999;12:85–88.

5 Schneider H, Streicher E: Mass transfer characterization of a new polysulfone membrane. Artif Organs 1985;2:180–183.

6 Block GA, Klassen PS, Lazarus JM, Ofsthun N, Lowrie EG, Chertow GM: Mineral metabolism, mortality and morbidity in maintenance hemodialysis. J Am Soc Nephrol 2004;15:2208–2218.

7 Zehnder C, Gutzwiller JP, Renggli K: Hemodiafiltration: a new treatment option for hyperphosphatemia in hemodialysis patients. Clin Nephrol 1999;52:152–159.

8 Maduell F, del Pozo C, Garcia H, Sanchez L, Hdez-Jaras J, Albero MD, Calvo C, Torregrosa I, Navarro V: Change from conventional haemodiafiltration to on-line haemodiafiltration. Nephrol Dial Transplant 1999;14:1202–1207.

9 Schiffl H, Lang SM, Bergner A: Ultrapure dialysate reduces dose of recombinant human erythropoietin. Nephron 1999;83:278–279.

10 Pizzarelli F, Cerrai T, Dattolo P, Tetta C, Maggiore Q: Convective treatments with on-line production of replacement fluid: a clinical experience lasting 6 years. Nephrol Dial Transplant 1998;13: 363–369.

11 Lin CL, Huang CC, Chang CT, Wu MS, Hung CC, Chien CC, Yang CW: Clinical improvement by increased frequency of on-line hemodiafiltration. Ren Fail 2001;23:193–206.

12 Altieri P, Sorba G, Bolasco P, Ledebo I, Ganadu M, Ferrara R, Menneas A, Asproni E, Casu D, Passaghe M, Sau G, Cadinu F, Sardinian Group on Hemofiltration On-Line: Comparison between hemofiltration and hemodiafiltration in a long-term prospective cross-over study. J Nephrol 2004; 17:414–422

13 Maggiore Q: Blood temperature and vascular stability during hemodialysis and hemofiltration. Trans Am Soc Artif Organs 1982;28:523–537.

14 Donauer J, Schweiger C, Rumberger B, Krumme B, Bohler J: Reduction of hypotensive side effects during online-haemodiafiltration and low temperature haemodialysis. Nephrol Dial Transplant 2003;18:1616–1622.

15 Wizemann V, Lotz C, Techert F, Uthoff S: On-line haemodiafiltration versus low-flux haemodialysis: a prospective randomized study. Nephrol Dial Transplant 2000;15(suppl 1):43–48.

16 Ward RA, Schmidt B, Hullin J, Hillebrand GF, Samtleben W: A comparison of on-line hemodiafiltration and high-flux hemodialysis: a prospective clinical study. J Am Soc Nephrol 2000;11: 2344–2350.

17 Arnadottir M, Berg AL, Hegbrant J, Hultberg B: Influence of haemodialysis on plasma total homocysteine concentration. Nephrol Dial Transplant 1999;14:142–146.

18 Guttormsen AB, Ueland PM, Svarstad E, Refsum H: Kinetic basis of hyperhomocysteinemia in patients with chronic renal failure. Kidney Int 1997;52:495–502.

19 Jones JD, Burnett PC: Creatinine metabolism in humans with decreased renal function: creatinine deficit. Clin Chem 1974;20:1204–1212.

20 House AA, Wells GA, Donnelly JG, Nadler SP, Hébert PC: Randomized trial of high-flux vs low-flux haemodialysis: effects on homocysteine and lipids. Nephrol Dial Transplant 2000;15: 1029–1034.

21 Van Tellingen A, Grooteman MPC, Bartels PCM, Van Limbeek J, Van Guldener C, ter Wee PM, Nubé MJ: Long-term reduction of plasma homocysteine levels by super-flux dialyzers in hemodialysis patients. Kidney Int 2001;59:342–347.

22 Locatelli F, Andrulli S, Memoli B, Maffei C, Del Vecchio L, Aterini S, De Simone W, Mandalari A, Brunori G, Amato M, Cianciaruso B, Zoccali C: Nutritional-inflammation status and resistance to erythropoietin therapy in hemodialysis patients. Nephrol Dial Transplant 2006;21:991–998.
23 Lin CL, Huang CC, Yu CC, Yang HY, Chuang FR, Yang CW: Reduction of advanced glycation end product levels by on-line hemodiafiltration in long-term hemodialysis patients. Am J Kidney Dis 2003;42:524–531.
24 Gerdemann A, Wagner Z, Solf A, Bahner U, Heidland A, Vienken J, Schinzel R: Plasma levels of advanced glycation end products during haemodialysis, haemodiafiltration and haemofiltration: potential importance of dialysate quality. Nephrol Dial Transplant 2002;17:1045–1049.
25 Canaud B, Bragg-Gresham JL, Marshall MR, Desmeules S, Gillespie BW, Depner T, Klassen P, Port FK: Mortality risk for patients receiving hemodiafiltration versus hemodialysis: European results from the DOPPS. Kidney Int 2006;69:2087–2093.
26 Locatelli F, Mastrangelo F, Redaelli B, Ronco C, Marcelli D, La Greca G, Orlandini G, the Italian Cooperative Dialysis Study Group: Effects of different membranes and dialysis technologies on patient treatment tolerance and nutritional parameters. Kidney Int 1996;50:1293–1302.
27 Hornberger JC, Chernew M, Petersen J, Garber AM: A multivariate analysis of mortality and hospital admission with high-flux dialysis. J Am Soc Nephrol 1992;3:1227–1237.
28 Locatelli F, Marcelli D, Conte F, Limido A, Malberti F, Spotti D: Comparison of mortality in ESRD patients on convective and diffusive extracorporeal treatments. The Registro Lombardo Dialisi e Trapianto. Kidney Int 1999;55:286–293.
29 Rabindranath KS, Strippoli GF, Roderick P, Wallace SA, MacLeod AM, Daly C: Comparison of hemodialysis, hemofiltration and acetate-free biofiltration for ESRD: systematic review. Am J Kidney Dis 2005;45:437–447.
30 Locatelli F: Comparison of hemodialysis, hemodiafiltration and hemofiltration: systematic review or systematic error? Am J Kidney Dis 2005;46:787–788.
31 Bolasco P, Altieri P, Andrulli S, Basile C, Di Filippo S, Feriani M, Pedrini L, Santoro A, Zoccali C, Sau G, Locatelli F: Convection versus diffusion in dialysis: an Italian prospective multicentre study. Nephrol Dial Transplant 2003;18(suppl 7):50–54.
32 Penne EL, Blankestijn PJ, Bots ML, Van den Dorpel MA, Grooteman MPC, Nubé MJ, ter Wee PM, on behalf of the CONTRAST Group: Resolving controversies regarding hemodiafiltration versus hemodialysis: the Dutch Convective Transport Study. Semin Dial 2005;18:47–51.
33 Cheung AK, Sarnak MJ, Yan G, Berkoben M, Heyka R, et al: Cardiac diseases in maintenance hemodialysis patients: results of the HEMO Study. Kidney Int 2004;65:2380–2389.

Prof. Francesco Locatelli, MD, FRCP
Divisione di Nefrologia e Dialisi, Azienda ospedaliera A. Manzoni
Via dell'Eremo 9–11
IT–23900 Lecco (Italy)
Tel. +39 034 148 9850, Fax +39 034 148 9860, E-Mail f.locatelli@ospedale.lecco.it

Ronco C, Canaud B, Aljama P (eds): Hemodiafiltration.
Contrib Nephrol. Basel, Karger, 2007, vol 158, pp 194–200

The Biological Response to Online Hemodiafiltration

V. Panichi[a], *C. Tetta*[b]

[a]Internal Medicine Department, University of Pisa, Pisa, Italy; [b]Fresenius Medical Care, International Research and Development, Bad Homburg, Germany

Abstract

The biologic response to uremia and to the associated chronic inflammation is an active area of research. Among the different modalities developed in the technology field of chronic renal replacement, hemodialfiltration has evolved consistently. On-line production of substitution fluid by 'cold sterilization' of dialysis fluid by ultrafiltration gives access to virtually an unlimited amount of sterile and non-pyrogenic intravenous grade solution. Today, on line HDF is already a widespread, accepted treatment. Here, we will review the main mechanisms through which on line hemodialfiltration acts and the biological response observed in relation to the immune system dysfunction and the anemia associated to chronic kidney disease.

Chronic kidney disease represents a complex mosaic of interwoven alterations at several levels: the cell, the microenvironment, the vasculature and the organ. Anemia, atherosclerosis and cardiovascular disease, immune dysfunction and alterations in bone metabolism are the clinical hallmarks. The biological response to uremia and to renal replacement therapy is at present an active area of research. The uremic syndrome is characterized by retention of solutes over a very large range of molecular weights. Despite its being elusive for several years, the uremic syndrome is the target of a major effort by the European Society for Artificial Organs, Uremic Toxins Group, to categorize uremic 'toxins' on the basis of molecular weight, protein binding and biological activity [1, 2]. These uremic retention solutes can be conveniently grouped into small water-soluble compounds of low molecular weight (less than 500 Da), middle molecules (greater than 500 Da), protein-bound solutes and low-molecular-weight proteins (5–35 kDa). Increasingly, evidence has been accumulating that both middle molecules (such as β_2-microglobulin) and largely protein-bound solutes (such as *p*-cresol and advanced glycosylation end products) may be important mediators of uremic toxicity. Standard hemodialysis (HD), which relies on diffusive solute clearance, has at best a moderate effect on removal of these larger-molecular-weight uremic retention products.

In recent years, it has become clear that the most important result of uremic toxicity not fully corrected by HD is vascular damage, characterized by the extraordinarily high rate of cardiovascular events in chronic kidney disease patients [3] and in the HD population [4]. While the pathogenesis of cardiovascular risk associated with uremia is not fully understood, it is clear that at least a component of this risk is due to 'nontraditional' cardiovascular risk factors, which include acute-phase inflammation, endothelial dysfunction, oxidative stress and insulin resistance [5–8]. Despite continuous technical improvement and better global patient care management, the annual mortality rate of patients with end-stage renal disease managed with 3 times weekly HD remains unacceptably high (10–22%) [9, 10], Factors affecting mortality include advanced age and comorbid conditions at the start of dialysis [11], the efficacy and quality of renal replacement therapy [12], practice patterns that may vary from region to region [13], different background atherosclerosis in the general population [14] and the intensity of chronic systemic inflammation. Chronic inflammation may play an important role in early morbidity and mortality in HD patients [15–18]. Several studies have attempted to address the question whether the type of the dialysis membrane, the quality of the dialysate or the uremic state may be responsible for the induction of a chronic inflammatory state [19–21].

It is known that among other nontraditional risk factors, the acute-phase reactants represent a class of proteins – mainly C-reactive protein and serum amyloid A – that are secreted primarily by hepatocytes under various appropriate stimuli such as interleukin 6 (IL-6). They are not merely biochemical markers of inflammation, but also act as modulators of the inflammatory response [22].

For years, standard low-flux HD has been the only treatment available. The introduction of high-permeability membranes has paved the way to high-flux HD and to hemodiafiltration (HDF).

Since the 80s there has been a steady growth in the technical development and clinical appraisal of HDF. Online production of substitution fluid by cold sterilization of dialysis fluid by ultrafiltration gives access to virtually an unlimited amount of sterile and nonpyrogenic intravenous-grade solution. Today, online HDF (OL-HDF) is already a widespread, accepted treatment. It is also the dialysis modality for which the most technology and inventiveness have been produced [23].

At present, HDF is a well-recognized treatment modality that offers a means of optimizing renal replacement therapy in chronic kidney disease patients [24]: by enhancing and enlarging the molecular-weight spectrum of uremic toxins removed, the convective clearance improves dialysis efficiency [25, 26]; by increasing the instantaneous solute flux of solutes including ions, HDF facilitates the restoration of the internal milieu; by improving the global hemocompatibility of the dialysis system (synthetic low-reactive membrane, ultrapurity of the dialysis fluid, protein coating of the membrane), HDF contributes to reducing the side effects and complications of long-term standard HD [for a review, see 27]. The incorporation of the infusion module into the dialysis proportioning machine hardware is also beneficial: first, it simplifies the handling procedure compared to bag HDF; second, it secures the process by enslaving the infusion module to the safety regulation of the HDF monitor, and third, it allows the physical integrity of the ultrafilters to be checked regularly by means of a built-in air pressure test. This low-cost production of substitution fluid has allowed the excellent convective and diffusive clearances of today's dialyzers to be exploited.

Parallel to further improvement in technical optimization for ever better efficiency, a great deal of published evidence has shown that OL-HDF induces a biological response from the host. This is intriguing, since it may be the link between some of the reported clinical effects. How strong this link might be is in general not easy to state, simply because of the fact that studies on the biological response were forcedly performed on relatively small patient cohorts. However, it has been clearly shown that from basic knowledge, the later extension of the determination of biomarkers, e.g. C-reactive protein, in large patient cohorts has spurred new trends in predictive risk analysis as it has been the case for the impact of chronic inflammation on overall mortality and that from cardiovascular disease. Figure 1 illustrates the possible aspects where convective-diffusive treatments could provide significant changes in patients with chronic kidney disease. We will focus on some findings that could provide the rational bases for future studies.

Immune Dysfunction and Online Hemodiafiltration

Studies on the ability of OL-HDF to modulate the immune response and systemic, chronic inflammation have disclosed an important potential for this technique. Ward et al. [26] and Beerenhout et al. [28] observed a reduction in plasma levels of complement D by postdilution HDF and predilution hemofiltration, respectively. Although the link to a clinically relevant outcome has yet to be shown, it should be remembered that complement D is a stimulant of the alternative route of complement and an inhibitor of the degranulation of polymorphonuclear leukocytes. More recent observations come from in-depth studies on the modulating role of OL-HDF on cells of the monocytic lineage. Circulating monocytes are heterogeneous in normal individuals. However, in

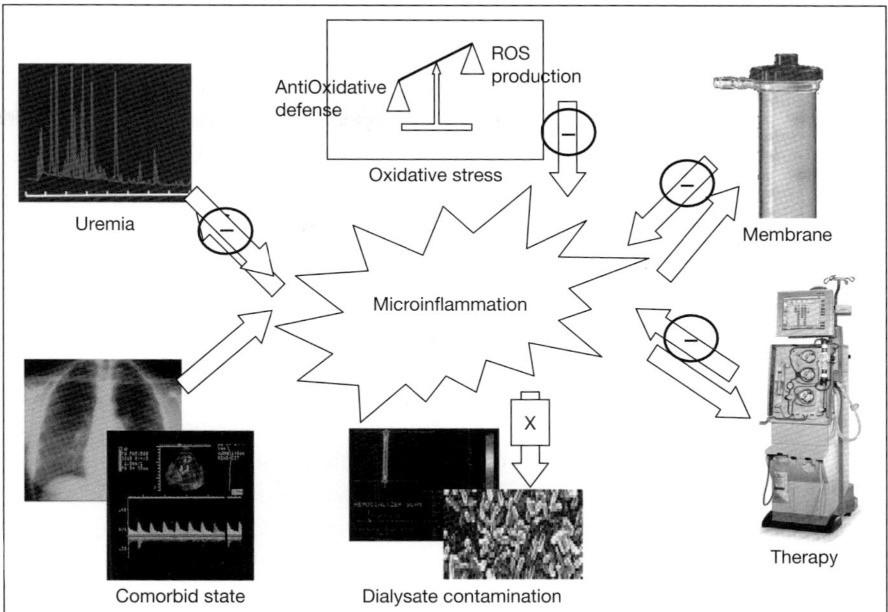

Fig. 1. Biological response to OL-HDF. Attenuation of microinflammation may occur due to the improved removal of retention solutes and of the uremic microenvironment, to improved biocompatibility of the membrane and the use of ultrapure reinfusion fluids leading to reduced monocyte activation and radical oxygen generation and finally to innovative OL-HDF monitors for absolute patient safety and long-term patient surveillance. ROS = Reactive oxygen species.

inflamed states such as in HD, the CD14+CD16+ subpopulation markedly increases, and this correlates with C-reactive protein levels. In a prospective, crossover study, Carracedo et al. [29] demonstrated that compared with high-flux HD, OL-HDF markedly reduced the number of proinflammatory CD14+CD16+ cells and the production of tumor necrosis factor α and IL-6. Future studies are needed to assess the possible therapeutic effect of convective transport on chronic inflammation that is associated with HD. In a subsequent study from the same group [30], the authors showed that the CD14+CD16+ subpopulation was correlated with the number of endothelial progenitor cells and microparticles. OL-HDF was able to reduce the levels of endothelial progenitor cells and microparticles and this reduction was paralleled by a significant decrease in the CD14+CD16+ subpopulation. OL-HDF attenuates endothelial dysfunction possibly by decreasing chronic inflammation. This effect may be directly caused by a modulatory effect of OL-HDF on proinflammatory cells or by a complex interaction that encompasses a wider removal of uremic toxins.

Anemia and Online Hemodiafiltration

In HD patients, erythropoietin resistance may be caused either by absorption of recombinant human erythropoietin by the membrane or an increased release of cytokines that inhibit erythropoiesis, such as IL-1β, tumor necrosis factor α and γ-interferon, or by a decrease in stimulatory cytokines such as IL-3, IL-6 and IL-10 [for a review, see 31]. These negative phenomena are reversed by the use of biocompatible dialysis techniques such as HDF. Other possible pathophysiological mechanisms for an improved regulation of anemia with OL-HDF have not yet been fully established. Uremic serum inhibits erythropoiesis, possibly by accumulation of protein-bound polyamines such as spermine or spermidine or the tetrapeptide mdN-acetyl-seryl-aspartyl-lysyl-proline (487 Da). Theoretically, protein-bound solutes are better removed during OL-HDF. It would be interesting to compare the effects of ultrafiltrate obtained by HD and HDF on erythropoiesis, and the effect of convective techniques on these potential inhibitors of erythropoiesis. To the best of our knowledge, such a study has not yet been performed.

In recent years, evidence has accumulated for the role of inflammatory cytokines in the inhibition of erythropoiesis in the anemia of HD patients. The most important mechanism for cytokine-induced anemia is the suppression of bone marrow erythropoiesis, but the extent to which increased cytokine levels and acute-phase response may contribute to resistance to erythropoietin-stimulating agent treatment is still not clear. Erythroid colony-forming units are inhibited by soluble factors in the sera from uremic patients. However, available results are conflicting, mainly because of differences in treatment modalities or membranes, lack of control groups and small numbers of enrolled patients.

Conclusions

There is accruing evidence for a biological response to OL-HDF. The increased awareness of its multiple advantages and technical advances have led to its widespread use. More studies will in the future provide the rational bases for its application in sicker and older patients.

References

1 Vanholder R, De Smet R, Glorieux G, et al: Review on uremic toxins: classification, concentration, and interindividual variability. Kidney Int 2003;63:1934–1943.

2 Vanholder R, De Smet R, Lameire N: Protein-bound uremic solutes: the forgotten toxins. Kidney Int 2001;78(suppl):S266–S270.

3 Levey AS, Coresh J, Balk E, et al: National Kidney Foundation practice guidelines for chronic kidney disease: evaluation, classification, and stratification. Ann Intern Med 2003;139:137–147.
4 Stenvinkel P, Pecoits-Filho R, Lindholm B: Coronary artery disease in end-stage renal disease: no longer a simple plumbing problem. J Am Soc Nephrol 2003;14:1927–1939.
5 Zoccali C, Tripepi G, Mallamaci F: Predictors of cardiovascular death in ESRD. Semin Nephrol 2005;25:358–362.
6 Himmelfarb J, Ikizler TA, Stenvinkel P, Hakim RM: The elephant in uremia: oxidant stress as a unifying concept of cardiovascular disease in uremia. Kidney Int 2002;62:1524–1538.
7 Morena M, Delbosc S, Dupuy AM, et al: Overproduction of reactive oxygen species in end-stage renal disease patients: a potential component of hemodialysis-associated inflammation. Hemodial Int 2005;9:37–46.
8 Brancaccio D, Tetta C, Gallieni M, Panichi V: Inflammation, CRP, calcium overload and a high calcium-phosphate product: a 'liaison dangereuse'. Nephrol Dial Transplant 2002;17:201–203.
9 Rayner HC, Pisoni RL, Bommer J, Canaud B, Hecking E, Locatelli F, et al: Mortality and hospitalization in haemodialysis patients in five European countries: results from the Dialysis Outcomes and Practice Patterns Study (DOPPS). Nephrol Dial Transplant 2004;19:108–120.
10 Ganesh SK, Hulbert-Shearon T, Port FK, et al: Mortality differences by dialysis modality among incident ESRD patients with and without coronary artery disease. J Am Soc Nephrol 2003;14: 415–424.
11 Goodkin DA, Bragg-Gresham JL, Koenig KG, et al: Association of comorbid conditions and mortality in hemodialysis patients in Europe, Japan, and the United States: the Dialysis Outcomes and Practice Patterns Study (DOPPS). J Am Soc Nephrol 2003;14:3270–3277.
12 Wolfe RA, Hulbert-Shearon TE, Ashby VB, et al: Improvements in dialysis patient mortality are associated with improvements in urea reduction ratio and hematocrit, 1999 to 2002. Am J Kidney Dis 2005;45:127–135.
13 Goodkin DA, Mapes DL, Held PJ: The Dialysis Outcomes and Practice Patterns Study (DOPPS): how can we improve the care of hemodialysis patients? Semin Dial 2001;14:157–159.
14 Yoshino M, Kuhlmann MK, Kotanko P, et al: International differences in dialysis mortality reflect background general population atheroslerotic cardiovascular mortality. J Am Soc Nephrol 2006; 17:3510–3519.
15 Ridker PM, Cushman M, Stampfer MJ, et al: Inflammation, aspirin and the risk of cardiovascular disease in apparently healthy men. N Engl J Med 1997;336:973–979.
16 Vasan RS, Sullivan LM, Roubenoff R, et al: Inflammatory markers and risk of heart failure in elderly subjects without prior myocardial infarction: the Framingham Heart Study. Circulation 2003;107:1486–1491.
17 Liuzzo G, Biasucci LM, Gallimore JR, et al: The prognostic value of C-reactive protein and serum amyloid A protein in severe unstable angina. N Engl J Med 1994;331:417–424.
18 Lagrand WK, Visser CA, Hermens WT, et al: C-reactive-protein as a cardiovascular risk: more than an epiphenomenon? Circulation 1999;100:96–102.
19 Carracedo J, Ramirez R, Madueno JA, et al: Cell apoptosis and hemodialysis-induced inflammation. Kidney Int Suppl 2002;80:89–93.
20 Lonnemann G: When good water goes bad: how it happens, clinical consequences and possible solutions. Blood Purif 2004;22:124–129.
21 Stenvinkel P, Ketteler M, Johnson RJ, et al: IL-10, IL-6, and TNF-α: central factors in the altered cytokine network of uremia – The good, the bad, and the ugly. Kidney Int 2005;67:1216–1233.
22 Schwendler SB, Filep JG, Galle J, et al: C-reactive protein: a family of proteins to regulate cardiovascular function. Am J Kidney Dis 2005;47:212–222.
23 Canaud B, Levesque R, Krieter D, et al: On line hemodiafiltration as routine treatment of end-stage renal failure: why pre- or mixed dilution mode is necessary in on line haemodiafiltration today? Blood Purif 2004;22(suppl 2):40–48.
24 Passlick-Deetjen J, Pohlmeier R: On-line hemodiafiltration: gold standard or top therapy? In Ronco C, La Greca G (eds): Hemodialysis Technology. Contrib Nephrol. Basel, Karger, 2002, vol 137, pp 201–211.
25 Kerr PB, Argiles A, Flavier JL, Canaud B, Mion CM: Comparison of hemodialysis and hemodiafiltration: a long-term longitudinal study. Kidney Int 1992;41:1035–1040.

26 Ward RA, Schmidt B, Hullin J, Hillebrand GF, Samtleben W: A comparison of on-line hemodiafiltration and high-flux hemodialysis: a prospective clinical study. J Am Soc Nephrol 2000;11: 2344–2350.

27 Van Laecke S, De Wilde K, Vanholder R: On line hemodiafiltration. Artif Organs 2006;30: 579–585.

28 Beerenhout CH, Luik AJ, Jeuken-Mertens SG, et al: Pre-dilution on-line haemodiafiltration vs low-flux haemodialysis: a randomized prospective study. Nephrol Dial Transplant 2005;20: 1155–1163.

29 Carracedo J, Merino A, Nogueras S, et al: CD14+CD16+ monocyte-derived dendritic cells: a prospective, crossover study. J Am Soc Nephrol 2006;17:2315–2321. DOI: 10.1681/.

30 Ramirez R, Carracedo J, Merino A, et al: Microinflammation induces endothelial damage in hemodialysis patients: the role of convective transport. Kidney Int 2007, E-pub ahead of print.

31 Locatelli F, Del Vecchio L, Pozzoni P, Andrulli S: Dialysis adequacy and response to erythopoiesis-stimulating agents: what is the evidence base? Semin Nephrol 2006;26;269–274.

Dr. Vincenzo Panichi
Internal Medicine Department, University of Pisa
Via Roma 57
IT–56100 Pisa (Italy)
Tel. +39 050 992 887, Fax +39 050 553 414, E-Mail vpanichi@med.unipi.it

Ronco C, Canaud B, Aljama P (eds): Hemodiafiltration.
Contrib Nephrol. Basel, Karger, 2007, vol 158, pp 201–209

Clearance of Beta-2-Microglobulin and Middle Molecules in Haemodiafiltration

James Tattersall

Department of Renal Medicine, St. James's University Hospital, Leeds, UK

Abstract

Middle molecules, consisting mostly of peptides and small proteins with molecular weight the range of 500–60,000 Da, accumulate in renal failure and contribute to the uraemic toxic state. β_2-Microglobulin (β_2-MG) with a molecular weight of 11,000 is considered representative of these middle molecules. These solutes are not well cleared by low-flux dialysis. High-flux dialysis will clear middle molecules, partly by internal filtration. This convective component of high-flux dialysis can be enhanced in a predictable way by haemodiafiltration (HDF). The convective and diffusive clearance rates of any middle molecule across any haemodiafilter can be predicted from known or measurable factors such as its sieving coefficient, bound fraction and molecular weight. The removal of middle molecules is also influenced by factors within the patient. β_2-MG is distributed within the extracellular fluid. During HDF, β_2-MG must transfer into the intravascular compartment across the capillary walls. This transcapillary transfer at a rate of approximately 100 ml/min slows β_2-MG removal from the body. Continuing transfer after the end of a treatment session results in a significant rebound of β_2-MG levels. This intercompartment transfer and its effect on β_2-MG clearance and concentration can be predicted by a 2-compartment model. By extrapolation, the behaviour of other middle molecules can be predicted. The 2-compartment model, which takes non-dialytic β_2-MG clearance at a rate of 3 ml/min and β_2-MG generation at a rate of 0.1 mg/min into account, can predict the effect of any HDF schedule on β_2-MG levels. Low-flux dialysis results in a β_2-MG level of around 40 mg/l. Three times weekly, 4-hour HDF can reduce β_2-MG levels to around 20 mg/l. Long (nocturnal) HDF can reduce β_2-MG levels to around 10 mg/l, compared to physiological levels of less than 5 mg/l.

One of the main motivations in performing haemodiafiltration (HDF) instead of haemodialysis is to enhance the removal of middle-molecular-weight toxins. To this end, new membranes have been developed to target removal of material of molecular weight in the range of 500–60,000 Da. These so-called middle molecules consist mostly of peptides and low-molecular-weight proteins with evidence of toxicity [1]. β_2-Microglobulin (β_2-MG) at 11,000 Da is considered representative of this material and is the most extensively studied [2]. This chapter reviews the techniques for quantifying and predicting the effect of HDF on the plasma levels of middle molecules.

Clearance of Middle Molecules in the Haemodiafilter

Diffusive Clearance

The rate of diffusion of solute through an aqueous fluid is inversely proportional to the square root of molecular weight (MW) [3]. Therefore, the diffusive clearance (K_D) can be estimated for any middle molecule from the equation below:

$$K_D = K_{Dref} \times \sqrt{\frac{MWref}{MW}}$$

where K_{Dref} is the diffusive clearance of a reference middle molecule of molecular weight $MWref$ (e.g. inulin), which can be read from the dialyser data sheet. For middle molecules, the relatively slow rate of diffusion and transfer through the membrane pores are the main limiting factors on K_D. Therefore, K_D is relatively independent of blood or dialysate flow rates as long as these are more than 200 ml/min. For β_2-MG (11,000 Da) K_D cannot exceed 12% of the mass transfer area coefficient (KoA) for urea (60 Da). K_D may be further reduced by resistance to passage through the pores, dependent on pore size and molecular weight.

Convective Clearance

In haemofiltration or HDF, the spontaneous filtration/backfiltration which occurs in high-flux dialysis is replaced by a controlled filtration and re-infusion which can be quantified precisely. As long as the solute is small enough to pass through the haemodiafilter membrane pores unimpeded, the clearance due to the filtration (convective clearance K_C) is equal to the filtration rate and will be the same for any solute.

In practice, larger solutes are somewhat impeded by the limited size of the membrane pores, resulting in a 'sieving' effect, where solute is retained on the blood side of the membrane, reducing clearance. This sieving effect is quantified for a specific solute and membrane as the sieving coefficient (SC). A sieving coefficient of 1 indicates no impediment, so clearance is equal to the filtration rate (Q_F). A sieving coefficient of zero means that the solute cannot pass through the membrane and the clearance is zero, regardless of filtration rate.

In the general case, for postdilution haemofiltration, convective clearance is given by the equation:

$$Kc = Qf \times S$$

Values for *SC* for representative middle molecules are known for any haemodiafilter [4]. *SC* is largely dependent on molecular weight and can be predicted or extrapolated. For β_2-MG, *SC* ranges from 0.6 to 0.9. The higher value is obtained from the so-called 'ultraflux' dialysers. It is worth noting that convective clearance is independent of blood flow, dialysate flow or membrane geometry.

Combining Convective and Diffusive Clearance

Convection and diffusion interact in a predictable way, depending on blood plasma flow (Q_{BP}) which is calculated from blood flow (Q_B), *Hct* and total protein in grams per litre (*Pt*) [5]:

$$Qbp = Qb \times (1 - Hct) \times (1 - 0.0107 \times Pt)$$

The clearance of any solute by HDF (*K*) in postdilution mode is given by the equation [6]:

$$K = Kd + \left(\frac{Qbp - Kd}{Qbp} \right) \times Qf \times S$$

For online HDF in predilution mode, dialysate flow (Q_D) is taken into account:

$$K = Kd + \left(\frac{\frac{Qbp + Qd}{Qbp \times Qd} - Kd}{Qd} \right) \times Qf \times S$$

In the case of middle molecules at the higher end of the molecular-weight range, where K_D is negligible, *K* is equal to K_C in postdilution mode. For other middle molecules, the contribution of K_D is fairly small, so any errors in its estimation have little impact on the calculation of *K*.

The above equations can be used to calculate small-solute clearance; in this case, blood water flow, instead of plasma water flow, should be used.

In practice, β_2-MG clearance of up to 100 ml/min is possible in a high-intensity postdialysis HDF with $Q_B = 450$ ml/min, $Q_F = 100$ ml/min, K_D for urea 320 ml/min and $SC = 0.8$.

Effect of Adsorption on Clearance

Peptides and low-molecular-weight proteins in the middle-molecule range are hydrophobic and are attracted to any non-aqueous material such as a dialyser membrane. This has the effect of causing some of the solute to be adsorbed onto the haemodiafilter membrane as it passes through. Most of this adsorption occurs in the supporting matrix material downstream from the rate-limiting pores so does not affect the clearance rate. Adsorption of solute onto the blood side of the membrane will tend to increase clearance, but by a limited and variable extent due to the relatively small area of the blood side surface and rapid saturation.

Effect of Protein Binding on Clearance

Some middle molecules bind to plasma proteins, particularly albumin [7, 8]. Only the unbound fraction (B) is able to cross the membrane either by diffusion or filtration. If there is significant binding, the clearance predictions should be multiplied by this unbound fraction.

Measuring Middle-Molecule Clearance

Adsorption of middle molecules will reduce solute concentration in the filtrate and prevent quantification of clearance by filtrate measurements. Cell membranes are effectively impermeable to middle molecules so plasma water flow (Q_{BP}) rather than blood water flow is used to calculate clearance on blood side measurements. Solute concentrations at the dialyser inlet (C_{in}) and downstream of the infusion line (C_{out}) are used in the following equation:

$$K = Qbp \times \left(\frac{Cin - Cout}{Cin} \right)$$

The Two-Compartment Model

In order to remove solute from the body, the solute must transfer from the far recesses of the body into the haemodiafilter. Factors delaying solute transfer within the body may have almost as much influence on the mass of solute removed as clearance at the haemodiafilter.

These factors within the body can be quantified and predicted using a 2-compartment model [9]. Solute is considered to be distributed within 2 aqueous compartments, the central and peripheral compartments. HDF clears solute from the central compartment only. Solute from the peripheral compartment must transfer into the central compartment before it can be cleared. After the end of the HDF, the concentration in the central compartment rebounds upwards due to continuing intercompartment transfer.

The rate of solute transfer between compartments is proportional to the difference in concentrations between compartments and a patient- and solute-specific intercompartment clearance rate (K_i).

During HDF the mass of solute (M_c, M_p), concentrations (C_c, C_p) and volumes (V_c, V_p) of the central and peripheral compartments can be computed by repeated solution of the following equations in small time increments (t). G_p and G_c are the solute generation rates, WG_p and WG_c are the rates of volume change in the peripheral and central compartments. The value K is the total clearance due to non-dialytic clearance plus HDF as appropriate. WG_c and WG_p will be negative during the HDF sessions and positive at other times.

$$Mp = Mp + \left(\left(Cc - Cp\right) \times Ki + Gp\right) \times t$$

$$Mc = Mc + \left(\left(Cp - Cc\right) \times Ki + Gc - Cc \times K\right) \times t$$

$$Cc = \frac{Mc}{Vc}$$

$$Cp = \frac{Mp}{Vp}$$

$$Vc = Vc + WGc \times t$$

$$Vp = Vp + WGp \times t$$

The 2-compartment model has been well studied for urea and creatinine. For these small solutes, V_c and V_p have volumes of approximately 25% of the body weight each and are considered to be the intracellular and extracellular water volumes. The mechanism of intercompartment transfer is diffusion across the cell membranes. K_i has a value of approximately 1,000 for urea and 500 for creatinine. Other small solutes such as phosphate and methylguanidine seem to be actively transported across the intercompartment boundary so their behaviour during dialysis is not well described by the 2-pool model [10].

β_2-Microglobulin Two-Compartment Kinetics

β_2-MG kinetics has now been well characterized and also reliably conforms to a 2-pool model [11, 12]. In the case of β_2-MG, the total volume of the 2 compartments (V) is approximately 14% of body weight and is considered to be the extracellular water. The 2 compartments are considered to be the plasma water and the extracellular, extravascular water. K_i for β_2-MG is approximately 100 ml/min. The plasma water compartment consists of about 25% of the total extracellular water volume [13]. Cell membranes are relatively impermeable to β_2-MG, and intracellular water appears to play no part in β_2-MG kinetics during HDF.

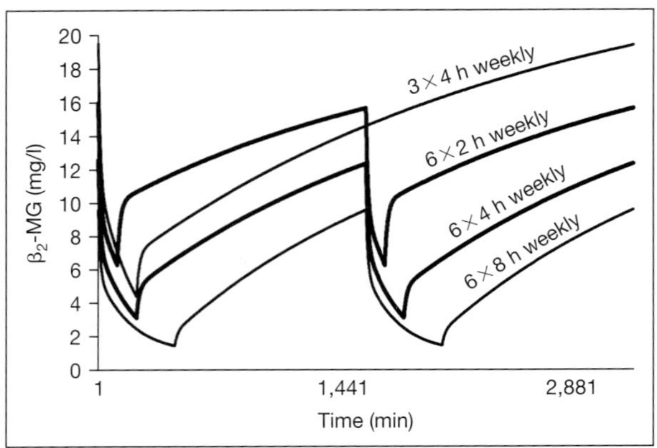

Fig. 1. Predicted blood β_2-MG concentrations over a 2-day cycle with different schedules. The model parameters are the same as indicated for table 1.

The generation rate for β_2-MG appears to be around 0.1 mg/min and is similar to subjects with normal renal function [14]. The non-dialytic β_2-MG clearance is around 3 ml/min in patients without renal function [15].

Kinetics of Other Middle Molecules

For middle molecules, the intercompartment boundary is the blood vessel walls, probably mostly the capillaries. The mechanism of transfer here is filtration and determined by capillary hemodynamics. This is likely to occur at a similar rate for all middle molecules (at least those which can be cleared by HDF) but this requires confirmation.

Equilibrated Kt/V

Urea removal is traditionally quantified as *Kt/V* where *K* is the total urea clearance, *t* is the treatment time and *V* the urea distribution volume. European guidelines recommend that *Kt/V* should take the postdialysis rebound and intercompartment effects into account. An equilibrated or rebound-corrected *Kt/V* (*eKt/V*) can be calculated using a postdialysis blood sample taken after the rebound is complete, at least 30 min after the end of dialysis [16].

For middle molecules (or at least β_2-MG), the rebound is more pronounced and takes longer. It is even more important to include rebound and intercompartment effects when considering middle molecules [17].

The 2-compartment model can be approximated by more simple mathematics using the patient clearance time (*tp*) which is closely related to K_i/V. The value *tp* can be used to calculate the postrebound concentration using the dialysis time in minutes (*t*), pre- and immediate postdialysis concentrations [18]:

$$rebound = pre \times \left(\frac{post}{pre} \right)^{\frac{t}{t+tp}}$$

A value for *eKt/V* can be calculated from the regular *Kt/V* using the immediate postdialysis blood sample:

$$eKt / V = Kt / V \times \frac{t}{t+tp}$$

For urea, *tp* is 35 min, for creatinine, 70 min.

In theory, this method should be equally suitable for predicting the rebound for β_2-MG and other middle molecules; in this case, a value for *tp* of 110 min is suggested by data in the literature and mathematical analysis.

Equivalent Renal Clearance

The equivalent renal clearance was originally described for urea as EKR [19]. It is defined as the generation rate (*G*) divided by the time-averaged concentration over the weekly cycle (TAC). EKR has the familiar units of millilitres per minute and can be normalized to a body water volume of 40 litres as EKRc. Values for β_2-MG *G* and TAC can be calculated using the 2-compartment model and used to calculate a β_2-MG or middle-molecule EKR.

EKR calculated in this way is particularly suitable for quantifying middle-molecule removal since it can be related to a physiological reference – normal renal function – and takes non-dialytic clearance, frequency and duration of dialysis into account. As far as we know, the toxicity of middle molecules relates to their TAC [20].

The Effect of Treatment Duration and Frequency

It is possible to use a 2-compartment model to predict the β_2-MG peak concentration and TAC for any dialytic schedule. Values for various dialysis schedules are shown in table 1. The results of the predictions in the table are in general agreement with β_2-MG levels reported in the literature.

With low-flux dialysis, the EKR for β_2-MG is 3 ml/min due to non-dialysis clearance, despite no β_2-MG clearance at the dialyser. HDF or high-efficiency, high-flux haemodialysis can reduce the peak β_2-MG levels to around 50% of the level seen with low-flux haemodialysis [21]. The reduction in β_2-MG TAC levels are not routinely measured but will be more impressive.

Table 1. Comparison between different dialysis strategies

Schedule	Duration h/treatment	Q_F ml/min	β_2-MG peak mg/l	β_2-MG TAC mg/l	EKR of β_2-MG ml/min	EKR of urea ml/min
3 times/week low-flux haemodialysis	4	0	40	40	3	14
3 times/week HDF	4	50	22	17	6	18
3 times/week HDF	4	100	19	14	7	18
6 times/week HDF	2	100	15	13	8	21
6 times/week HDF	4	100	12	9	11	37
6 times/week HDF	8	50	10	7	14	60
6 times/week HDF	8	100	10	6	17	60
Normal renal function			<5	<5	>20	80

Data were computed using a 2-compartment model as described in the text. For HDF, a 2.2-m^2 surface area dialyser with a urea dialytic clearance of 340 ml/min at 450 ml/min blood flow and an SC of 0.8 for β_2-MG is used. For low-flux HD, there is no dialytic β_2-MG clearance and urea clearance of 250. Volumes of 10.2 and 40 litres were assumed for β_2-MG and urea, respectively.

Due to the considerable rebound associated with short treatments, moving from 3×4 to 6×2 h per week results in only minimal further decrease in the peak β2-MG level [22].

It is possible to approach physiological TAC levels for both urea and β_2-MG found with normal renal function using extended, high-intensity daily treatments. This would have to be delivered by nocturnal or continuous dialysis [23].

References

1 Winchester JF, Audia PF: Extracorporeal strategies for the removal of middle molecules. Semin Dial 2006;19:110–114.

2 Winchester JF, Salsberg JA, Levin NW: Beta-2 microglobulin in ESRD: an in-depth review. Adv Ren Replace Ther 2003;10:279–309.

3 Ofsthun NJ: Limitations of membrane structure and dialyzer design on large solute removal in dialysis. Blood Purif 2000;18:264–266.

4 Klingel R, Ahrenholz P, Schwarting A, Rockel A: Enhanced functional performance characteristics of a new polysulfone membrane for high-flux hemodialysis. Blood Purif 2002;20:325–333.

5 Padrini R, Canova C, Conz P, Mancini E, Rizzioli E, Santoro A: Convective and adsorptive removal of beta2-microglobulin during predilutional and postdilutional hemofiltration. Kidney Int 2005;68:2331–2337.

6 Ficheux A, Argiles A, Mion H, Mion CM: Influence of convection on small molecule clearances in online HDF. Kidney Int 2000;57:1755–1763.

7 Bammens B, Evenepoel P, Verbeke K, Vanrenterghem Y: Removal of the protein-bound solute *p*-cresol by convective transport: a randomized crossover study. Am J Kidney Dis 2004;44:278–285.

8 Dhondt A, Vanholder R, Van BW, Lameire N: The removal of uremic toxins. Kidney Int Suppl 2000;76:S47–S59.

9 Sargent JA, Gotch FA: Mathematic modeling of dialysis therapy. Kidney Int Suppl 1980;10:S2–S10.

10 Eloot S, Torremans A, De Smet R, Marescau B, De Wachter D, De Deyn PP, Lameire N, Verdonck P, Vanholder R: Kinetic behavior of urea is different from that of other water-soluble compounds: the case of the guanidino compounds. Kidney Int 2005;67:1566–1575.

11 Ward RA, Greene T, Hartmann B, Samtleben W: Resistance to intercompartmental mass transfer limits beta2-microglobulin removal by post-dilution HDF. Kidney Int 2006;69:1431–1437.

12 David S, Bottalico D, Tagliavini D, Mandolfo S, Scanziani R, Cambi V: Behaviour of beta2-microglobulin removal with different dialysis schedules. Nephrol Dial Transplant 1998;13(suppl 6):49–54.

13 Leypoldt JK, Cheung AK, Deeter RB, Goldfarb-Rumyantzev A, Greene T, Depner TA, Kusek J: Kinetics of urea and beta-microglobulin during and after short hemodialysis treatments. Kidney Int 2004;66:1669–1676.

14 Floege J, Bartsch A, Schulze M, Shaldon S, Koch KM, Smeby LC: Clearance and synthesis rates of beta 2-microglobulin in patients undergoing hemodialysis and in normal subjects. J Lab Clin Med 1991;118:153–165.

15 Xu XQ, Gruner N, Al-Bashir A, Trutt-Ibing CH, Melzer H, Fassbinder W, Stiller JS, Manm H: Determination of extra renal clearance and generation rate of beta2-microglobulin in hemodialysis patients using a kinetic model. ASAIO J 2001;47:623–627.

16 Leypoldt JK, Cheung AK: Revisiting the hemodialysis dose. Semin Dial 2006;19:96–101.

17 Leypoldt JK, Cheung AK, Deeter RB: Rebound kinetics of beta2-microglobulin after hemodialysis. Kidney Int 1999;56:1571–1577.

18 Tattersall JE, De Takats D, Chamney P, Greenwood RN, Farrington K: The post-hemodialysis rebound: predicting and quantifying its effect on Kt/V. Kidney Int 1996;50:2094–2102.

19 Casino FG, Lopez T: The equivalent renal urea clearance: a new parameter to assess dialysis dose. Nephrol Dial Transplant 1996;11:1574–1581.

20 Maduell F, del Pozo C, Garcia H, Sanchez L, Hdez-Jaras J, Albero MD, Calvo C, Torregrosa I, Navarro V: Change from conventional haemodiafiltration to on-line haemodiafiltration. Nephrol Dial Transplant 1999;14:1202–1207.

21 Pickett TM, Cruickshank A, Greenwood RN, Taube D, Davenport A, Farrington K: Membrane flux not biocompatibility determines beta-2-microglobulin levels in hemodialysis patients. Blood Purif 2002;20:161–166.

22 Canaud B, Assounga A, Kerr P, Aznar R, Mion C: Failure of a daily haemofiltration programme using a highly permeable membrane to return beta 2-microglobulin concentrations to normal in haemodialysis patients. Nephrol Dial Transplant 1992;7:924–930.

23 Raj DS, Ouwendyk M, Francoeur R, Pierratos A: Beta-2-microglobulin kinetics in nocturnal haemodialysis. Nephrol Dial Transplant 2000;15:58–64.

James Tattersall
Department of Renal Medicine, St. James's University Hospital
Leeds LS9 7TF (UK)
Tel. +44 113 206 4119, Fax +44 113 206 4696, E-Mail jamestattersall@doctors.org.uk

Ronco C, Canaud B, Aljama P (eds): Hemodiafiltration.
Contrib Nephrol. Basel, Karger, 2007, vol 158, pp 210–215

Inflammation and Hemodiafiltration

Rafael Ramirez, Alejandro Martin-Malo, Pedro Aljama

Department of Nephrology, Hospital Reina Sofia, Cordoba, Spain

Abstract

Atherosclerosis and the subsequent cardiovascular diseases are the most important causes of morbidity and mortality in patients with chronic kidney disease (CKD). CKD atherosclerosis is closely associated with the inflammatory status which is chronically present in these patients. Hemodiafiltration (HDF) is a highly effective dialysis modality expanding the spectrum of removed uremic toxins from small to middle-sized molecular solutes. In addition, the online (OL) HDF using high fluid substitution allows a greater clearance of large uremic toxins. We have shown that OL-HDF markedly reduces the number of CD14+CD16+ monocyte-derived dendritic cells and their proinflammatory potential in CKD patients without clinical evidence of inflammatory disease. Moreover, we have also reported that OL-HDF improved endothelial dysfunction with a decrease in the number of endothelial microparticles (EMP) in peripheral blood and an increase in the percentage of endothelial progenitor cells (EPC) as compared with high-flux hemodialysis (HF-HD). The results obtained showed in both studies a reduction of CD14+CD16+ dendritic cells, EMP and ECP in comparison with HF-HD. These data strongly suggest that the microinflammation status observed in CKD patients is associated with endothelial damage and that amelioration of the chronic microinflammation using high convective transport appears to reduce endothelial damage and promote endothelial repair. Future studies will have to assess the mechanisms of these immunological changes and their relevance in the reported improved survival of patients treated with OL-HDF.

Inflammation is a physiological phenomenon necessary to maintain tissue integrity against injury. However, when the inflammatory response is inappropriate or excessively activated, it may lead to a chronic inflammatory state with harmful consequences. In fact, an activated acute-phase response has been shown to be a predictor of cardiovascular disease in the general population. Chronic kidney disease (CKD) has been associated with a high prevalence of cardiovascular complications [1]. However, classic risk factors for atherosclerosis such as hypertension, dyslipidemia, obesity and smoking seem to be less important than other additional factors such as uremic toxins or inflammation. Several papers have reported that most CKD patients have a subclinical microinflammatory state with high serum levels of some proinflammmatory/proatherogenic cytokines and accumulation in peripheral blood of activated mononuclear cells that prolong their lifespan. Markers of inflammation such as C-reactive protein and cytokines are independent predictors of all-cause and cardiovascular mortality in these patients [2, 3].

The potential for reversal of established vascular disease is unknown in hemodialysis (HD) patients since cardiovascular disease in CKD stage V is already well established. The quality and technology of HD have improved in relation to the biocompatibility of the materials used and the ability to remove larger uremic toxin molecules. The question of whether the use of convective transport may have an impact on the combined process of inflammation, endothelial damage and repair is of paramount importance. By combining ultrafiltration (convective clearances for removing larger solutes) with diffusion (for removal of small solutes), hemodiafiltration (HDF) offers a highly effective dialysis modality expanding the spectrum of removed uremic toxins from small to middle-sized molecular solutes. The online (OL) HDF using high fluid substitution allows a greater clearance of large uremic toxins [4, 5].

The mortality of dialysis patients remains elevated despite advances in dialysis technology, significant improvement in dialysis quality and better global care of patients. On one side, it is interesting to note that a preliminary report from the international Dialysis Outcomes and Practice Patterns Study has shown that patients undergoing HDF had a reduced risk of death compared to those treated by conventional HD [6]. This is a unique report that deserves further analysis showing for the first time that high-efficiency convective therapies are associated with a reduced death risk accounting for comorbid conditions of patients and dialysis dose. The spectrum of eliminated uremic toxins together with the adoption of ultrapure dialysate may all contribute to explain the reduction of the chronic inflammation. The latter has been associated with an elevated number of circulating monocytes, an increased percentage of mature proinflammatory monocytes and an overproduction of interleukin (IL) 1, tumor necrosis factor α and IL-6, without the ability to synthesize the anti-inflammatory cytokine IL-10 [7]. Overt signs of chronic inflammation as evidenced by high plasma levels of the acute-phase response proteins such as C-reactive protein have been recognized as an independent risk factor of gross and cardiovascular mortality in CKD patients [7–9].

In a recent paper of our group we have shown for the first time that the convective component of OL-HDF reduces the number of proinflammatory CD14+CD16+ cells (fig. 1), the intracellular production of tumor necrosis

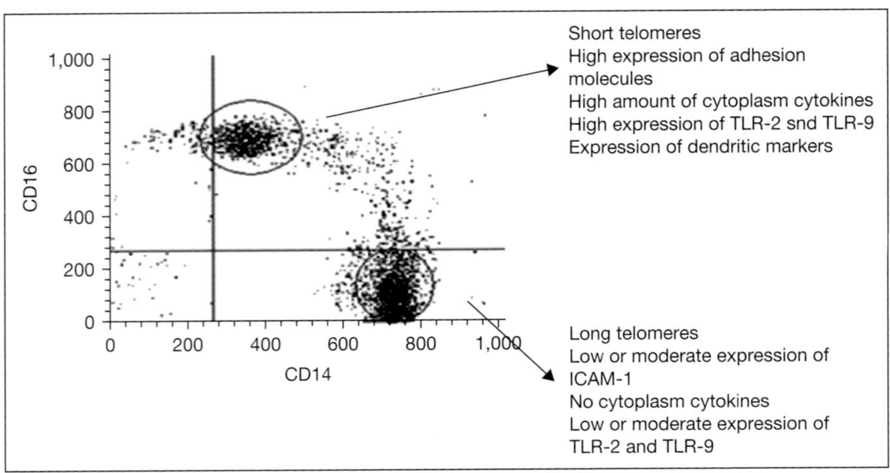

Fig. 1. Characteristics of CD14+CD16+ cells in HD patients. TLR = Toll-like receptor; ICAM = intercellular adhesion molecule.

factor α and IL-6 as compared with high-flux HD (HF-HD) [10]. Both dialysis modalities HF-HD and OL-HDF were in fact equal for the membrane used and water quality. The study was performed in patients treated in one single center to insure uniform procedures and standards of ultrapure dialysis fluids during the whole duration of the study. The patients included in this study showed low plasma levels of C-reactive protein, had normal plasma albumin and showed no evidence of otherwise clinically evident inflammatory disease. Therefore, the observed changes in the CD14+CD16+ cell population were observed in well-nourished patients with very mild inflammation. Obviously, further studies will be needed to assess whether these observations may be confirmed in an HD population with overt inflammation as well. In addition, we have observed a shortened telomere in CD14+CD16+ activated cells. The percentage of CD14+CD16+ activated cells with a short telomere was higher in HF-HD than in OL-HDF. These data strongly suggest that there was a higher percentage of senescent cells in HF-HD as compared with OL-HDF. The main drawback of this study was that we did not evaluate the biological response with respect to different volume exchanges, which might give a more precise information on the relative role of convective transport.

Several studies have shown evidence of endothelial damage and endothelial dysfunction in HD patients [11]. Research in the biology of the endothelium has provided new targets to examine endothelial damage and repair in human pathology. Circulating endothelial cells have recently been recognized as useful markers of vascular injury and angiogenesis [12]. Upon a noxious insult,

Table 1. Biomarkers (%) of endothelial injury and repair in HF-HD and OL-HDF

	EMP	EPC	CD14+CD16+ cells
Healthy subjects	9 ± 4.3	5.8 ± 4.7	5 ± 3
HF-HD	21.2 ± 6.8[a]	13.2 ± 3.4[b]	23 ± 7.8[a]
OL-HDF	14.9 ± 3.6[a, b]	9.7 ± 1.9[a]	12 ± 9.2[a, b]

n = 16. [a] $p < 0.05$ versus healthy subjects; [b] $p < 0.05$ versus HF-HD.

endothelial cells may undergo vesiculation releasing 'endothelial microparticles' (EMP) into the bloodstream. EMP harbor cell surface proteins and cytoplasmic elements and express endothelial-specific surface markers. In addition, EMP are currently viewed as a new pathway that can be used by endothelial cells to exchange information. Endothelial progenitor cells (EPC) which originate from the bone marrow, rather than from vessel walls, can be identified through their expression of CD34 (a surface marker common to hematopoietic stem cells and mature endothelial cells) and vascular endothelial cell growth factor receptor 2 (or kinase-domain-related receptor). EPC are considered to have a role in the repair of vascular injury, angiogenesis and tissue vascularization [13].

Patients undergoing HD show a high number of circulating CD31+/annexin V+ EMP as compared to healthy human subjects. Taking into account that the elevated number of EMP was associated with a remarkably high number of EPC [14], we designed a prospective crossover study to examine whether OL-HDF may not only improve microinflammation, as indicated by CD14+CD16+ dendritic cells, but also EMP and EPC numbers, as biomarkers of endothelial injury and repair in comparing OL-HDF with HF-HD (table 1). Both circulating EMP and EPC were reduced after 4 months of OL-HDF [15]. However, EPC did not reach the circulating levels observed in the control group (table 1). Interest has emerged from recent human studies underscoring the tight association of EMP with endothelial dysfunction and arterial dysfunction in CKD. By a linear regression analysis, we found in this report a significant correlation between proinflammatory CD14+CD16+ cells and the number of EMC and EPC. Therefore, it is possible to speculate that CD14+CD16+ monocyte-derived dendritic cells may have an additional effect on endothelial activation and injury leading to release of EMP into the circulation, and stimulation of the bone marrow to increase the production of circulating EPC. However, we were unable to claim a direct cause-and-effect relationship between microinflammation, formation of EMP and increased numbers of circulating EPC.

There was no increase in EMP in postdialysis blood samples from OL-HDF. In contrast, a marked increase in EMP was observed in all patients during the HF-HD period. However, in both dialysis modalities, EPC decreased significantly in the postdialysis blood samples compared with the predialysis values. Why EPC increase in HF-HD and diminish in OL-HDF is not clear. Recent studies also suggest that circulating detached endothelial cells and stimulated EPC from the bone marrow may reflect endothelial injury. In our paper [15], we did not assess the plasma levels of vascular endothelial growth factor, a stimulus for EPC release from bone marrow. Obviously, the potential role played by vascular endothelial growth factor could not be excluded from our study. Another potential confounding factor is the effect of erythropoietin therapy, a strong stimulus for EPC release; however, it is important to highlight that there was no significant change in the erythropoietin dose in the course of the study.

In summary, OL-HDF seems to improve microinflammation and endothelial injury and repair, as indicated by a reduction of CD14+CD16+ dendritic cells, EMP and ECP in comparison with HF-HD. Future studies will have to assess the mechanisms of these immunological changes, and their relevance in the reported improved survival of patients treated with OL-HDF.

Acknowledements

This work was supported by grants from: Instituto de Salud Carlos III (FIS 03/0946, 05/0896, 06/0724, 06/0747 and RETIC RD06/006L/0007 – FEDER) and Fundación Nefrologica.

References

1 Reiss AB, Glass AD: Atherosclerosis: immune and inflammatory aspects. J Invest Med 2006;54: 123–131.
2 Roberts MA, Hare DL, Ratnaike S, Ierino FL: Cardiovascular biomarkers in CKD: pathophysiology and implications for clinical management of cardiac disease. Am J Kidney Dis 2006;48: 341–360.
3 Zoccali C: Traditional and emerging cardiovascular and renal risk factors: an epidemiologic perspective. Kidney Int 2006;70:26–33.
4 Ward RA, Schmidt B, Hullin J, Hillebrand GF, Samtleben W: A comparison of on-line hemodiafiltration and high-flux hemodialysis: a prospective clinical study. J Am Soc Nephrol 2000;11: 2344–2350.
5 Locatelli F, Manzoni C, Di Filippo S: The importance of convective transport. Kidney Int 2002; 61(suppl 80):S115–S120.
6 Canaud B, Bragg-Gresham JL, Marshall MR, Desmeules S, Gillespie BW, Depner T, Klassen P, Port FK: Mortality risk for patients receiving hemodiafiltration versus hemodialysis: European results from the DOPPS. Kidney Int 2006;69:2087–2093.
7 Kaysen GA: The microinflammatory state in uremia: causes and potential consequences. J Am Soc Nephrol 2001;12:1549–1557.
8 Rostaing L, Peres C, Tkaczuk J, Charlet JP, Bories P, Durand D, Ohayon E, de Preval C, Abbal M: Ex vivo flow cytometry determination of intracytoplasmic expression of IL-2, IL-6, IFN-γ and TNF-α in monocytes and T lymphocytes, in chronic hemodialysis patients. Am J Nephrol 2000; 20:18–26.

9 Carracedo J, Ramirez R, Madueño JA, Soriano S, Rodríguez-Benot A, Rodriguez M, Martin-Malo A, Aljama P: Cell apoptosis and hemodialysis-induced inflammation. Kidney Int 2002;80:89–93.
10 Carracedo J, Merino A, Nogueras S, Carretero D, Berdud I, Ramirez R, Tetta C, Rodriguez M, Martin-Malo A, Aljama P: On-line hemodiafiltration reduces the proinflammatory CD14+CD16+ monocyte-derived dendritic cells: a prospective, crossover study. J Am Soc Nephrol 2006;17: 2315–2321.
11 Locatelli F, Pozzoni P, Tentori F, del Vecchio L: Epidemiology of cardiovascular risk in patients with chronic kidney disease. Nephrol Dial Transplant 2003;18(suppl 7):vii2–9.
12 Jimenez JJ, Jy W, Mauro LM, et al: Endothelial microparticles (EMP) as vascular disease markers. Adv Clin Chem 2005;39:131–157.
13 Masuda H, Kalka C, Asahara T: Endothelial progenitor cells for regeneration. Hum Cell 2000;13: 153–160.
14 Herbrig K, Pistrosch F, Oelschlaegel U, et al: Increased total number but impaired migratory activity and adhesion of endothelial progenitor cells in patients on long-term hemodialysis. Am J Kidney Dis 2004;44:840–849.
15 Ramirez R, Carracedo J, Merino A, Nogueras S, Alvarez-Lara MA, Rodriguez M, Martin-Malo A, Tetta C, Aljama P: Microinflammation induces endothelial damage in hemodialysis patients: the role of convective transport. Kidney Int 2007, in press.

Prof. Pedro Aljama
Department of Nephrology, Hospital Reina Sofia
Avda. Menendez Pidal, 1
ES–14004 Cordoba (Spain)
Tel. +34 57010143, E-Mail Pedro.aljama.sspa@juntadeandalucia.es

Ronco C, Canaud B, Aljama P (eds): Hemodiafiltration.
Contrib Nephrol. Basel, Karger, 2007, vol 158, pp 216–224

Effect of Online Hemodiafiltration on Morbidity and Mortality of Chronic Kidney Disease Patients

Bernard Canaud

Nephrology, Dialysis and Intensive Care Unit, Aider and Renal Research and Training Institute, Lapeyronie University Hospital, Montpellier, France

Abstract

Conventional diffusion-based dialysis modalities including high-flux hemodialysis (HD) are limited in their capacity to clear uremic toxins. Moreover they are associated with a relatively high incidence of morbidity and mortality. Online hemodiafiltration (ol-HDF) combining the use of a high-flux membrane dialyzer, ultrapure dialysis fluid and high convective fluid exchange is highly efficient with the lowest bioreactive profile in renal replacement therapy methods. Regular use of high-efficiency ol-HDF is associated with reduced morbidity (hypotension incidence, better blood pressure control, improved hemocompatibility, reduced inflammation profile, improved lipid profile, improved anemia correction, reduced incidence of β_2-microglobulin amyloidosis and hospitalization). More recently, several cohort studies have shown that high-efficiency ol-HDF is associated with a 35% reduced risk of mortality in an unselected dialysis population. ol-HDF has been proven to be a safe and very efficient renal replacement therapy. ol-HDF has come of age and should be considered now as the new standard for highly efficient renal replacement therapy.

Introduction

Conventional diffusion-based dialysis modalities including high-flux hemodialysis (HD) are limited in their capacity to clear middle and large-size uremic toxins [1, 2]. Moreover, dialysis-related complications, including β_2-microglobulin amyloidosis, accelerated atherosclerosis, left ventricular hypertrophy, inflammation, malnutrition and ageing, are as many clinical manifestations showing the limits of conventional HD methods. Mixed diffusive and convective methods such as hemodiafiltration (HDF), mimicking glomerular filtration of native kidneys, are then required for enlarging the molecular-weight spectrum of uremic toxins removed by dialysis and for enhancing the overall efficacy of the renal replacement therapy in order to improve the outcome for patients with chronic kidney disease stage 5 (CKD-5) [3–6].

Worldwide clinical experience has proven for several thousand CKD patients treated with online (ol) HDF that the method was safe, reliable and economically viable [7]. Safety and reliability of ol-HDF machines is now certified by European notified bodies under the EC label (European Community).

The enhanced efficiency of high-flux convective therapies is one of the best-documented aspects of the method. HDF provides significantly higher instantaneous clearances than high-flux HD both for small- and middle-molecule solutes [8–10]. Inorganic phosphate and β_2-microglobulin are two major uremic markers with high clinical relevance that can be used to support this fact. Phosphate removal is increased with HDF methods reaching up 30–35 mmol/session [11]. Based on 3 sessions a week, total phosphate removal is still not adequate to restore phosphate balance in CKD patients. Phosphatemia control requires however a reduced dose of phosphate binders [12]. β_2-Microglobulin removal is also increased with high-flux ol-HDF [13, 14]. The reduction ratio of β_2-microglobulin averages usually 70–80%. β_2-Microglobulin mass removal ranges between 150 and 200 mg/session [15]. Several prospective controlled studies have confirmed that HDF treatment was accompanied by a significant decline in blood β_2-microglobulin concentrations on a mid-term period [16, 17]. High circulating β_2-microglobulin concentrations have been shown recently to be associated with an increased relative risk of mortality in CKD-5 HD-treated patients.

ol-HDF combining the use of a high-flux membrane dialyzer, ultrapure dialysis fluid and high convective fluid exchange provides the lowest bioreactive profile in the field of extracorporeal renal replacement therapy. This property is quite beneficial for CKD patients, since by reducing dialysis-induced cell and protein activation, ol-HDF contributes also to the prevention or cure of inflammation, a major actor in the dialysis-related pathology.

Online Hemodiafiltration Reduces Morbidity in Patients with Chronic Kidney Disease Stage 5

The regular use of high-efficiency ol-HDF is associated with several clinically beneficial effects contributing to reduce the overall morbidity of CKD-5 patients. They are summarized in this section.

The *incidence of hypotensive episodes* is reduced with HDF methods permitting to achieve more easily dry weight while restoring the sodium fluid balance [18]. Indeed, this is particularly interesting in cardiac-compromised patients and/or in hypotension-prone patients. This beneficial effect has been related to a vasomodulation effect involving a negative thermal balance (increased peripheral vascular resistance and venous tone), a high sodium concentration of the substitution fluid (increased osmolality) and removal of vasodilating mediators (reduced endothelial dysfunction) [19, 20]. HD intolerance (nausea, vomiting, cramps and headache) is reduced with high-efficiency HDF compared to conventional HD. Postdialysis fatigue is less frequently observed with convective therapies [21]. Such properties are particularly suitable in elderly, diabetics and cardiac patients.

Better blood pressure control is generally observed in HDF-treated patients. This beneficial cardiac effect is mainly due to the preservation of intradialytic hemodynamic stability permitting to correct easily the extracellular fluid overload. Increased treatment time or frequency combined with a better compliance to sodium diet restriction may facilitate the achievement of this goal [22]. Regular application of high-efficiency ol-HDF has been associated with a reduction of left ventricular hypertrophy contributing to a better preservation of cardiac function [23].

Recent studies have suggested that high-flux therapies including ol-HDF might contribute to a longer and better *preservation of residual renal function*. Interestingly, this positive effect appears now comparable to that observed in peritoneal dialysis patients [24]. Although this phenomenon is not completely understood or proved, it might result from a reduction of the inflammation state of HD patients and from a reduced incidence of intradialytic hypotension episodes [25].

Improved hemocompatibility and reduced inflammation is commonly reported with ol-HDF. Based on sensitive markers of the acute-phase reaction (C-reactive protein, interleukins 1 and 6, interleukin 1 and 6 receptor antibodies, albumin) or on proinflammatory cell populations such as monocytes-derived CD14+ and CD16+ cells, several prospective studies have shown that the behavior of these markers remains stable over time in ol-HDF [26–29]. More recently in a prospective randomized study, it has been shown that ol-HDF was associated with less damaging and better repair effects on the endothelial cells [30]. These positive effects result from the combined use of a synthetic biocompatible membrane, ultrapure dialysis fluid and increased removal of some putative uremic toxins. Prevention of inflammation is a crucial concern for reducing the incidence of dialysis-related complications in long-term dialysis patients [31].

Renal anemia commonly observed in HD patients requires erythropoietin use in 80–100% of patients. Although this fact remains still controversial, high-efficiency ol-HDF has been shown to improve anemia control and to reduce erythropoietin needs in HD patients [32]. This positive effect has been particularly noted when patients were switched from low-flux HD to high-flux HDF or to HD with protein-leaking high-flux membranes [21]. These observations suggest that convective methods might remove some protein-bound erythropoietic inhibitor substance. It is also worth noting that the improvement in anemia is associated with a reduced inflammation state of the patient [33].

Caloric and/or protein malnutrition is observed in about one third of dialysis patients. Several recent studies have shown that the use of high-flux methods including HDF may have a positive impact on the nutritional state when compared to low-flux membranes [17, 34]. Anthropometric parameters, such as dry weight and body mass index, and albumin tend to increase over time in patients treated with convective therapies [35]. This is associated with an increase in dietary protein intake as evaluated by the urea generation rate [8]. One must recognize that this positive effect might result from combined effects of the use of high-flux membranes with ultrapure dialysate and more speculatively with the removal of anorexia-inducing uremic toxins [33].

Dyslipidemia profile, oxidative stress and advanced glycation end products reported in dialysis patients contribute to accelerate the atheromatosis and atherosclerotic process. The regular use of convective therapies has been shown to improve lipid profile [36] and to reduce oxidative stress and advanced glycation end product concentrations [37, 38]. Such a beneficial effect may be partly due to the improved biocompatibility of the dialyzer and the ultrapurity of the dialysate [39]. Note that the increased loss of natural antioxidant substances (vitamin C, vitamin E, selenium) may abolish in part the beneficial effect of high-efficiency convective modalities [40]. In contrast, a recent study has shown that asymmetric dimethylarginine concentrations were similar in high-flux and HDF-treated patients [41]. The regular oral supplementation in natural antioxidants appears highly desirable in both HD- and ol-HDF-treated patients.

β_2-Microglobulin amyloidosis has become a major complication of long-term HD therapy. Using carpal tunnel syndrome as crude and first manifestation of β_2-microglobulin amyloidosis in HD patients, it is commonly accepted that its incidence reaches 50% at 10 years and 100% at 20 years when conventional low-flux HD treatment is applied. Several cohort studies indicate that the extended use of high-flux membranes has a beneficial impact on the development of β_2-microglobulin amyloidosis reducing its incidence [42]. Indeed, almost all studies report a 50% reduction of the incidence of carpal tunnel syndrome when combining the use of convective methods and ultrapure dialysis fluid [43].

Growth retardation is a major concern in children with CKD-5. Conventional HD alone has not been able to reverse this development retardation. A recent study based on daily Ol-HDF has shown that this schedule is able to correct growth retardation in children with CKD [44]. This beneficial effect is achieved by combining the improvement of treatment efficacy, the enhancement of dietary and caloric intakes and the better correction of internal milieu disturbances (acidosis, calcium and phosphate control) [45]. The combined use of growth hormone, erythropoietic stimulating agents and ol-HDF provides now the opportunity to normalize growth rate in CKD kids [46, 47].

Hospitalization, used as a global marker of renal replacement therapy morbidity, is similar to conventional-HD-treated patients [48]. Few cohort studies addressing this issue have not found significant differences of morbidity and mortality in the convective-mode-treated group of patients [49]. Large cohort studies such as the United States Renal Data System have shown a significant reduction of morbidity and mortality in patients treated with high-flux methods as compared to those treated with low-flux dialyzers [50, 51]. These positive results were not confirmed in the large prospective and controlled HEMO study recently reported [52]. Indeed, it must be underlined that in the HEMO study dialyzer reuse may have blunted beneficial effects of high-flux methods by altering some performances. In summary, no significant difference in terms of frequency and duration of hospitalization stay has been reported neither in high-flux methods nor in high-efficiency ol-HDF. In other words, this observation means that high-efficiency ol-HDF is not harmful for CKD patients.

Online Hemodiafiltration Improves Survival in Patients with Chronic Kidney Disease Stage 5

Mortality is the most robust primary endpoint used to compare the efficacy of renal replacement therapy modalities. Few cohort studies have shown that mortality was reduced in HDF-treated groups [49, 53–55]. Meanwhile, the negative results of the HEMO study reported recently with patients either receiving a high dialysis dose or using a high-flux membrane were relatively disappointing [56]. It is however interesting to note that in the high-flux-treated group the incidence of cardiovascular events was nevertheless reduced. A recent reappraisal analysis of the HEMO study has shown that high predialysis β_2-microglobulin concentrations were strong and independent predictors of mortality in HD patients [57]. This observation strongly supports the fact that enhanced removal of middle uremic toxins is beneficial for CKD patients.

The European section of the international Dialysis and Outcomes Practice Patterns Study has shown that high-efficiency-HDF-treated patients had a better survival than regularly HD-treated patients accounting for age, sex, dialysis dose, comorbid conditions and country specificities [58]. Despite the fact that the relative risk of death was reduced in both HDF-treated groups, only the high-efficiency HDF group (substitution volume 15–25 l/session) had a significant benefit marked by a 35% reduction of death risk compared to patients treated with low-flux HD. Independent investigators have recently confirmed this positive finding when analyzing a large European database (Euclid). The relative risk of death was reduced in this study by 36% in HDF-treated patients [59]. It has also been observed in a retrospective US study that high-efficiency HDF based on 2 filters in series was able to reduce mortality in HDF by 65% [60].

Conclusions

High-efficiency ol-HDF has been proven to be the most efficient renal replacement therapy for CKD-5 patients. By combining diffusive and convective clearances, ol-HDF offers the highest removal rates for both small- and middle-molecule uremic toxins. By combining ultrapure dialysis fluid and synthetic hemocompatible membranes, ol-HDF improves considerably the hemocompatibility of the HD system. Clinical studies indicate that regular use of ol-HDF tends to reduce dialysis-related morbidity. Large cohort studies have shown that the survival of CKD-5 HDF-treated patients was significantly improved. By customizing the dialysis schedule to the patient's needs and tolerance, either by increasing session frequency (e.g. daily HDF) or by lengthening treatment duration (longer dialysis session), it has to be proven that ol-HDF may again expand this beneficial effect on dialysis outcomes [61, 62].

References

1 Henderson LW: Dialysis in the 21st century. Am J Kidney Dis 1996;28:951–957.

2 Clark WR, Gao D. Low-molecular weight proteins in end-stage renal disease: potential toxicity and dialytic removal mechanisms. J Am Soc Nephrol 2002;13:S41–S47.

3 Vanholder R, Glorieux G, De Smet R, et al: New insights in uremic toxins. Kidney Int Suppl 2003; 84:S6.

4 Vanholder R, Glorieux GL, De Smet R: Back to the future: middle molecules, high flux membranes, and optimal dialysis. Hemodial Int 2003;7:52.

5 Henderson LW, Clark WR, Cheung AK: Quantification of middle molecular weight solute removal in dialysis. Semin Dial 2001;14:294–299.

6 Leypoldt JK, Cheung AK, Carroll CE, Stannard DC, Pereira BJ, Agodoa LY, Port FK: Effect of dialysis membranes and middle molecule removal on chronic hemodialysis patient survival. Am J Kidney Dis 1999;33:349–355.

7 Canaud B, Bosc JY, Leray-Moragues H, Stec F, Argiles A, Leblanc M, Mion C: On-line haemodiafiltration: safety and efficacy in long-term clinical practice. Nephrol Dial Transplant 2000;15(suppl 1):60–67.

8 Canaud B, Bosc JY, Leblanc M, Garred LJ, Vo T, Mion C. Evaluation of high-flux hemodiafiltration efficiency using an on-line urea monitor. Am J Kidney Dis 1998;31:74–80.

9 Maduell F: Hemodiafiltration. Hemodial Int 2005;9:47–55.
10 Shinzato T, Kobayakawa H, Maeda K: Comparison of various treatment modes in terms of beta 2-microglobulin removal: hemodialysis, hemofiltration, and push/pull HDF. Artif Organs 1989;13: 66–70.
11 Lornoy W, De Meester J, Becaus I, Billiouw JM, Van Malderen PA, Van Pottelberge M. Impact of convective flow on phosphorus removal in maintenance hemodialysis patients. J Ren Nutr 2006; 16:47–53.
12 Zehnder C, Gutzwiller JP, Renggli K: Hemodiafiltration – A new treatment option for hyperphosphatemia in hemodialysis patients. Clin Nephrol 1999;52:152.
13 Krieter DH, Lemke HD, Canaud B, Wanner C: Beta-2-microglobulin removal by extracorporeal renal replacement therapies. Biochim Biophys Acta 2005;1753:146–153.
14 Ward RA, Greene T, Hartmann B, Samtleben W. Resistance to intercompartmental mass transfer limits beta2-microglobulin removal by post-dilution hemodiafiltration. Kidney Int 2006;69: 1431–1437.
15 Lornoy W, Becaus I, Billiouw JM, et al: On-line haemodiafiltration: remarkable removal of beta2-microglobulin – Long-term clinical observations. Nephrol Dial Transplant 2000;15(suppl 1):49.
16 Locatelli F, Mastrangelo F, Redaelli B, et al: Effects of different membranes and dialysis technologies on patient treatment tolerance and nutritional parameters. The Italian Cooperative Dialysis Study Group. Kidney Int 1996;50:1293.
17 Basile C: The effect of convection on the nutritional status of haemodialysis patients. Nephrol Dial Transplant 2003;18(suppl 7):vii46–49.
18 Altieri P, Sorba G, Bolasco P, Ledebo I, Ganadu M, Ferrara R, Menneas A, Asproni E, Casu D, Passaghe M, Sau G, Cadinu F, Sardinian Study Group on Hemofiltration On-line. Related comparison between hemofiltration and hemodiafiltration in a long-term prospective cross-over study. J Nephrol 2004;17:414–422.
19 Donauer J, Schweiger C, Rumberger B, Krumme B, Bohler J: Reduction of hypotensive side effects during online-haemodiafiltration and low temperature haemodialysis. Nephrol Dial Transplant 2003;18:1616–1622.
20 van der Sande FM, Rosales LM, Brener Z, Kooman JP, Kuhlmann M, Handelman G, Greenwood RN, Carter M, Schneditz D, Leunissen KM, Levin NW: Effect of ultrafiltration on thermal variables, skin temperature, skin blood flow, and energy expenditure during ultrapure hemodialysis. J Am Soc Nephrol 2005;16:1824–1831.
21 Maduell F, del Pozo C, Garcia H, Sanchez L, Hdez-Jaras J, Albero MD, Calvo C, Torregrosa I, Navarro V: Change from conventional haemodiafiltration to on-line haemodiafiltration. Nephrol Dial Transplant 1999;14:1202–1207.
22 Stegmayr BG: Ultrafiltration and dry weight – What are the cardiovascular effects? Artif Organs 2003;27:227–229.
23 Maduell F, Navarro V, Torregrosa E, Rius A, Dicenta F, Cruz MC, Ferrero JA: Change from three times a week on-line hemodiafiltration to short daily on-line hemodiafiltration. Kidney Int 2003;64:305–313.
24 McKane W, Chandna SM, Tattersall JE, et al: Identical decline of residual renal function in high-flux biocompatible hemodialysis and CAPD. Kidney Int 2002;61:256.
25 Pozzoni P, Filippo S, Manzoni C, Locatelli F: The relevance of convection in clinical practice: a critical review of the literature. Hemodial Int 2006;10(suppl 1):S33–S38.
26 van Tellingen A, Grooteman MP, Schoorl M, et al: Intercurrent clinical events are predictive of plasma C-reactive protein levels in hemodialysis patients. Kidney Int 2002;62:632.
27 Canaud B, Wizemann V, Pizzarelli F, et al: Cellular interleukin-1 receptor antagonist production in patients receiving on-line haemodiafiltration therapy. Nephrol Dial Transplant 2001;16:2181.
28 Olsson J, Dadfar E, Paulsson J, Lundahl J, Moshfegh A, Jacobson SH: Preserved leukocyte CD11b expression at the site of interstitial inflammation in patients with high-flux hemodiafiltration. Kidney Int 2007;71:582–588.
29 Carracedo J, Merino A, Nogueras S, Carretero D, Berdud I, Ramirez R, Tetta C, Rodriguez M, Martin-Malo A, Aljama P: On-line hemodiafiltration reduces the proinflammatory CD14+CD16+ monocyte-derived dendritic cells: a prospective, crossover study. J Am Soc Nephrol 2006;17: 2315–2321.

30 Ramirez R, Carracedo J, Merino A, Nogueras S, Alvarez-Lara MA, Rodriguez M, Martin-Malo A, Tetta C, Aljama P. Microinflammation induces endothelial damage in hemodialysis patients: the role of convective transport. Kidney Int 2007, E-pub ahead of print.
31 Deppisch RM, Beck W, Goehl H, et al: Complement components as uremic toxins and their potential role as mediators of microinflammation. Kidney Int Suppl 2001;78:S271.
32 Vaslaki L, Major L, Berta K, Karatson A, Misz M, Pethoe F, Ladanyi E, Fodor B, Stein G, Pischetsrieder M, Zima T, Wojke R, Gauly A, Passlick-Deetjen J: On-line haemodiafiltration versus haemodialysis: stable haematocrit with less erythropoietin and improvement of other relevant blood parameters. Blood Purif 2006;24:163–173.
33 Schiffl H, Lang SM, Stratakis D, et al: Effects of ultrapure dialysis fluid on nutritional status and inflammatory parameters. Nephrol Dial Transplant 2001;16:1863.
34 Lindsay RM, Spanner E, Heidenheim AP, et al: A multicenter study of short hour dialysis using AN69S: preliminary results. ASAIO Trans 1991;37:M465.
35 Savica V, Ciolino F, Monardo P, Mallamace A, Savica R, Santoro D, Bellinghieri G: Nutritional status in hemodialysis patients: options for on-line convective treatment. J Ren Nutr 2006;16: 237–240.
36 Blankestijn PJ, Vos PF, Rabelink TJ, et al: High-flux dialysis membranes improve lipid profile in chronic hemodialysis patients. J Am Soc Nephrol 1995;5:1703.
37 Chun-Liang L, Chiu-Ching H, Chun-Chen Y, et al: Reduction of advanced glycation end products levels by on-line hemodiafiltration in long-term hemodialysis patients. Am J Kidney Dis 2003;42: 524.
38 Calo LA, Naso A, Carraro G, Wratten ML, Pagnin E, Bertipaglia L, Rebeschini M, Davis PA, Piccoli A, Cascone C: Effect of haemodiafiltration with online regeneration of ultrafiltrate on oxidative stress in dialysis patients. Nephrol Dial Transplant 2007, E-pub ahead of print.
39 Ward RA, McLeish KR: Oxidant stress in hemodialysis patients: what are the determining factors? Artif Organs 2003;27:230.
40 Morena M, Cristol JP, Bosc JY, et al: Convective and diffusive losses of vitamin C during haemodiafiltration session: a contributive factor to oxidative stress in haemodialysis patients. Nephrol Dial Transplant 2002;17:422.
41 Kalousova M, Kielstein JT, Hodkova M, Zima T, Dusilova-Sulkova S, Martens-Lobenhoffer J, Bode-Boger SM: No benefit of hemodiafiltration over hemodialysis in lowering elevated levels of asymmetric dimethylarginine in ESRD patients. Blood Purif 2006;24:439–444.
42 Locatelli F, Manzoni C, Di Filippo S: The importance of convective transport. Kidney Int Suppl 2002;80:115.
43 Lonnemann G, Koch KM: Beta(2)-microglobulin amyloidosis: effects of ultrapure dialysate and type of dialyzer membrane. J Am Soc Nephrol 2002;13(suppl 1):S72.
44 Fischbach M, Terzic J, Laugel V, Dheu C, Menouer S, Helms P, Livolsi A: Daily on-line haemodiafiltration: a pilot trial in children. Nephrol Dial Transplant 2004;19:2360–2367.
45 Fischbach M, Terzic J, Menouer S, Dheu C, Soskin S, Helmstetter A, Burger MC: Intensified and daily hemodialysis in children might improve statural growth. Pediatr Nephrol 2006;21:1746–1752.
46 Kari JA, Rees L: Growth hormone for children with chronic renal failure and on dialysis. Pediatr Nephrol 2005;20:618–621.
47 Boehm M, Riesenhuber A, Winkelmayer WC, Arbeiter K, Mueller T, Aufricht C: Early erythropoietin therapy is associated with improved growth in children with chronic kidney disease. Pediatr Nephrol 2007, E-pub ahead of print.
48 Locatelli F, Pozzoni P, Manzoni C, Di Filippo S: High-flux hemodialysis and hemodiafiltration: impact on outcome; in Ronco C, La Greca G (eds): Hemodialysis Technology. Contrib Nephrol. Basel, Karger, 2002, vol 137, pp 193–200.
49 Locatelli F, Marcelli D, Conte F, Limido A, Malberti F, Spotti D. Comparison of mortality in ESRD patients on convective and diffusive extracorporeal treatments. The Registro Lombardo Dialisi E Trapianto. Kidney Int 1999;55:286–293.
50 Port FK, Wolfe RA, Hulbert-Shearon TE, Daugirdas JT, Agodoa LY, Jones C, Orzol SM, Held PJ: Mortality risk by hemodialyzer reuse practice and dialyzer membrane characteristics: results from the USRDS dialysis morbidity and mortality study. Am J Kidney Dis 2001;37:276–286.

51 Chauveau P, Nguyen H, Combe C, Chene G, Azar R, Cano N, Canaud B, Fouque D, Laville M, Leverve X, Roth H, Aparicio M, French Study Group for Nutrition in Dialysis: Dialyzer membrane permeability and survival in hemodialysis patients. Am J Kidney Dis 2005;45:565–571.
52 Eknoyan G, Beck GJ, Cheung AK, et al: Effect of dialysis dose and membrane flux in maintenance hemodialysis. N Engl J Med 2002;19:347.
53 Santoro A, Panzetta G, Tessitore N, Atti M, Mancini E, Esteban J, London G, Ara JM, Miguel JL, Neumann KH, Opatrny K, Perez R, Perrone B, Wizemann V, Zucchelli P: A prospective randomised European multicentre study of medium-long run mortality and morbidity comparing acetate-free biofiltration and bicarbonate dialysis. J Nephrol 1999;12:375–382.
54 Wizemann V, Lotz C, Techert F, Uthoff S: On-line haemodiafiltration versus low-flux haemodialysis: a prospective randomized study. Nephrol Dial Transplant 2000;15(suppl 1):43–48.
55 Schiffl H. Prospective randomized cross-over long-term comparison of online haemodiafiltration and ultrapure high-flux haemodialysis. Eur J Med Res 2007;12:26–33.
56 Eknoyan G, Beck GJ, Cheung AK, et al: Effect of dialysis dose and membrane flux in maintenance hemodialysis. N Engl J Med 2002;19:347.
57 Cheung AK, Rocco MV, Yan G, Leypoldt JK, Levin NW, Greene T, Agodoa L, Bailey J, Beck GJ, Clark W, Levey AS, Ornt DB, Schulman G, Schwab S, Teehan B, Eknoyan G: Serum beta-2 microglobulin levels predict mortality in dialysis patients: results of the HEMO study. J Am Soc Nephrol 2006;17:546–555.
58 Canaud B, Bragg-Gresham JL, Marshall MR, Desmeules S, Gillespie BW, Depner T, Klassen P, Port FK: Mortality risk for patients receiving hemodiafiltration versus hemodialysis: European results from the DOPPS. Kidney Int 2006;69:2087–2093.
59 Jirka T, Cesare S, Di Benedetto A, Perera Chang M, Ponce P, Richards N, Tetta C, Vaslaky L: Mortality risk for patients receiving hemodiafiltration versus hemodialysis. Kidney Int 2006;70: 1524.
60 Bosch JP, Lew SQ, Barlee V, Mishkin GJ, von Albertini B: Clinical use of high-efficiency hemodialysis treatments: long-term assessment. Hemodial Int 2006;10:73–81.
61 Canaud B, Morena M, Leray-Moragues H, Chalabi L, Cristol JP: Overview of clinical studies in hemodiafiltration: what do we need now? Hemodial Int 2006;10(suppl 1):S5–S12.
62 Penne EL, Blankestijn PJ, Bots ML, van den Dorpel MA, Grooteman MP, Nube MJ, ter Wee PM, CONTRAST Group: Resolving controversies regarding hemodiafiltration versus hemodialysis: the Dutch Convective Transport Study. Semin Dial 2005;18:47–51.

Prof. B. Canaud
Department of Nephrology, Dialysis and Intensive Care Unit, Lapeyronie Hospital,
University of Montpellier
371, avenue du Doyen-Gaston-Giraud
FR–34295 Montpellier Cedex 5 (France)
Tel. +33 4 67 33 89 55, Fax +33 4 67 60 37 83, E-Mail b-canaud@chu-montpellier.fr

Ronco C, Canaud B, Aljama P (eds): Hemodiafiltration.
Contrib Nephrol. Basel, Karger, 2007, vol 158, pp 225–231

Optimizing the Prescription of Hemodiafiltration

Francisco Maduell

Department of Nephrology, Hospital Clínic Barcelona, Barcelona, Spain

Abstract

Hemodiafiltration with larger amounts of substitution fluid offers an optimal way to remove uremic substances. Hemodiafiltration could be indicated for all hemodialysis patients. Large observational studies have shown an association of a lower mortality risk with hemodiafiltration using more than 15 liters of substitution fluid. Specific indications should be considered because hemodiafiltration has been reported to be effective against hyperphospatemia, malnutrition, insomnia, irritability, restless-leg syndrome, polyneuropathy, anemia, itching and joint pain, and may prevent dialysis-associated amyloidosis. In this chapter, hemodiafiltration prescriptions concerning blood and dialysate flow, infusion rate, vascular access and frequency are detailed.

Hemodialysis can be considered a routine renal replacement therapy that guarantees reasonable short-term outcomes. The long-term clinical outcomes, however, could be improved. Malnutrition is common, hyperphosphatemia, hypertension and heart failure control is poor, rehabilitation and quality of life are suboptimal, and hospitalization and mortality rates are high. The most common cause of mortality in chronic hemodialysis patients is cardiovascular disease, which is the attributed cause of death in approximately 50% of patients. Depner [1] defined this situation as 'residual syndrome', which includes susceptibility to infection, reduced maximal oxygen consumption during exercise, sleep disturbances, depression, impaired mental concentration, reduced stamina and markedly increased susceptibility to cardiovascular complications. Possible causes of residual syndrome are accumulation of dialyzable solutes that are incompletely removed and aggregation of large-molecular-weight solutes that are difficult to remove by dialysis.

Various complications in hemodialysis patients may be related to an accumulation of larger uremic substances difficult to remove by conventional hemodialysis. Hemodiafiltration with larger amounts of substitution fluid offers an optimal way to remove uremic substances ranging widely in molecular size from small solutes to low-molecular-weight proteins [2, 3].

Hemodiafiltration Prescriptions: Patient Indication

Hemodiafiltration could be indicated in all hemodialysis patients. High-volume hemodiafiltration techniques mark a new step towards mimicking the blood purification of the native kidney. These techniques offer superior uremic substance removal over a wider range of molecular sizes, yet require the use of biocompatible membranes and ultrapure dialysate, which has been related to additional clinical benefits. Recent large observational studies with robust adjustments for demographic and comorbid confounding factors have shown an association of a lower mortality risk with hemodiafiltration using more than 15 liters of substitution fluid [4, 5].

A number of studies have addressed the potential role played by larger solutes or low-molecular-weight proteins in dialysis-related complications and the potential clinical advantages offered by high-convection therapies. Specific indications should be considered because hemodiafiltration has been reported to be effective against hyperphosphatemia, malnutrition, insomnia, irritability, restless-leg syndrome, polyneuropathy, anemia, itching and joint pain, and may prevent dialysis-associated amyloidosis.

Hyperphosphatemia

Hemodiafiltration improves phosphate elimination and could be considered as a treatment option for hyperphosphatemia [6]. Lornoy et al. [7] reported that treatment with online hemodiafiltration in postdilution mode resulted in higher phosphorus removal than hemodialysis.

Malnutrition

Anorexia in uremic patients has been related to an accumulation of uremic substances. In uremic rats, Anderstam et al. [8] identified toxins in the range of 1,000–5,000 Da, which led to suppression of food intake. Leptin, with a molecular weight of 16,000 Da, may have an appetite-suppressing effect and could accumulate in dialysis patients [9].

Anemia

Online hemodiafiltration could improve erythropoietin response as a result of the increased removal of medium- and large-sized molecules. Bonforte et al.

[10] showed an improvement in anemia in 32 patients with high-volume online replacement fluid. Osawa et al. [11] were able to lower the erythropoietin dose with pull/push hemodiafiltration. Maduell et al. [12] reported improved correction of anemia in 37 patients with lower erythropoietin doses when conventional hemodiafiltration (4 liters) was switched to online hemodiafiltration (24 liters). Ward et al. [13] and Wizemann et al. [14] could not confirm these observations in 24 and 23 patients, respectively, treated with online hemodiafiltration compared with 21 patients treated with high-flux hemodialysis and 21 patients treated with low-flux hemodialysis.

Infectious Complications

Uremic patients have a significant risk of infectious complications. Indeed, these complications are the first cause of hospitalization and the second cause of death in hemodialysis patients. Several granulocyte-inhibiting proteins are present in uremic patients, which may contribute to the high incidence of infectious complications. Degranulation-inhibiting protein I and granulocyte inhibitory protein II inhibit in vitro glucose uptake and chemotaxis of polymorphonuclear leukocytes. Factor D decreases the complement-mediated clearance of immune complexes and inhibits granulocyte degranulation. All these uremic toxins are better removed with high-volume hemodiafiltration [13, 15].

Joint Pain

Maeda et al. [16] observed a significant increase in upper arm movement range and alleviation of shoulder joint pain in 30 patients after switching treatment from hemodialysis to push/pull hemodiafiltration (30 liters of convective volume). The clinical observations of Kim et al. [17] support the hypothesis that joint-pain-related substances may have a molecular size larger than β_2-microglobulin. These authors investigated the relationship between joint pain relief and the removal pattern of low-molecular-weight proteins, and observed higher removal rates of α_1-microglobulin and α_1-acid glycoprotein with online hemodiafiltration than with high-flux hemodialysis. Sato and Koga [18] also observed a decrease in joint pain and significant improvements in the range of upper arm adduction and abduction movements when 6 patients undergoing hemodialysis were changed to online hemodiafiltration.

Dialysis-Related Amyloidosis

Using data from a Japanese dialysis patient registry, Nakai et al. [19] investigated which of a number of treatment modes was most effective for the treatment of dialysis-related amyloidosis in 1,196 patients. When the risk of a worse therapeutic effect for low-flux hemodialysis was stated as 1, the risk for patients using high-flux hemodialysis was 0.489, while that for online hemodiafiltration was 0.013.

Cardiovascular Stability

Convective treatments have been reported to provide superior cardiovascular stability, thereby reducing intradialysis hypotension even in patients with increased cardiovascular risk [20]. Donauer et al. [21] reported a reduction of hypotensive side effects during online hemodiafiltration and low-temperature hemodialysis. In some patients with severe hypotension, we have observed [unpubl. data] an improvement in predialysis blood pressure with high convective treatments.

Neurological Complications

Insomnia, irritability, restless-leg syndrome, polyneuropathy and pruritus can be due to accumulation of medium-sized or large molecules. Hemodiafiltration with high-volume replacement fluid improves these symptoms due to improved blood purification [22, 23].

Blood and Dialysate Flow

The main limiting factors for infusion flow (Q_I) are blood flow (Q_B) and transmembrane pressure, which rise in proportion to Q_I. Although some monitors have a Q_I one third of the Q_B value, the maximum recommended Q_I is 25% of the Q_B value in postdilution mode. Although online hemodiafiltration can be performed with every Q_B, a prescription of Q_B between 360 and 500 ml/min allows a Q_I of between 80 and 125 ml/min.

In a routine 3 times weekly session, the recommended dialysate flow is 700–800 ml/min, although lower flows are possible.

Infusion Rate

Postdilution hemodiafiltration is the most efficient infusion mode for obtaining maximum clearances of small and larger solutes, even though this mode can increase the frequency of technical problems (hemoconcentration and high transmembrane pressure). The predilution mode, while partially preventing technical problems, reduces the cumulative solute transfer as a consequence of the diluted concentration [14, 24].

Simultaneous pre- and postdilution, i.e. mixed, hemodiafiltration, could be a highly effective technique to remove uremic toxins, while avoiding the disadvantages of the traditional infusion modes [25].

Vascular Access

A native fistula is the best option for all hemodialysis modalities as well as for hemodiafiltration. However, the use of a native fistula or graft has decreased over the last decade, due to greater patient age and the increased prevalence of cardiovascular disease and diabetes. For this reason, the use of permanent tunneled catheters has increased in the last few years (20–25% in our dialysis unit), and the possibility of performing hemodiafiltration with permanent catheters has been considered.

In 1998, Canaud et al. [26] reported 7 patients with double-lumen permanent catheters who underwent online hemodiafiltration. During the last year, we have treated 8 patients, aged 65 years or older, 3 men and 5 women, with online hemodiafiltration with a new generation of permanent tunneled catheters. Dialysis parameters were a helixone dialyzer of 1.8 m^2 surface area, blood flow of 372 ml/min (range 300–450), dialysate flow of 800 ml/min, dialysis time of 289 min and bicarbonate-buffered dialysate. The mean reinfusion volume was 20.1 ± 4 liters (range 18–25 liters).

Frequency

Daily dialysis experiences have shown excellent clinical results because a higher frequency of dialysis is more physiological and decreases fluctuations in liquids, solutes and electrolytes. Improvements in comfort during and between dialysis, as well as in clinical and biochemical parameters, anemia correction, hypertension control, nutritional status and quality of life have been reported.

In a previous study, we combined the more physiological and effective dialysis schedule (daily dialysis) with online hemodiafiltration. Patients on standard 4- to 5-hour 3 times weekly online hemodiafiltration were changed to 2- to 2.5-hour 6 times weekly online hemodiafiltration. The principal advantages observed were excellent patient clinical tolerance, disappearance of postdialysis fatigue, improvement of sleep disorders, reduction of phosphate binders, improvement of nutritional status (body weight increased by more than 3 kg after 1 year), better control of blood pressure without antihypertensive medications and partial regression of left ventricular hypertrophy [27].

In a pilot trial in children with daily online hemodiafiltration [28], 5 children were switched from standard online hemodiafiltration (4 h, 3 times/week) to daily online hemodiafiltration (3 h, 6 times/week). This strategy led to a reduction in blood pressure and an improvement in left ventricular size and function, normalization of predialytic plasma phosphorus and improvements in general well-being and dialysis acceptance.

References

1 Depner TA: Uraemic toxicity: urea and beyond. Semin Dial 2001;14:246–251.

2 Clark WR, Gao D: Low-molecular weight proteins in end-stage renal disease: potential toxicity and dialytic removal mechanism. J Am Soc Nephrol 2002;13(suppl 1):S41–S47.

3 Henderson LW, Clark WR, Cheung AK: Quantification of middle molecular weight solute removal in dialysis. Semin Dial 2001;14:294–299.

4 Canaud B, Bragg-Gresham JL, Marshall MR, Desmeules S, Gillespie BW, Depner T, Klassen P, Port FK: Mortality risk for patients receiving hemodiafiltration versus hemodialysis: European results from the DOPPS. Kidney Int 2006;69:2087–2093.

5 Jirka T, Cesare S, Di Benedetto, Chang MP, Ponce P, Richards N, Tetta C, Vaslaky L: Mortality risk for patients receiving hemodiafiltration versus hemodialysis. Kidney Int 2006;70:1524.

6 Zehnder C, Gutzwiller JP, Renggli K: Hemodiafiltration – A new treatment option for hyperphosphatemia in hemodialysis patients. Clin Nephrol 1999;52:152–159.

7 Lornoy W, De Meester JD, Becaus I, Billiouw JM, Van Malderen PA, Van Pottelberge: Impact of convective flow on phosphorus removal in maintenance hemodialysis patients. J Ren Nutr 2006; 16:47–53.

8 Anderstam B, Mamoun A, Södersten P, Bergström J: Middle-sized molecule fractions isolated from uremic ultrafiltrate and normal urine inhibit ingestive behavior in the rat. J Am Soc Nephrol 1996;7:2453–2460.

9 Merabet E, Dagogo-Jack S, Coyne DW, Klein S, Santiago JV, Hmiel SP, Landt M: Increased plasma leptin concentrations in end stage renal disease. J Clin Endocrinol Metab 1997;82:847–850.

10 Bonforte G, Grillo P, Zerbi S, Surian M: Improvement of anemia in hemodialysis patients treated by hemodiafiltration with high-volume on-line prepared substitution fluid. Blood Purif 2002;20: 357–363.

11 Osawa S, Sakuraba N, Yamamoto H, Hisajima S. Clinical evaluation of HDF: especially effects on EPO administration in HDF patients. Clin Pharmacol Ther 1997;7:1159–1162.

12 Maduell F, Pozo C, Garcia H, Sanchez L, Hdez-Jaras J, Albero D, Calvo C, Torregrosa l, Navarro V: Change from conventional haemodiafiltation to on-line haemodiafiltration. Nephrol Dial Transplant 1999;14:1202–1207.

13 Ward RA, Schmidt B, Hullin J, Hillebrand GF, Samtleben W: A comparison of on-line hemodiafiltration and high-flux hemodialysis: a prospective clinical study. J Am Soc Nephrol 2000;11: 2344–2350.

14 Wizemann V, Lotz C, Techert F, Uthoff S: On-line haemodiafiltration versus low-flux hemodialysis: a prospective randomized study. Nephrol Dial Transplant 2000;15(suppl 1):S43–S48.

15 Haag-Weber M, Cohen G, Hörl WH: Clinical significance of granulocyte-inhibiting proteins. Nephrol Dial Transplant 2000;15(suppl 1):15–16.

16 Maeda K, Kobayakawa H, Fujita Y, Takai I, Morita H, Emoto Y, Miyazaki T, Shinzato T: Effectiveness of push/pull hemodiafiltration using large-pore membrane for shoulder joint pain in long-term dialysis patients. Artif Organs 1990;14:321–327.

17 Kim ST, Yamamoto C, Asabe H, Sato T, Takamiya T: Online haemodiafiltration: effective removal of high molecular weight toxins and improvement in clinical manifestations of chronic haemodialysis patients. Nephrology 1996;2(suppl 1):S183–S186.

18 Sato T, Koga N: Centralized on-line hemodiafiltration system utilizing purified dialysate as substitution fluid. Artif Organs 1998;22:285–290.

19 Nakai S, Iseki K, Tabei K, Kubo K, Masakane I, Fushimi K, Kikuchi K, Shinzato T, Sanaka T, Akiba T: Outcomes of hemodiafiltration based on Japanese dialysis patient registry. Am J Kidney Dis 2001;38(suppl 1):S212–S216.

20 Mion M, Kerr PG, Argiles A, Canaud B, Flavier JL, Mion CM: Hemodiafiltration in high-cardiovascular-risk patients. Nephrol Dial Transplant 1992;7:453–455.

21 Donauer J, Schweiger C, Rumberger B, Krumme B, Böhler J: Reduction of hypotensive side effects during online-haemodiafiltration and low temperature haemodialysis. Nephrol Dial Transplant 2003;18:1616–1622.

22 Mucsi I, Molnar MZ, Ambrus C, Szeifert L, Kovacs AZ, Zoller R, Barotfi S, Remport A, Novak M: Restless legs syndrome, insomnia and quality of life in patients on maintenance dialysis. Nephrol Dial Transplant 2005;20:571–577.
23 Zakrzewska-Pniewska B, Jedras M: Is pruritus in chronic uremia patients related to peripheral somatic and autonomic neuropathy? Study by R-R interval variation test (RRIV) and by sympathetic skin response (SSR). Neurophysiol Clin 2001;31:181–193.
24 Maduell F, García H, Hdez-Jaras J, Calvo C, Navarro V: Comparación de la infusión predilucional versus postdilucional en HDF en línea. Nefrología 1998;18(suppl 3):49.
25 Pedrini L, De Cristofaro V, Pagliari B, Samà F: Mixed predilution and postdilution online hemodiafiltration compared with traditional infusion modes. Kidney Int 2000;58:2155–2165.
26 Canaud B, Bosc JY, Leray H, Stec F, Argiles A, Leblanc M, Mion C: On-line haemodiafiltration: state of the art. Nephrol Dial Transplant 1998;13(suppl 5):3–11.
27 Maduell F, Navarro V, Torregrosa E, Rius A, Dicenta F, Cruz MC, Ferrero JA: Change from thrice weekly on-line hemodiafiltration to short daily on-line hemodiafiltration. Kidney Int 2003;64:305–313.
28 Fischbach M, Terzic J, Laugel V, Dheu C, Menouer S, Helms P, Livolsi A: Daily on-line haemodiafiltration: a pilot trial in children. Nephrol Dial Transplant 2004;19:2360–2367.

Francisco Maduell Canals, MD
Servicio de Nefrología, Hospital Clínic Barcelona
C/Villarroel, 170
ES–08006 Barcelona (Spain)
Tel. +34 93 227 5400, Fax +34 93 454 6033, E-Mail fmaduell@clinic.ub.es

Author Index

Subject Index